CURRENT NEURO-OPHTHALMOLOGY
Volume 2

CURRENT

NEURO-
OPHTHALMOLOGY

VOLUME 2

Edited by

Simmons Lessell, M.D.
Professor of Ophthalmology
Harvard Medical School
Director of Neuro-Ophthalmology
Department of Ophthalmology
Massachusetts Eye and Ear Infirmary
Boston, Massachusetts

and

J. T. W. van Dalen, M.D., Ph.D.
Associate Professor of Ophthalmology
Department of Ophthalmology
The University of Arizona Health Sciences Center
Tucson, Arizona

YEAR BOOK MEDICAL PUBLISHERS, INC.
Chicago • London • Boca Raton • Littleton, Mass.

International Standard Serial Number: 0893-0147
International Standard Book Number: 0-8151-5389-9

Sponsoring Editor: Christopher W. Freiler
Associate Managing Editor, Serial Publications Editing: Denise Dungey
Assistant Director, Manuscript Services: Frances M. Perveiler
Production Coordinator: Max Perez
Proofroom Supervisor: Barbara M. Kelly

Contributors

Myles Behrens, M.D.
Professor of Clinical Ophthalmology
Columbia Presbyterian Medical Center
New York, New York

Hans Bynke, M.D., Ph.D.
Associate Professor
Neuro-ophthalmology Unit
Department of Ophthalmology
University Hospital of Lund
Lund, Sweden

Jeffrey L. Cummings, M.D.
Dementia Research Program
Department of Neurology
Department of Psychiatry and Biobehavioral Sciences
UCLA School of Medicine
Neurobehavior Unit
West Los Angeles Veterans Administration Medical Center (Brentwood
Division)
Los Angeles, California

Jon Currie, M.B., B.S., F.R.A.C.P.
The Mental Health Research Insitute of Victoria
Parkville, Victoria, Australia
The Save Sight and Eye Health Institute
University of Sydney
Sydney, New South Wales, Australia

L. F. Dell'Osso, Ph.D.
Professor
Departments of Neurology and Biomedical Engineering
Case Western Reserve University
Director
Ocular Motor Neurophysiology Laboratory
Veterans Administration Medical Center
Cleveland, Ohio

Joel S. Dunnington, M.D.
Assistant Professor of Radiology
Department of Radiology
Texas Tech University Health Sciences Center
Lubbock, Texas

Carl Ellenberger, Jr., M.D.
Good Samaritan Hospital
Lebanon, Pennsylvania

Thomas A. Gardner, M.D.
Fellow
Department of Ophthalmology
Allegheny General Hospital
Pittsburgh, Pennsylvania

John W. Gittinger, Jr., M.D.
Professor of Surgery and Neurology
University of Massachusetts Medical School
Worcester, Massachusetts

Joel S. Glaser, M.D.
Professor
Ophthalmology and Neurologic Surgery
Bascom Palmer Eye Institute
Department of Ophthalmology
University of Miami
Miami, Florida

G. P. M. Horsten, M.D., Ph.D.
Eye Clinic
Academic Medical Center
Amsterdam, The Netherlands

Mandes R. Kates, M.D., Ph.D.
Clinical Assistant
Manhattan Eye, Ear, and Throat Hospital
New York, New York

John S. Kennerdell, M.D.
Clinical Professor of Ophthalmology
University of Pittsburgh School of Medicine
Chairman of Ophthalmology
Allegheny General Hospital
Pittsburgh, Pennsylvania

Martin L. Leib, M.D.
Director
Orbit and Ophthalmic Plastic Surgery Service
The Edward S. Harkness Eye Institute
Columbia-Presbyterian Medical Center
Assistant Professor of Clinical Ophthalmology
Columbia University College of Physicians and Surgeons
New York, New York

Jin S. Leo, M.D.
Professor of Radiology
Texas Tech University Health Sciences Center
Lubbock, Texas

George M. McCormick, M.D.
Department of Neurology
Bowman Gray School of Medicine
Wake Forest University
Winston-Salem, North Carolina

Ekkehard Mehdorn, M.D.
Professor of Ophthalmology
Medical University of Lübeck
Lübeck, Federal Republic of Germany

Jeffrey G. Odel, M.D.
Instructor of Clinical Ophthalmology
Columbia Presbyterian Medical Center
New York, New York

Joseph Rizzo, M.D.
Massachusetts Eye and Ear Infirmary
Department of Ophthalmology
Harvard Medical School
Boston, Massachusetts

Peter J. Savino, M.D.
Neuro-Ophthalmology Service
Wills Eye Hospital
Philadelphia, Pennsylvania

Dieter Schmidt, M.D.
Universitäts-Augenklinik
Freiburg, Federal Republic of Germany

Patrick A. Sibony, M.D.
Associate Professor of Ophthalmology
State University of New York at Stony Brook
Stony Brook, New York

H. Stanley Thompson, M.D.
Professor
Ophthalmology
Department of Ophthalmology
University of Iowa
Iowa City, Iowa

Jonathan D. Trobe, M.D.
Departments of Ophthalmology and Neurology
University of Michigan Medical Center
Ann Arbor, Michigan

B. Todd Troost, M.D.
Department of Neurology
Bowman Gray School of Medicine
Wake Forest University
Winston-Salem, North Carolina

Ronald J. Tusa, Ph.D.
Department of Neurology
The Johns Hopkins University School of Medicine
Baltimore, Maryland

J. T. W. van Dalen, M.D., Ph.D
Associate Professor of Ophthalmology
The University of Arizona Health Sciences Center
Tucson, Arizona

W. I. M. Verhagen, M.D., Ph.D.
Department of Neurology and Clinical Neurophysiology
Canisius Wilhelmina Hospital
Nijmegen, The Netherlands

David S. Zee, M.D.
Departments of Neurology and Ophthalmology
The Johns Hopkins University School of Medicine
Baltimore, Maryland

Preface

The purpose of *Current Neuro-ophthalmology* is to provide an in depth, biannual review of the neuro-ophthalmology literature from the past 2 years. Neuro-ophthalmology topics will be reviewed by experts in their fields; each chapter has a wealth of references.

The series started in 1980. Three volumes were published by Elsevier (1980-1984) before publication was taken over by Year Book Medical Publishers. Under their aegis, the first review, *Current Neuro-ophthalmology,* was published in the fall of 1987. The present publication, therefore, is the fifth review of the neuro-ophthalmology world literature. It is remarkable that many of the original contributing reviewers are still willing to take this heavy review task on their shoulders. The proliferation of the neuro-ophthalmology literature is still continually making review an almost impossible task. As editors, we are thankful that we have such an excellent group of experts who have done such a tremendously good job.

One of the most profound changes in the world of neuro-ophthalmology was the advent of neural imaging techniques. Computed tomography (CT) was introduced in 1972 and the clinical use of magnetic resonance imaging (MRI) is spreading rapidly.

Chapters on computed tomography (Drs. M.L. Leib and M.R. Kates) and on neuroradiology (Dr. J.S. Leo et al.) describe threse methods in detail. It should not be surprising however that CT and MRI play a big role in other chapters, too. Other areas that have received much attention in the recent neuro-ophthalmology literature are reviewed, such as Alzheimer's disease (Dr. J.L. Cummings), botulinum toxin therapy (Dr. P.A. Sibony) and stroke-carotid artery endarterectomy (Dr. J.D. Trobe). Also the more classic neuro-ophthalmology entities such as anterior ischemic optic neuropathy (Dr. M.M. Behrens), migraine therapy (Dr. B.T.

Troost) and myasthenia gravis therapy (Dr. D. Schmidt) are discussed at length. Concerning nystagmus-nestor, Dr. L. Dell'Osso has "discovered" two new types of nystagmus. His list now contains 45 different types of nystagmus and 16 saccadic oscillations/intrusions.

These post-publication peer reviews of the neuro-ophthalmology literature give you a current assessment of the present status of neuro-ophthalmology. We hope that this book will be of benefit to you and to your patients.

Simmons Lessell, M.D.
J.T.W. van Dalen, M.D., Ph.D.

Contents

PART ONE

THE VISUAL SYSTEM

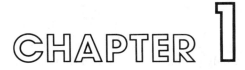

CHAPTER 1

Optic Neuritis

Jon Currie, M.B., B.S., F.R.A.C.P

The Mental Health Research Institute of Victoria, Parkville, Victoria, Australia; The Save Sight and Eye Health Institute, University of Sydney, Sydney, New South Wales, Australia

DIFFERENTIAL DIAGNOSIS OF OPTIC NEURITIS

Neuroretinitis

One form of optic neuritis (ON) needs to be distinguished from idiopathic or demyelinating ON: neuroretinitis, an inflammatory (vascular?) condition of the optic disk and retina characterized by optic disk swelling and the development of a "macular star figure" in the outer plexiform layer of the retina around the macula by lipid exudates derived from leaking optic disk capillaries. Parmley et al.[1] studied 50 patients with neuroretinitis and followed up 10 prospectively for 1 to 2 years and 13 retrospectively for a mean of 8 years. On follow-up, no patient with neuroretinitis either had developed symptoms or signs of multiple sclerosis (MS) or had oligoclonal bands in the cerebrospinal fluid (CSF). Thus, the clinical sign of a macular star in the presence of ON or disk swelling ("papillitis") distinguishes neuroretinitis from the ON of MS and carries an excellent prognosis in comparison with demyelinating ON. A number of variations occur in the presentation of neuroretinitis: in particular, the macular star may not develop until 1 or 2 weeks after the initial symptoms of visual loss. Therefore, Parmley et al. suggest that patients who have signs and symptoms of ON without a macular star should be reexamined after 2 weeks for the development of such a star, with its consequent improvement in prognosis.

Curr Neuro Ophthalmol 2:3–16, 1990
© 1990, Year Book Medical Publishers, Inc.
0893–0147/89/02-003-016-$04.00

3

Infective-Parainfective ON

Jones et al.[2] reported severe ON as the only prominant finding in a 61-year-old man with infectious mononucleosis (Epstein-Barr virus). Visual function recovered nearly completely. The authors also discussed seven other well-documented cases of ON associated with infectious mononucleosis. Purvin et al.[3] described chiasmal ON associated with Epstein-Barr virus infection in a 13-year-old boy, again with good recovery of vision. A 14-year-old girl developed severe bilateral ON, 1 week after a typical varicella vesicular eruption.[4] Visual loss was rapid and accompanied by photopsia and eye pain and proceeded to total blindness. Visual recovery in one eye was very poor, contrary to previous reports,[5, 6] and the authors speculate as to whether treatment with steroids may have *worsened* the visual prognosis. Tunis and Tapert[7] reported a case of unilateral ON occurring 24 days after an episode of herpes zoster ophthalmicus, with the usual poor visual recovery. A useful literature review accompanies this report. Weber and Mikulis[8] reviewed inflammatory disorders of the paranasal sinuses that can cause ON, with emphasis on the diagnostic use of the computed tomographic (CT) scan. Holder et al.[9] described a case of malignant external otitis in a diabetic man that progressed to cause multiple cranial nerve palsies and finally sudden, total monocular visual loss. In a culture from a biopsy of the involved optic nerve, *Pseudomonas aeruginosa* grew.

Margo et al.[10] reported severe unilateral visual loss and neuroretinitis associated with the systemic symptoms of visceral larva migrans. Markedly elevated serum enzyme-linked immunosorbent assay titers for *Toxocara canis* were useful in making the diagnosis, but the visual loss did not respond to treatment with thiabendazole. Farris and Webb[11] reported a classic picture of unilateral ON that developed 15 days after completion of "adequate" antibiotic treatment for Lyme disease *(Borrelia burgdorferi)*. Initial visual loss was severe (light perception), and recovery over several months was incomplete. The patient's initial presentation with Lyme disease had included fever and rash, followed by aseptic meningitis, radicular sensory neuropathy, transverse myelitis, and partial bilateral sixth-nerve palsies.

Pall and Williams[12] reported two complex cases in which ON and hearing loss occurred in association with the Guillain-Barré syndrome, following an otherwise trivial influenzalike illness. In the first patient, ON occurred sequentially in each eye and progressed to total blindness. The second patient had complete unilateral loss of vision. The appearance of the optic disks was normal in the acute stages of visual loss, but optic atrophy later supervened. Auditory function recovered rapidly and completely in both patients. Visual function remained at no light perception for 3 months in the first patient before slowly recovering to 6/9 bilaterally. The second patient remained completely blind in the involved eye. Steroid therapy did not appear to halt progression or accelerate recovery of visual loss in either patient. These two cases are also important in documenting combined involvement of both central and peripheral nervous systems in the Guillain-Barré syndrome.

However, the award for the year's most exotic paper must go to Rebhun et al.,[13] who described the development of varying degrees of ON, retinal vasculitis, retinitis, and chorioretinitis in 21 alpacas and one llama over a 30-day period. Four of the animals also developed neurologic dysfunction. A herpes virus (probably equine herpesvirus I) was isolated from four of the affected animals, and diagnostic antibody titers for equine herpesvirus I were found in the serum of all but one of the animals. This may prove a useful animal model as we try to treat our immunocompromised patients and patients with acquired immunodeficiency syndrome (AIDS) with blinding retinal and optic nerve disease of unknown etiology.

AIDS and Syphilis

As expected, there has been an increasing number of case reports of ON associated with AIDS.[14-19] The majority of these cases still seem to be caused by cytomegalovirus (CMV) infection of the retina and optic nerve,[14-16] with CMV inclusions in the glial cells of the optic nerve. However, there has also been a concomitant increase in the number of cases of syphilitic ON reported with[17-19] or without[20-22] human immunodeficiency virus (HIV) infection. Surprisingly, no cases have yet been reported of visual dysfunction due to direct HIV infection of the optic nerve, despite the neurotrophic propensity of the virus. Cytomegalovirus involvement of the optic nerve appears to have a very poor visual prognosis, even when antiviral therapy, such as with dihydroxy propoxymethyl guanine (DHPG), leads to regression of CMV retinitis.[15, 23, 24] Optic nerve involvement often progresses to total blindness.[15, 24] However, Robinson et al.[25] did show improvement in visual acuity and reversal of an afferent pupillary defect after treatment with DHPG in one patient with CMV ON, when treatment was commenced before visual loss was extreme. Intravitreal DHPG therapy may offer some benefits in selected cases and requires further evaluation.[24, 26]

The rising prevalence of both HIV infection and syphilis has led to the suggestion that all patients infected with HIV be tested for syphilis and vice versa.[24, 27] This is emphasized in three recent case reports of syphilitic ON in HIV antibody-positive patients.[17-19] In this setting, syphilitic ON often seems to be bilateral and visual loss is usually profound. However, with high-dose penicillin therapy, useful visual recovery often occurs, making this an important differential diagnosis to consider in patients with ON.

Optic perineuritis is characterized by a swollen optic disk or disks, normal visual function except for enlarged blind spots on visual field testing, and normal CSF pressure. When unilateral, it must be considered as one of the differential diagnoses in the "big blind spot syndrome."[28] Optic perineuritis is recognized as an uncommon complication of secondary or meningovascular syphilis, and a typical, bilateral case is reported by Toshniwal,[22] with a useful literature review. Unilateral involvement in syphilitic optic perineuritis is uncommon, and two cases reported by McBurney and Rosenberg[20] are therefore of interest. Resolution with penicillin therapy is to be expected and is also of diagnostic value.

Inflammatory and Autoimmune Optic Neuritis

Oppenheimer and Hoffbrand[29] described a case of ON associated with systemic lupus erythematosus (SLE), in which anticardiolipin antibodies and a circulating lupus anticoagulant helped to differentiate this vasculitic ON from idiopathic demyelinating ON. They reemphasize that differentiation of SLE from MS can often be difficult, since ON may be a presenting symptom of SLE and myelopathy can often occur during its course. This was illustrated in the reports of three additional cases of SLE causing ON and transverse myelitis,[30, 31] one in which the spinal cord lesion was demonstrated by magnetic resonance imaging (MRI) scan.[30]

Four cases of neuromyelitis optica with 3 to 7 years of follow-up[32] confirm many of the previously reported features: subacute onset, association of ON and myelitis within several weeks or months, absence of relapse over prolonged follow-up, lack of immunologic abnormalities, good prognosis for paraplegia but poor prognosis for visual loss, and corticosteroid therapy useful for spinal cord involvement but not for visual dysfunction. Less common features in these four cases were unilateral visual loss (one case), onset following acute lymphocytic meningitis (one case), childhood onset (one case), and corticosteroid dependence (two cases). The authors suggest that because of the poor visual prognosis, absence of relapse, and high CSF cell and protein levels, neuromyelitis optica is not just a variant of MS and should be differentiated from it.

The association of recurrent ON with myasthenia gravis was reported three times.[33-35] The first episode of ON occurred 7 years after the development of myasthenia, and there were subsequently at least four episodes of ON involving one or both eyes. There was no clinical or serologic evidence of SLE or MS.

In extensive review of the ocular and systemic manifestations of 112 patients with relapsing polychondritis,[36] one patient had ON at presentation and five developed ON during the course of the disease. In one patient, ON was associated with anterior uveitis and episcleritis.

Bilateral ON may follow envenomation by multiple wasp[37] or bee stings.[38]

Neoplastic-Paraneoplastic ON

Optic neuritis may occur as a nonmetastatic complication of malignant neoplasia. Bennet[39] reported a case of bilateral ON, which was the presenting feature of a squamous cell carcinoma of the lung. The ON resolved following dexamethasone therapy and resection of the primary tumor. In another pathologically confirmed case, unilateral ON developed 4 months after presentation of a paraneo-plastic brain-stem encephalomyelitis with ophthalmoplegia.[40] Histologic examina-tion of the optic nerves showed mild chronic perivascular inflammation, with moderate gliosis and mild central demyelination and axonal loss.

Rapid visual loss caused by bilateral involvement of the optic nerves was re-ported in three patients with high-grade non-Hodgkin's lymphoma.[41] In two cases, optic nerve involvement was the only neurologic complication. All three patients responded to high-dose corticosteroid therapy and/or radiotherapy.

Petersen et al.[42] provide an interesting report of three cases in which apoplexy in a pituitary adenoma produced acute clinical signs and symptoms mimicking ON. They speculate that this unusual presentation was caused by compression of a post-fixed chiasm by acute upward bulging of the sellar diaphragm. In each case, the pituitary tumor was easily identified by CT scan; this again emphasizes the need to perform a CT scan in any case of ON where there is diagnostic uncer-tainty.

A case in which idiopathic inflammation of the optic nerve mimicked an optic nerve sheath meningioma or optic nerve glioma on CT scan was reported twice.[43, 44] As discussed by McCrary et al.,[45] ON can cause diffuse enlargement of the optic nerve and chiasm on CT and MRI scan. The clinical history and neuro-ophthalmic examination remain the best diagnostic tools to prevent unnecessary surgical inter-vention.

ON AND MS

Pathogenesis

In a superb review of the pathogenesis of ON associated with MS, Sergott and Brown[46] discuss in detail the evidence for viral, cell-mediated, and antibody-me-diated etiologies. Patients with acute idiopathic ON have elevated CSF levels of free antimyelin basic protein antibodies, similar to those of patients with MS with acute relapses.[47] There is also intrathecal synthesis of oligoclonal IgG antibodies to one or more viruses during the early development of MS from isolated ON, possibly suggesting recruitment of B-cell clones producing viral antibodies of dif-ferent specificities.[48] However, no evidence for infection with human retroviruses HTLV-I, II, or III was found in serum or CSF of patients with ON or MS.[49]

Considerable controversy still surrounds the question of whether retinal vascular abnormalities and vitritis occur in ON. Although reported by ophthalmologists for over 40 years, most neurologists have rarely seen these changes for themselves and have therefore been reluctant to accept that they occur in the ON of MS. This controversy has been well addressed by Lightman et al.[50] in a recent publication. In 50 consecutive patients presenting with isolated ON and no history or signs suggestive of MS, each patient's pupils were dilated, the fundus was examined by indirect ophthalmoscopy, and a fluorescein angiogram was performed. All but three patients were examined within 8 weeks of the onset of ON. Fourteen (28%) of the 50 patients showed evidence of retinal vascular abnormalities and/or exudation of cells into the vitreous. Perivenous sheathing with fluorescein leakage on angiography was the commonest abnormality. Of note, in only one patient were these abnormalities visible with a direct ophthalmoscope through the undilated pupil. Since most neurologists do not perform a dilated-pupil examination with indirect ophthalmoscopy or fluorescein angiography, this may explain why such lesions have been so rarely reported in the neurologic literature. Multiple sclerosis developed in eight (57%) of the 14 patients with these changes but in only five (16%) of those 32 without such changes. The authors, therefore, suggest that the presence of retinal vascular sheathing and/or inflammation is of predictive value in assessing the risk for progression of isolated ON to clinical MS and may be equivalent to finding evidence (clinical or laboratory) of lesions in the central white matter outside the optic nerve. It has long been known that the cerebral venules are abnormal in the lesions of MS, with the demyelinating plaque oriented around the vessel and perivenous cuffing being a prominent feature of the active lesion. These vascular changes have often been considered just to be a consequence of myelin breakdown. However, the retinal vascular changes occur in areas free of myelin or oligodendrocytes, which argues strongly against this interpretation. The authors postulate that such vascular changes in MS may, in fact, be the primary event leading to the formation of a new demyelinating lesion.

Rate of Conversion From ON to MS

Two excellent long-term follow-up studies[51, 52] provide much-needed and remarkably similar answers to the question: How often after an initial attack of ON will a patient subsequently progress to develop MS? Two particular strengths of the study published by Rizzo and Lessell[51] are that it is prospective in nature and that the initial cohort of patients with ON was extremely carefully defined at the beginning of the study.[53] Between 1966 and 1972, 421 patients with possible ON were evaluated to obtain the final cohort of 60 definite ON cases. All patients were examined by the one experienced neuro-ophthalmologist to establish the diagnosis of ON. All patients had only isolated ON, with no clinical evidence of MS on examination before entering the study. In the follow-up study of this cohort, 6 of the 60 original patients had died, with none developing MS before death. The remaining 54 patients were all available for reassessment, with a mean length of follow-up of 15 years and a range of 5 to 20.5 years. Thirty-five (58%) of the 60 patients with ON had developed MS (69% of the women and 33% of the men). Life table analysis methods probably provide the most realistic assessment of risk in a prospective study. Using the Kaplan-Meier life table analysis, this study suggests that 74% of the women and 34% of the men will have developed MS within

15 years of their initial attack of isolated ON. After 20 years of individual follow-up, it is predicted that 91% of women and 45% of men will develop MS.

The risk of developing MS does not decline after the first few years following the initial attack of ON, and the proportion of patients developing MS steadily increases. Women who have their attack of ON between the ages of 21 and 40 years appear to have the highest risk for developing MS, and the risk is 3.4 times greater for women than for men. Recurrence of ON does not increase the risk of developing MS if the effects of age and sex are taken into account. In the past, some authors considered that the MS that develops after an initial presentation with ON is less severe than with other modes of presentation. However, 6 (17%) of the 35 patients with MS in this study were either moderately or severely disabled after 15 years of follow-up.

Despite some methodologic limitations, Francis et al.[52] found very similar results in their long-term follow-up study. At a mean follow-up interval of 11.3 years (range, 5.8 to 30.5 years), 58 (57%) of the 101 patients available for review had developed MS. Actuarial analysis of these data predicts that 15 years after the initial episode of ON, 75% of patients will develop MS. Some limitations in this study are that it began retrospectively, with 58 of the initial 146 patients already having developed MS before entering the study[54]; that only 101 (69%) of the initial 146 patients reported in 1978[54] were available for follow-up; and, most importantly, that no distinction was made between male and female subjects. This study also found a significantly raised frequency of HLA-DR2 both in patients with isolated ON and in patients with ON/MS, but this did not appear to influence the long-term progression from ON to MS. However, HLA-DR3 was increased in the patient group with ON/MS but not in the group with ON only. Based on actuarial analysis, over 95% of DR3-positive patients with ON will have developed MS within 15 years, while in patients with ON with both DR2 and DR3, the likelihood is even greater. In view of such a high risk of developing MS after ON, the authors suggest that if an effective treatment for MS is developed, patients with DR2 and DR3 may benefit from its institution during the presenting episode of ON.

Diagnosis of MS

The "gold standard" for the diagnosis of MS remains *clinically* definite MS, demonstrated by white matter dysfunction disseminated in time and place. However, with recent advances in immunologic, electrophysiologic, and neuroimaging techniques, emphasis has changed to include "paraclinical" or laboratory-supported diagnosis for definite MS. Different psychophysical and electrophysiologic tests continue to be evaluated in the search for "silent" optic nerve lesions; in addition to evoked potentials, these have included contrast sensitivity,[55–58] Aulhorn flicker test,[59] pupil cycling,[60] pattern electroretinogram,[61–64] and a renewed interest in abnormalities of color vision.[65-69] With varying degrees of effectiveness, a number of studies have utilized multimodel test batteries, including evoked potentials and MRI, in the continuing quest for earlier and more definitive diagnosis of MS.[70-75] Paty et al.[71] undertook a prospective evaluation of 200 patients with suspected MS, using such a multimodel battery. In 38 patients presenting with ON, the visual evoked potential (VEP) was abnormal in 87% of cases, while MRI scan abnormalities were present in 66% to 76% of cases. Cerebrospinal fluid oligoclonal bands (61%), abnormal somatosensory evoked potentials (SEPs; 34%), and CT scan abnormalities (21%) proved less useful in diagnosis. In general, it appears that MRI is the procedure of choice for investigating patients presenting with ON, followed sequentially by CSF studies for oligoclonal bands, SEPs, and CT scans only if each preceding test is negative.

On MRI scan, Kinnunen et al.[72] found that four (40%) of ten patients with ON that was still clinically isolated after 9 to 14 years had silent periventricular or central white matter lesions compatible with MS. The clinical significance of this observation is uncertain. Only one patient had an abnormal SEP or brain-stem evoked potential (BAEP), but eight (80%) of ten patients had abnormal VEPs. These authors also conclude that MRI is more sensitive than evoked potentials in detecting other CNS lesions in patients with ON. The frequency of HLA-B12 and DR2 was significantly increased in ON compared with normal subjects, suggesting a possible common predisposing factor for MS and ON.

Similarly, in children with ON and MS, MRI was more sensitive than evoked potentials in showing disseminated lesions.[73] Central white matter lesions were present at follow-up in two (40%) of five children with bilateral isolated ON and five (71%) of seven of children with ON and MS. Also, HLA-DR2 was increased in childhood ON.

An extensive study by Ormerod et al.[76] provides some of the most comprehensive information to date on MRI scanning in ON and MS. Characteristic periventricular and discrete white matter abnormalities were seen in 99% of patients with clinically definite MS. Using postmortem MRI scans, the authors have been able to demonstrate histologically that the white matter lesions seen on MRI scan originate from chronic plaques of MS. The study included 57 patients with isolated ON (no previous neurologic disease), 42 of whom were adults presenting with their first episode of acute isolated unilateral ON. Twenty-nine (69%) of these 42 patients, scanned 1 to 40 weeks (mean, 9 weeks) after the onset of ON, had multiple brain lesions. In 28 patients these were periventricular, and 21 (50%) of the 42 patients showed additional discrete lesions elsewhere in the cerebral white matter. Eight (28%) of 29 patients tested had SEP and/or BAEP abnormalities, in comparison with 61% with abnormal MRI scans. However, VEPs were abnormal in 100% of optic nerves with ON. These authors also emphasize that it is not yet justified, on the basis of a single MRI scan, to conclude that patients found to have multiple MRI lesions on presentation with isolated ON already have MS. Twenty-five adults with isolated ON were rescanned after 5 to 20 months. Five (20%) of these had new MRI lesions, fulfilling the criteria for clinically probable

MS. However, 6 (35%) of 17 of those with an abnormal initial scan experienced a clinical relapse attributable to a lesion outside the optic nerve, without showing new lesions on MRI scan. None of the patients with a normal initial MRI scan had further clinical symptoms.

In a study of ten patients with isolated ON, Johns et al.[77] found seven (70%) had intracranial MRI abnormalities, with a pattern of lesions in the periventricular white matter similar to that seen in MS. In a follow-up period of 2 months to 2 years (mean, 13.6 months), one patient with an abnormal scan developed MS and one patient had recurrent ON, while none of the three patients with normal scans had further symptoms. In common with several previous studies,[78, 79] this report suggests that in isolated ON there is often more extensive white matter involvement than just the optic nerves, but these reports are unable to distinguish whether this is a monophasic disorder or a sequential demyelination such as occurs in MS.

Despite the sensitivity of the MRI scan to detect CNS white matter lesions in patients with MS, efforts to detect the symptomatic lesion in the optic nerve of patients with ON have been less successful. Miller et al.[80] have developed an MRI technique using a short time inversion recovery sequence that largely overcomes the problems of differentiating between the signals from optic nerve and orbital fat. Thirty-seven patients with ON were studied, 29 with clinically isolated ON and 8 with clinically diagnosed MS. Focal MRI lesions were seen in 37 (84%) of 44 symptomatic optic nerves and in 6 (20%) of 30 asymptomatic nerves. However, VEPs were abnormal in 100% of symptomatic optic nerves and 27% of asymptomatic optic nerves and remain the investigation of choice in suspected demyelinating disease of the optic nerve. Of interest, MRI lesions were frequently seen in the anterior (45%), midintraorbital (61%), or intracanalicular (34%) portions of the optic nerve, but rarely in the intracranial portion (5%) or chiasm (2%). Poor or slow recovery of vision occurred more often with lesions involving the optic canal, supporting the suggestion that by rapidly reducing inflammatory swelling and edema of the optic nerve at this critical site, high-dose steroid therapy may improve visual outcome.[81] Not surprisingly, marked swelling of the optic disk was associated with anterior lesions of the optic nerve, but mild disk swelling also occurred with lesions more posteriorly situated in the nerve.

Treatment of ON and Recovery of Visual Function

Two studies challenge the common clinical doctrine that vision returns to "normal" (20/30 or better) in most patients with ON.[82, 83] Sanders et al.[82] reexamined 53 patients more than 6 months after their episode of ON, measuring contrast sensitivity, color vision, and visual fields (automated perimetry). Abnormalities of one or more of these measures were found in 100%, 55%, 43%, respectively, of nonrecovered (acuity, >1.0), recovered (acuity, >1.0), and unaffected eyes. Taking into account clinical examination and patient symptoms, abnormalities rose to

100%, 88%, and 67%. These abnormalities correlated with the amplitude of the VEP but not with its latency, suggesting that the VEP amplitude provides information about visuospatial perception, while the VEP latency is more related to the extent of demyelination.[83]

Fleishman et al.[84] found similar results using a slightly more extensive test battery in 27 patients (35 eyes), all with recovery to 20/30 or better in Snellen acuity. Abnormalities included relative afferent pupillary defect (95%), light brightness sense (89%), subjective abnormality of vision (85%), stereopsis defect (84%), optic disc pallor (77%), contrast sensitivity (72%), FM 100 Hue (57%), automated perimetry (26%), and Ishihara color plates (11%). Contrast sensitivity was also abnormal in 33% of asymptomatic eyes.

These two studies suggest that symptomatic visual dysfunction is common and optic nerve damage is virtually universal after resolution of ON, even when Snellen acuity has returned to normal. In the past, several studies found little benefit for visual outcome in treating acute demyelinating ON with corticosteroids, although the clinical course to recovery may be shortened. Since such trials normally had Snellen visual acuities as their end point, it is perhaps time to reopen the question of corticosteroid therapy for acute ON and to investigate what effects such intervention would have on these more subtle residual visual deficits that actually appear to be common.

In challenging conventional teaching, Dutton et al.[85] in 1982 described three cases of acute, severe visual loss that they ascribed to "autoimmune ON" and that responded dramatically to early, intensive, intravenous (IV) pulse methylprednisolone therapy. This raised the possibility that such patients formed one end of the spectrum of what we currently call "idiopathic" ON. Spoor[86] subsequently reported the beneficial results of short-term high-dose IV steroid therapy in 6 patients with "optic neuropathy of uncertain etiology." Spoor and Rockwell[81] have now added to this growing controversy with a further report of IV methylprednisolone therapy in ON. Nineteen consecutive patients with ON of uncertain etiology were evaluated: 7 patients were excluded when a cause for the ON became evident (MS, SLE, syphilis, Leber's optic neuropathy, disk drusen). The 12 remaining patients were treated with IV methylprednisolone (250 to 500 mg every 6 hours) for 3 to 7 days, after which the corticosteroid treatment was either abruptly discontinued or a rapidly tapering oral dose was administered. Initial visual loss was often profound in these 12 patients (finger counting or worse in 8 patients). Eleven of the 12 patients had "a gratifying response to IV megadose corticosteroids"; 8 improved rapidly and dramatically to near-normal visual acuity during the course of treatment, despite documented progressive visual loss before the onset of treatment in 5 of these cases. The degree of optic disk swelling did not correlate with the response to treatment, and 2 patients with optic disk atrophy also had a good response. Results such as these suggest that a multicenter, placebo-controlled, randomized study is required to determine the role of high-dose corticosteroid therapy in ON; such a study has now commenced in the United States.

REFERENCES

1. Parmley VC, Schiffman JS, Maitland CG, et al: Does neuroretinitis rule out multiple sclerosis? *Arch Neurol* 1987; 44:1045–1048.

2. Jones J, Gardner W, Newman T: Severe optic neuritis in infectious mononucleosis. *Ann Emerg Med* 1988; 17:361–364.

3. Purvin V, Herr GJ, De Myer W: Chiasmal neuritis as a complication of Epstein-Barr virus infection. *Arch Neurol* 1988; 45:458–460.

4. Purvin V, Hrisomalos N, Dunn D: Varicella optic neuritis. *Neurology* 1988; 38:501–503.

5. Selbst RG, Selhorst JB, Harbison JW, et al: Parainfectious optic neuritis. *Arch Neurol* 1983; 40:347–350.

6. Miller DH, Kay R, Schon F, et al: Optic neuritis following chickenpox in adults. *J Neurol* 1986; 233:182–184.

7. Tunis SW, Tapert MJ: Acute retrobulbar neuritis complicating herpes zoster ophthalmicus. *Ann Ophthalmol* 1987; 19:453–460.

8. Weber AL, Mikulis DK: Inflammatory disorders of paraorbital sinuses and their complications. *Radiol Clin North Am* 1987; 25:615–630.

9. Holder CD, Gurucharri M, Bartels LJ, et al: Malignant external otitis with optic neuritis. *Laryngoscope* 1986; 96:1021–1023.

10. Margo CE, Sedwick LA, Rubin ML: Neuroretinitis in presumed visceral larva migrans. *Retina* 1986; 6:95–98.

11. Farris BK, Webb RM: Lyme disease and optic neuritis. *J Clin Neurol Ophthalmol* 1988; 8:73–78.

12. Pall HS, Williams AC: Subacute polyradiculopathy with optic and auditory nerve involvement. *Arch Neurol* 1987; 44:885–887.

13. Rebhun WC, Jenkins DH, Riis RC, et al: An epizootic of blindness and encephalitis associated with a herpesvirus indistinguishable from equine herpesvirus I in a herd of alpacas and llamas. *J Am Vet Med Assoc* 1988; 192:953–956.

14. Grossniklaus HE, Frank KE, Tomsak RL: Cytomegalovirus retinitis and optic neuritis in acquired immune deficiency syndrome: Report of a case. *Ophthalmology* 1987; 94:1601–1604.

15. Hooymans JM, Sprenger HG, Weits J: Treatment of cytomegalovirus retinitis with DHPG in a patient with AIDS. *Doc Ophthalmol* 1987; 67:5–12.

16. Hansen LL, Wiecha I, Witschel H: Initial diagnosis of acquired immunologic deficiency syndrome (AIDS) by the ophthalmologist. *Klin Monatsbl Augenheilkd* 1987; 191:1133–1136.

17. Carter JB, Hamill RJ, Matoba AY: Bilateral syphilitic optic neuritis in a patient with a positive test for HIV. *Arch Ophthalmol* 1987; 105:1485–1486.

18. Zambrano W, Perez GM, Smith JL: Acute syphilitic blindness in AIDS. *J Clin Neuro Ophthalmol* 1987; 7:1–5.

19. Zaidman GW: Neurosyphilis and retrobulbar neuritis in a patient with AIDS. *Ann Ophthalmol* 1986; 18:260–261.

20. McBurney J, Rosenberg ML: Unilateral syphilitic optic perineuritis presenting as the big blind spot syndrome. *J Clin Neuro Ophthalmol* 1987; 7:167–169.

21. Barthelmess-Mosler S, Volcker HE: Iritis and optic nerve meningitis: Initial symptoms of latent syphilis. *Klin Monatsbl Augenheilkd* 1987; 190:196–198.

22. Toshniwal P: Optic perineuritis with secondary syphilis. *J Clin Neuro Ophthalmol* 1987; 7:6–10.

23. Palestine AG, Stevens G, Lane HC, et al: Treatment of cytomegalovirus retinitis with dihydroxy propoxymethyl guanine. *Am J Ophthalmol* 1986; 101:95–101.

24. Buchi ER, Fitting PL, Michel AE, et al: Long-term intravitreal ganciclovir for cytomegalovirus retinitis in a patient with AIDS. *Arch Ophthalmol* 1988; 106:1349–1350.

25. Robinson MR, Streeten BW, Hampton GR, et al: Treatment of cytomegalovirus optic neuritis with dihydroxy propoxymethyl guanine. *Am J Ophthalmol* 1986; 102:533–534.

26. Henry K, Cantrill H, Fletcher C, et al: Use of intravitreal ganciclovir (dihydroxy propoxymethyl guanine) for cytomegalovirus retinitis in a patient with AIDS. *Am J Ophthalmol* 1987; 103:17–23.

27. Tramont EC: Syphilis in the AIDS era. *N Engl J Med* 1987; 316:1600–1601.

28. Miller NR: The big blind spot syndrome: Unilateral optic disc edema without visual loss or increased intracranial pressure, in Smith JL (ed): *Neuro-ophthalmology Update*. New York, Masson Publishers USA Inc, 1977, pp 163–169.

29. Oppenheimer S, Hoffbrand BI: Optic neuritis and myelopathy in systemic lupus erythematosus. *Can J Neurol Sci* 1986; 13:129–132.

30. Kenik JG, Krohn K, Kelly RB, et al: Transverse myelitis and optic neuritis in systemic lupus erythematosus: A case report with magnetic resonance imaging findings. *Arthritis Rheum* 1987; 30:947–950.

31. Tamaoka A, Murayama S, Sonoh M, et al: Two cases of retrobulbar neuritis and transverse myelopathy as the initial symptoms suggestive of systemic lupus erythematosus (SLE): Case report and review of literature. *Rinsho Shinkeigaku* 1986; 26:483–489.

32. Leys D, Petit H, Block AM, et al: Neuromyelite optique de Devic: Quatre cas. *Rev Neurol* 1987; 143:722–728.

33. Mapelli G, De Palma P, Franco F, et al: Myasthenia gravis and recurrent retrobulbar optic neuritis: An unusual combination of diseases. *Ophthalmologica* 1986; 192:234–237.

34. Mapelli G, De Palma P, Franco F, et al: Optic neuritis with an autoimmune disease (myasthenia gravis). *Acta Neurol* 1986; 8:141–144.

35. Mapelli G: Concurrence of myasthenia gravis and optic neuritis. *J Neurol* 1986; 233:190–191.

36. Isaak BL, Liesegang TJ, Michet CJ Jr: Ocular and systemic findings in relapsing polychondritis. *Ophthalmology* 1986; 93:681–689.

37. Singh I, Chaudhary U: Bilateral optic neuritis following multiple wasp stings. *J Indian Med Assoc* 1986; 84:251–252.

38. Breen LA, Burde RM, Mendelsohn GE: Beesting papillitis. *J Clin Neuro Ophthalmol* 1983; 3:97–100.

39. Bennet WM: Bronchial carcinoma presenting with non-metastatic bilateral papillitis. *Br J Dis Chest* 1986; 80:189–190.

40. Boghen D, Sebag M, Michaud J: Paraneoplastic optic neuritis and encephalomyelitis: Report of a case. *Arch Neurol* 1988; 45:353–356.

41. Holte H, Saeter G, Dahl IM, et al: Progressive loss of vision in patients with high-grade non-Hodgkin's lymphoma. *Cancer* 1987; 60:2521–2523.

42. Petersen P, Christiansen KH, Lindholm J: Acute monocular disturbances mimicking optic neuritis in pituitary apoplexy. *Acta Neurol Scand* 1988; 78:101–103.

43. Zhang TL, Shao SF, Zhang T, et al: Idiopathic inflammation of optic nerve simulating optic nerve sheath meningioma. *Chin Med J Engl* 1987; 100:541–542.

44. Zhang TL, Shao SF, Zhang T, et al: Idiopathic inflammation of optic nerve simulating optic nerve sheath meningioma: CT demonstration. *J Comput Assist Tomogr* 1987; 11:360–361.

45. McCrary JA, Demer JL, Friedman DI, et al: Computed tomography and magnetic resonance imaging in the diagnosis of inflammatory disease of the optic nerve. *Surv Ophthalmol* 1987; 31:352–355.

46. Sergott RC, Brown MJ: Current concepts of the pathogenesis of optic neuritis associated with multiple sclerosis. *Surv Ophthalmol* 1988; 33:108–116.

47. Warren KG, Catz I, Bauer C: Cerebrospinal fluid antibodies to myelin basic protein in acute idiopathic optic neuritis. *Ann Neurol* 1988; 23:297–299.

48. Sandberg-Wollheim M, Vandvik B, Nadj C, et al: The intrathecal immune response in the early stage of multiple sclerosis. *J Neurol Sci* 1987; 81:45–53.

49. Madden DL, Mundon FK, Tzan NR, et al: Serologic studies of MS patients, controls, and patients with neurologic diseases: Antibodies to HTLV-I, II, III. *Neurology* 1988; 38:81–84.

50. Lightman S, McDonald WI, Bird AC, et al: Retinal venous sheathing in optic neuritis: Its significance for the pathogenesis of multiple sclerosis. *Brain* 1987; 110:405–414.

51. Rizzo JF, Lessell S: Risk of developing multiple sclerosis after uncomplicated optic neuritis: A long-term prospective study. *Neurology* 1988; 38:185–190.

52. Francis DA, Compston DAS, Batchelor JR, et al: A reassessment of the risk of multiple sclerosis developing in patients with optic neuritis after extended follow-up. *J Neurol Neurosurg Psychiatry* 1987; 50:758–765.

53. Cohen MM, Lessell S, Wolf PA: A prospective study of the risk of developing multiple sclerosis in uncomplicated optic neuritis. *Neurology* 1979; 29:208–213.

54. Compston DAS, Batchelor JR, Earl CJ, et al: Factors influencing the risk of multiple sclerosis developing in patients with optic neuritis. *Brain* 1978; 101:495–511.

55. Nordmann JP, Saraux H, Roullet E: Contrast sensitivity in multiple sclerosis: A study in 35 patients with or without optic neuritis. *Ophthalmologica* 1987; 195:199–204.

56. Lorance RW, Kaufman D, Wray SH, et al: Contrast visual testing in neurovisual diagnosis. *Neurology* 1987; 37:923–929.

57. Plant GT, Hess RF: Regional threshold contrast sensitivity within the central visual field in optic neuritis. *Brain* 1987; 110:489–515.

58. Wright CE, Drasdo N, Harding GF: Pathology of the optic nerve and visual association areas: Information given by the flash and pattern visual evoked potential, and the temporal and spatial contrast sensitivity function. *Brain* 1987; 110:107–120.

59. Christ TH, Pillunat LE, Stodmeister R: The "Flicker test" according to Aulhorn in the diagnosis of acute optic neuritis. *Ophthalmologica* 1986; 192:220–227.

60. Milton JG, Longtin A, Kirkham TH, et al: Irregular pupil cycling as a characteristic abnormality in patients with demyelinative optic neuropathy. *Am J Ophthalmol* 1988; 105:402–407.

61. Dodt E: The electrical response of the human eye to patterned stimuli: Clinical observations. *Doc Ophthalmol* 1987; 65:271–286.

62. Veagan, Billson FA: The differential effects of optic nerve disease on pattern and focal electroretinograms. *Doc Ophthalmol* 1987; 65:45–55.

63. Porciatti V: Non-linearities in the focal ERG evoked by pattern and uniform-field stimulation: Their variation in retinal and optic nerve dysfunction. *Invest Ophthalmol Vis Sci* 1987; 28:1306–1313.

64. Ringens PJH, van Lith GHM, van der Poel H: The pattern-elicited electroretinogram. *Ophthalmologica* 1986; 192:217–219.

65. Jaeger W: Diagnostic value of pseudoprotanomaly for differential diagnosis between retinal and optic nerve disease. *Klin Monatsbl Augenheilkd* 1987; 191:427–429.

66. Engell T, Trojaborg W, Raun NE: Subclinical optic neuropathy in multiple sclerosis: A neuroophthalmological investigation by means of visually evoked response, Farnworth-Munsell 100 Hue test and Ishihara test and their diagnostic value. *Acta Ophthalmol* 1987; 65:735–740.

67. Harrison AC, Becker WJ, Stell WK: Color vision abnormalities in multiple sclerosis. *Can J Neurol Sci* 1987; 14:279–285.

68. Sellers KL, Chioran GM, Dain SJ, et al: Red-green mixture thresholds in congenital and acquired color defects. *Vision Res* 1986; 26:1083–1097.

69. Frederiksen J, Larsson H, Olesen J, et al: Evaluation of the visual system in multiple sclerosis: II. Color vision. *Acta Neurol Scand* 1986; 74:203–209.

70. Hume AL, Waxman SG: Evoked potentials in suspected multiple sclerosis: Diagnostic value and prediction of clinical course. *J Neurol Sci* 1988; 83:191–210.

71. Paty DW, Oger JJ, Kastrukoff LF, et al: MRI in the diagnosis of MS: A prospective study with comparison of clinical evaluation, evoked potentials, oligoclonal banding and CT. *Neurology* 1988; 38:180–185.

72. Kinnunen E, Larsen A, Ketonen L, et al: Evaluation of central nervous system involvement in uncomplicated optic neuritis after prolonged follow-up. *Acta Neurol Scand* 1987; 76:147–151.

73. Riikonen R, Ketonen L, Sipponen J: Magnetic resonance imaging, evoked responses and cerebrospinal fluid findings in a follow-up study of children with optic neuritis. *Acta Neurol Scand* 1988; 77:44–49.

74. Sola P, Merrelli E, Schoenhuber R, et al: Neurophysiological and CSF immunological study of 19 patients affected by acute idiopathic optic neuritis. *Acta Neurol Scand* 1987; 75:140–144.

75. Fischer C, Mauguiere F, Ibanez V, et al: Visual, early auditory and somatosensory evoked potentials in multiple sclerosis (917 cases). *Rev Neurol* 1986; 142:517–523.

76. Ormerod IE, Miller DH, McDonald WI, et al: The role of NMR imaging in the assessment of multiple sclerosis and isolated neurological lesions: A quantitative study. *Brain* 1987; 110:1579–1616.

77. Johns K, Lavin P, Elliot JH, et al: Magnetic resonance imaging of the brain in isolated optic neuritis. *Arch Ophthalmol* 1986; 104:1486–1488.

78. Ormerod IEC, McDonald WI, du Boulay EPGH, et al: Disseminated lesions at presentation in patients with optic neuritis. *J Neurol Neurosurg Psychiatry* 1986; 49:124–127.

79. Jacobs L, Kinkel PR, Kinkel WR: Silent brain lesions in patients with isolated idiopathic optic neuritis: A clinical and nuclear magnetic resonance imaging study. *Arch Neurol* 1986; 43:452–455.

80. Miller DH, Newton MR, van der Poel JC, et al: Magnetic resonance imaging of the optic nerve in optic neuritis. *Neurology* 1988; 38:175–179.

81. Spoor TC, Rockwell DL: Treatment of optic neuritis with intravenous megadose corticosteroids. *Ophthalmology* 1988; 95:131–134.

82. Sanders EA, Volkers AC, van der Poel JC, et al: Estimation of visual function after optic neuritis: A comparison of clinical tests. *Br J Ophthalmol* 1986; 70:918–924.

83. Sanders EA, Volkers AC, van der Poel JC, et al: Visual function and pattern visual evoked response in optic neuritis. *Br J Ophthalmol* 1987; 71:602–608.

84. Fleishman JA, Beck RW, Linares DA, et al: Deficits in visual function after resolution of optic neuritis. *Ophthalmology* 1987; 94:1029–1035.

85. Dutton JJ, Burde RM, Klingele TG: Autoimmune retrobulbar optic neuritis. *Am J Ophthalmol* 1982; 94:11–17.

86. Spoor TC: Treatment of optic neuritis with megadose corticosteroids. *J Clin Neuro Ophthalmol* 1986; 6:137–143.

CHAPTER 2

Tumors of the Optic Nerve

John S. Kennerdell, M.D.
Clinical Professor of Ophthalmology, University of Pittsburgh School of Medicine; Chairman of Ophthalmology, Allegheny General Hospital, Pittsburgh, Pennsylvania

Thomas A. Gardner, M.D.
Fellow, Department of Ophthalmology, Allegheny General Hospital, Pittsburgh, Pennsylvania

Tumors of the optic nerve include optic nerve gliomas, chiasmal gliomas, and optic nerve sheath meningiomas. Management of optic nerve and chiasmal gliomas has been controversial for some time. Numerous articles continue to support some response of these tumors to radiotherapy. Optic nerve sheath meningiomas also appear to respond to radiotherapy, which is especially useful after subtotal surgical excision. New treatment modalities being investigated include chemotherapy for gliomas and hormonal therapy for meningiomas.

Diagnosis of these tumors has continued to improve with the rapidly advancing technology of magnetic resonance imaging (MRI). Higher magnetic field strength, faster scanning times, and the new gadolinium contrast agent provide increased sensitivity and specificity.

DIAGNOSTIC IMAGING

Magnetic resonance imaging and computed tomography (CT) can provide complementary information about orbital tumors. When knowledge of calcification is

Curr Neuro Ophthalmol 2:17–22, 1990
© 1990, Year Book Medical Publishers, Inc.
0893–0147/89/02-017-022-$04.00

important in the differential diagnosis, CT should be used because MRI does not image calcium. However, this provides MRI an advantage when imaging intracanalicular tumors and intracanalicular extension of orbital tumors; MRI does not have the artifacts from the surrounding bone seen with CT scans. The tumor and any surrounding edema can be easily seen on MRI T_2-weighted images. Magnetic resonance imaging can show early infiltration into the canal before any mass effect would be seen with CT; MRI can scan coronal and sagittal views without repositioning the patient or using computer reformatting. Also, MRI has no associated ionizing radiation.

Brown et al.[1] report a series of patients with neurofibromatosis who had CT and MRI (0.35-tesla) scans. Of 21 patients, 13 were found to have optic pathway lesions. Both CT and MRI were found to be equivalent in detecting optic nerve and chiasmal lesions. However, MRI showed posterior extension much better than contrast-enhanced CT. Haik et al.[2] and Patronas et al.,[3] both using 0.5-tesla scanners, showed some improvement in detecting chiasmal lesions with the MRI.

Magnetic resonance imaging has also been shown to visualize the arachnoidal gliomatosis typical of optic nerve gliomas associated with neurofibromatosis. Seiff et al.[4] reported the MRI and CT scans of such a patient. On T_2-weighted MRI scans, the intraneural and perineural glial proliferation could be easily differentiated.

Eidelberg et al.[5] used a short TI inversion (STIR) pulse sequence to image intraneural abnormalities when evaluating patients with chronic optic neuropathy. The STIR sequence has the advantage of suppressing the signal from the orbital fat, which can cause volume averaging and chemical shift artifacts.

OPTIC NERVE GLIOMA

The definitive management of optic nerve glioma remains unclear. Further studies continue in the use of radiotherapy and chemotherapy.

Continuing analysis of patients in the well-known Hoyt and Baghdassarian[6] report has shown increased morbidity and mortality according to Imes and Hoyt.[7] Of note, in patients with neurofibromatosis, there were 6 of 9 deaths attributable to other tumors and only two to the chiasmal gliomas. Of the 7 mortalities in patients without neurofibromatosis, 3 were due to the chiasmal tumor, 2 were perioperative, and 2 were due to medical illnesses. The surviving patients have been followed up for 14 to 44 years with a good quality of life and no noticeable decrease in vision. Unfortunately, the only long-term ophthalmologic follow-up information is entirely subjective.

The effect of radiotherapy on optic nerve gliomas has been debated for many years. Montgomery et al.[8] reported a series of 16 patients diagnosed by biopsy or observation at craniotomy. Vision was reported to improve or remain stable in all of the surviving patients. No information was given on the exact visual acuity or visual fields. They noted that no recurrences occurred after treatment with 5,000 rad or more. Follow-up ranged from 1 to 14 years, with 4 deaths attributed to growth or recurrence of the gliomas.

Horwich and Bloom[9] reported on 29 patients treated with radiotherapy for progressive disease, 87% of whom had tumor involving the chiasm. Ninety percent had no progression. Of the 23 patients in whom the visual acuity and visual fields were evaluated (the other six were infants), there was initial improvement in visual acuity in 43%, and 48% remained stable. The visual fields initially improved in 18% and remained stable in the remaining 82%. It is not clear how much time had elapsed after radiotherapy when the acuity and visual fields were reexamined. There was a 93% survival at 10 and 15 years of follow-up. Thirty-three percent of the patients had some amount of endocrine dysfunction. Fifty gray of radiation is recommended for adults and 45 Gy for children, preferably waiting until the child is older than 2 years.

Wong et al.[10] found improved visual acuity in six (35%) of 17 patients with chiasmal gliomas and a decreased recurrence rate with radiotherapy. Flickinger et al.[11] reported visual stabilization and 87% progression-free survival at 15 years in 36 patients with optic nerve or chiasmal gliomas. Weiss et al.[12] also reported improvement in visual acuity and visual field and recommend treatment of chiasmal gliomas at the initial time of diagnosis rather than waiting for any increase in symptoms. All recommend treatment with 50 Gy.

Fletcher et al.[13] noted that tumor appearance on CT scans did not correlate with visual function in follow-up examinations. The tumor can grow without visual deterioration, and there can be decreased visual function with no observable tumor expansion. They also had five tumors decrease in size after radiotherapy.

Rosenstock et al.[14] presented a preliminary report of chemotherapy treatment of chiasmal gliomas with vincristine and dactinomycin. The 4 initial patients remained stable, and 6 of 12 of the more recent patients had tumor shrinkage documented on CT. Further follow-up is anxiously awaited as it may provide an alternative to radiotherapy, especially in younger children.

Wolter[15] reported on 2 patients who underwent optic nerve glioma excision, with a 10-year follow-up. There was remarkably little external sign of the surgery. Long-term effects of the surgical excision of the optic nerve glioma included retinal and iris atrophy.

In our opinion, optic nerve glioma management remains surgical, with complete excision through a craniotomy if function is poor and the tumor is large. Observation is justified in patients with fair to good function and acceptable proptosis. Chiasmal gliomas should be observed unless function is deteriorating or significant growth is seen, at which time radiotherapy or possible chemotherapy should be considered.

MENINGIOMA

Radiotherapy can also be effective in the treatment of optic nerve sheath meningioma. Smith et al.[16] reviewed 5 patients with primary optic nerve sheath meningiomas who were treated with radiotherapy. They noted improved visual acuity and visual fields along with regression of optic ciliary shunt vessels.

Kennerdell et al.[17] reviewed the overall management of optic nerve sheath meningiomas in 38 patients in conjunction with their typical clinical progression. All of the patients observed with initial acuity of 20/40 or better had visual deterioration within 5 years. Tumor growth was not seen in these patients with CT or MRI scanning. Observation or surgical excision was offered to patients with little or no vision, and radiotherapy was offered to patients with primary intraorbital meningiomas with progressive visual loss. Six patients were treated with 5,500 rad for progressive visual loss. All of these patients had improvement in their visual acuity and visual fields, which has been maintained on minimum follow-up of 3 years. No change in tumor size was observed. Radiation is also recommended following subtotal excision. Attempted total excision of the tumor with preservation of the optic nerve is no longer recommended.

Guyer et al.[18] reported long-term follow-up after optic canal decompression for a variety of causes of compressive optic neuropathy. They reported that ten (66.7%) of 15 eyes had an improvement of visual acuity, but only 4 eyes (26.7%) actually improved to better than 20/200, and 1 eye decreased from 20/20 with full visual field to no light perception. No controls were included for comparison. Surgical decompression may provide both the diagnosis and treatment in patients with an intracanalicular tumor, which is not seen with neuroimaging. Surgery may also stop progressive visual loss, but it is not to be taken lightly or considered definitive.

Barbaro et al.[19] Petty et al.[20] and Kupersmith et al.[21] have shown good response with radiotherapy after subtotal excision of intracranial meningiomas. Kupersmith et al. included pathology of a recurrent meningioma after radiotherapy, which showed hyalinized necrotic tissue.

Olson et al.[22] reported an interesting in vivo study of responses of meningioma cells in tissue culture to various hormonal agonists and antagonists. A progesterone antagonist was the only one to decrease the cell growth significantly. We hope this will become a useful adjunct in future therapeutic protocols.

It is becoming clear to us that radiation has a role in optic nerve meningioma management, but treatment must be carefully individualized.

OTHER OPTIC NERVE TUMORS

Wojno et al.[23] presented an interesting patient with bilateral optic nerve sheath enlargement of unknown cause. A complete serologic and radiologic workup including spinal fluid analysis was unremarkable. The patient underwent bilateral optic nerve sheath decompression with stabilization of his vision, with 9 months of follow-up. Microscopic examination of the optic nerve sheath showed no abnormality.

REFERENCES

1. Brown EW, Riccardi VM, Mawad M, et al: MR imaging of optic pathways in patients with neurofibromatosis. *AJNR* 1987; 8:1031–1036.
2. Haik BG, St Louis L, Bierly J, et al: Magnetic resonance imaging in the evaluation of optic nerve gliomas. *Ophthalmology* 1987; 94:709–717.
3. Patronas NJ, Dwyer AJ, Papathanasiou M, et al: Contributions of magnetic resonance imaging in the evaluation of optic gliomas. *Surg Neurol* 1987; 28:367–371.
4. Seiff SR, Brodsky MC, MacDonald G, et al: Orbital optic glioma in neurofibromatosis. *Arch Ophthalmol* 1987; 105:1689–1692.
5. Eidelberg D, Newton MR, Johnson G, et al: Chronic unilateral optic neuropathy: A magnetic resonance study. *Ann Neurol* 1988; 24:3–11.
6. Hoyt WG, Baghdassarian SA: Optic glioma of childhood: Natural history and rationale for conservative management. *Br J Ophthalmol* 1969; 53:793–798.
7. Imes RK, Hoyt WF: Childhood chiasmal gliomas: Update on the fate of patients in the 1969 San Francisco study. *Br J Ophthalmol* 1986; 70:179–182.
8. Montgomery AB, Griffin T, Parker RG, et al: Optic nerve glioma: The role of radiation therapy. *Cancer* 1977; 40:2079–2080.
9. Horwich A, Bloom HJG: Optic gliomas: Radiation therapy and prognosis. *Radiat Oncol Biol* 1985; 11:1067–1079.
10. Wong JYC, Uhl V, Wara WM, et al: Optic gliomas. *Cancer* 1987; 60:1847–1855.
11. Flickinger JC, Torres C, Deutsch M: Management of low grade gliomas of the optic nerve and chiasm. *Cancer* 1988; 61:635–642.
12. Weiss L, Sagerman RH, King GA, et al: Controversy in the management of optic nerve glioma. *Cancer* 1987; 59:1000–1004.
13. Fletcher WA, Imes RK, Hoyt WF: Chiasmal gliomas: Appearance and long-term changes demonstrated by computerized tomography. *J Neurosurg* 1986; 65:154–159.
14. Rosenstock JG, Packer RJ, Bilaniuk L, et al: Chiasmatic optic glioma treated with chemotherapy. *J Neurosurg* 1985; 63:862–866.
15. Wolter JR: Ten years without orbital optic nerve: Late clinical results after removal of retrobulbar gliomas with preservation of blind eyes. *J Pediatr Ophthalmol Strabismus* 1988; 25:55–59.
16. Smith JL, Vuksanovic MM, Yates BM, et al: Radiation therapy for primary optic nerve meningiomas. *Clin Neuro Ophthalmol* 1981; 1:85–99.
17. Kennerdell JS, Maroon JC, Malton M, et al: The management of optic nerve sheath meningiomas. *Am J Ophthalmol* 1988; 106:450–457.
18. Guyer DR, Miller NR, Long DM, et al: Visual function following optic canal decompression via craniotomy. *J Neurosurg* 1985; 62:631–638.
19. Barbaro NM, Gutin PH, Wilson CB, et al: Radiation therapy in the treatment of partially resected meningiomas. *Neurosurgery* 1987; 20:525–528.
20. Petty AM, Kun LE, Meyer GA: Radiation therapy for incompletely resected meningiomas. *J Neurosurg* 1985; 62:502–507.

21. Kupersmith MJ, Warren FA, Newall J, et al: Irradiation of meningiomas of the intracranial anterior visual pathway. *Ann Neurol* 1987; 21:131–137.

22. Olson JJ, Beck DW, Schlechte J, et al: Hormonal manipulation of meningiomas in vitro. *J Neurosurg* 1986; 65:99–107.

23. Wojno T, Beck RW, Grosserode R: Bilateral optic nerve sheath enlargement. *Ophthalmic Surg* 1986; 17:584–588.

CHAPTER 3

Other Optic Nerve Disorders

Myles Behrens, M.D.

Professor of Clinical Ophthalmology, Columbia Presbyterian Medical Center, New York, New York

Jeffrey G. Odel, M.D.

Instructor of Clinical Ophthalmology, Columbia Presbyterian Medical Center, New York, New York

Repka and Miller found the causes of optic atrophy in 89% of 218 children.[1] Tumor (most gliomas or craniopharyngiomas) accounted for 29%, inflammation 17%, trauma 11%, heredity 9%, perinatal events 9%, hydrocephalus 6%, neurodegenerative diseases 5%, toxic and metabolic causes 1%, and miscellaneous causes 3%. They considered that the high incidence of tumors in their series probably reflected the fact that the series came from a referral center and that the incidence of neurodegenerative diseases in their study may be misleadingly low, since optic atrophy may develop late in the course of neurodegenerative disease. Neuroimaging is indicated in any child with optic atrophy if the history fails to provide an obvious explanation.

Advances in neuroimaging continue. Short inversion time inversion recovery (STIR) sequences in magnetic resonance imaging (MRI) of the optic nerves[2] can demonstrate a high signal in the optic nerve in optic neuritis.[3] The technique also shows the edema in acute optic neuritis. Compressive and infiltrative lesions are also well defined by MRI.[4] In perioptic orbital mass lesions, MRI can clarify the relation of the tumor to the optic nerve.

Peli et al. reported on the various techniques for retinal nerve fiber layer photography.[5] The Canon CF-60Z camera was preferred over the Zeiss FF-111, Pana-

Curr Neuro Ophthalmol 2:23–42, 1990
© 1990, Year Book Medical Publishers, Inc.
0893–0147/89/02-023-042-$04.00

tomic-X film over Plus-X film, and the Standard SE-40 blue filter over the green Spectrotech 540 filter. Filter choice was affected by specific circumstances: the blue filter provided better contrast for examining patients with lightly pigmented fundi; the green filter was preferred in the presence of light-scattering opacities in the media.

Newman et al. documented evidence of retinal nerve fiber layer loss in diseases of the outer retinal layers.[6] Diffuse or local changes were shown in cone-rod dystrophies, rod-cone dystrophies, juvenile macular degeneration, fundus flavimaculatus, vitelliform macular dystrophy, and Leber's congenital amaurosis. Progression of nerve fiber layer defects correlated with progression of the disease. These findings suggest that there is transsynaptic degeneration or primary involvement of the inner retinal layers in diseases of the outer layers. We have observed an inordinant degree of disk pallor in patients with the fundus findings and electroretinographic abnormalities of Leber's congenital amaurosis. The authors suggest that electroretinography (ERG) may be useful in the evaluation of patients with defects in the retinal nerve fiber layer but who do not have obvious optic nerve disease. They also noted an abnormal pattern ERG (PERG) in Stargardt's disease (juvenile macular degeneration). In their opinion, this suggests some inner retinal involvement in this disease.

Shortly thereafter, Holder clarified the relation of the abnormal PERG to the site of the lesions.[7] He cited selective involvement of the main positive (P50) component in dysfunction of the retina/macula and of the late negative (N95) component in optic nerve diseases. This wave is most likely generated by the ganglion cells and is affected by retrograde degeneration. One study has reported using the PERG and visually evoked potential (VEP) in cases of multiple sclerosis.[8] It helps to distinguish demyelination from axonal damage. In demyelination the PERG is normal but the VEP is delayed. With axonal damage, both the PERG and the VEP are abnormal. A subsequent report evaluated the PERG in patients with ocular hypertension and glaucoma.[9] It showed reduction in the second negative wave in patients with optic nerve dysfunction.

Drucker et al. evaluated contrast grading sensitivity (using Regan's low-contrast letter charts) in 35 eyes of 31 patients with optic neuropathies.[10] All had Snellen acuities of at least 20/30. A 93% sensitivity was found. Color vision tests using the Ishihara plates showed abnormalities in only 49% of the eyes.

Browning and Buckley tested brightness comparison with a swinging 6-V test light and with the patient's eyes closed.[11] Not surprisingly, they were able to predict relative afferent pupillary defects in 62% of 206 unselected patients in subgroups of patients with glaucoma and with other optic neuropathies. Correct predictions were made in 92% of the former group and 83% of the latter. This may be a useful test in patients for whom conventional pupillary testing is not possible.

Sadun and others documented seven human retinofugal pathways using the paraphenylene-diamine staining method.[12-14] There are pathways to the geniculate, pretectum, superior colliculus and pulvinar, and three pathways to the hypothalamus. As indicated, this would suggest parallel visual systems that most likely serve different visual tasks. This is further support for parallel processing within the anterior visual pathway.

CONGENITAL ANOMALIES

A fine review of optic nerve hypoplasia was published by Lambert et al.[15] It emphasized the role of supranormal regression of optic nerve axons in the pathogenesis of this disorder. In normal fetal human optic nerve there is overproduction of axons and then subsequent regression.[16] Another review examined levels within the nervous system at which lesions may be associated with optic nerve hypoplasia.[17] Six illustrative cases were included. Case 1 was an interesting example of temporal sector hypoplasia in association with macular coloboma.

Optic nerve hypoplasia was present in 48% of cases of fetal alcohol syndrome.[18] A study by Cook et al. indicated that the "insult" in the fetal alcohol syndrome occurs at a very specific period in the mouse embryo, which corresponds to the third fetal week in humans.[19] Katz et al. reported a case of an infant with the nevus sebaceous of Jadassohn associated with a porencephalic cyst and dysplastic right cerebral hemisphere, who also had optic nerve hypoplasia.[20] The more commonly recognized chorioretinal colobomas were also present.

Lincoff et al. reported the results of a multicenter study in which retinoschisis was found as the primary basis for retinal separations found in continuity with optic disk pits.[21] There were further reports reviewing the treatment of serous macular detachments associated with optic disk pits or colobomas.[22-24] A- and B-scan ultrasonography were reported in patients with optic nerve head colobomas.[25] These demonstrated excavation and thickening of the distal optic nerve. The pattern was somewhat distinct from that seen in glaucomatous cupping. The computed tomographic (CT) findings in optic nerve colobomas and in the related morning glory syndrome were reported.[26, 27] Widening of the retrobulbar optic nerve with funnel-shaped or craterlike excavation, with prolapse of ocular contents and scleral ectasia, were demonstrated. Figure 1 demonstrates the MRI appearance of such a colobomatous defect in a patient with visual impairment with a large elongated optic nerve head and a suggestion of a filled-in pit. The MRI helped to allay initial concern that there was a mass lesion of the distal optic nerve.

TRAUMA AND DECOMPRESSION

The surprising recovery of vision after loss of light perception from presumed direct optic nerve trauma from shotgun injury was reported by Feist et al.[28] The VEP was absent on the seventh day following injury and the first suggestion of a pupillary response to light was at 12 days. Light perception appeared at 15 days,

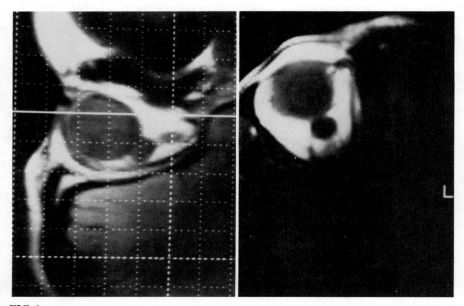

FIG 1.
MRI scans, sagittal and axial, showing colobomatous enlargement of distal optic nerve shadow. Initially a mass lesion had been suspected.

and by 4 months, without any surgical or medical therapy, the patient could see 20/100 in the superior field!

An interesting case of indirect optic nerve injury was reported by Purvin.[29] The patient was a weight lifter who suffered visual loss from a 270 pound barbell that rested on his brow, presumably deforming his orbit. This apparently distorted his optic canal without any blow or impact, and represented the clinical equivalent of Anderson and co-workers' experiments on skull trauma.[30]

Another case of optic nerve avulsion was reported; however, the diagnosis was difficult because the patient was evaluated a year after injury.[31]

Manor et al. reported a case of indirect optic nerve trauma complicated by increased intracranial pressure.[32] The patient developed bilateral papilledema more prominently in the contralateral eye. It persisted in the contralateral eye, but progressively decreased as optic atrophy supervened on the side of the injured optic nerve. This was recognized as being compatible with the experimental observation of Quigley et al. of retention of slow axoplasmic flow 2 weeks after optic nerve transection, but abnormal flow at 3 weeks when axonal degeneration supervened.[33]

Carter and Nerad reported another instance of visual loss from orbital emphysema.[34] The typical fluctuation (from a one-way valve phenomenon associated with expiration) was present. There was also a report of an optic neuropathy from compressed air injury from a truck tire whose air stem had penetrated the orbit.[35]

There was some improvement in vision following bilateral optic nerve decompression in a case of osteopetrosis[36] and the authors emphasized the need to widely unroof the canal. Since some primary retinopathy may be present in this disease, ERG would be of value to help understand the basis for the visual loss.

Leone and Wissinger discussed their experience with transcranial surgical approaches to the orbit.[37] They removed the superior rim and the roof, a procedure indicated mainly for masses in the orbital apex that are not fully accessible by other techniques. Of course, this technique is also useful for the management of optic nerve tumors that require canal and intracranial exposure, as well. The authors used a modification of the technique of Maroon and Kennerdell[38] with a controlled break across the anterior roof and exposure of the optic nerve, after techniques by Housepian et al.[39, 40]

TOXIC NEUROPATHIES

Hayasaka et al. found optic atrophy without evidence of retinal pigment degeneration in six of nine children with lactic acidosis.[41] Etiologies included Leigh subacute necrotizing encephalomyelopathy, mitochondrial myopathy, pyruvate decarboxylase deficiency, and cytochrome oxidase deficiency.

Spaide et al. studied optic nerve function in 32 patients with cystic fibrosis.[42] They found that visually asymptomatic patients who have used chloramphenicol may have color vision and VEP abnormalities. They also found that contrast grating sensitivity was decreased in patients with cystic fibrosis as compared to controls, even if chloramphenicol had not been used. It may be that there are factors other than chloramphenicol that play a role in impairment of optic nerve function in patients with cystic fibrosis.

Snebold et al. reported the case of a 32-year-old man with ornithine transcarbamoylase deficiency and hyperammonemia.[43] He had episodic bilateral visual impairment and confusion, presumably consequent to his disease. It was uncertain whether the metabolic visual impairment resulted from dysfunction at the level of the optic nerve or the cerebral hemispheres.

Severe bilateral optic atrophy was reported in an infant with primary oxalosis.[44] There was marked attenuation of retinal arterioles in addition to the characteristic yellow dots scattered throughout the posterior pole and midperiphery and pigmented macular lesons. The optic atrophy was attributed to widespread loss of axons in the inner retinal layers. The authors cited evidence of oxalate deposit at that location. The VEP was abnormal; an ERG was not done. This is unfortunate, since the retinal findings suggest the possibility of primary *outer* retinal involvement, perhaps with secondary loss of ganglion cells and nerve fiber layer (see previous section). His end-stage renal failure might also have played a role, although there was no hypertension.

HEREDITARY OPTIC NEUROPATHIES

Nikoskelainen et al. continued their clarification of the inheritance of Leber's hereditary optic neuropathy.[45] They reported a study of four families and included not only affected individuals but also asymptomatic subjects with peripapillary microangiopathy. A fundus photograph of a patient with typical peripapillary changes present for 7 years without loss of vision was included. Nikoskelainen et al. showed that every daughter and son of a female carrier inherits the trait. This confirmed the presumption of maternal or cytoplasmic inheritance. They also reported that a high percentage of patients have electrocardiographic abnormalities. Forty of 79 in the descending female lines, but only 1 of 20 in the descending male lines, showed abnormalities. Most were asymptomatic. Fourteen of the 40 abnormalities in the female line were preexcitation syndromes with shortened P–R interval—either the Wolff-Parkinson-White or the Lown-Ganong-Levine syndrome. Cardiac dysfunction was found in both males and females but did not necessarily correlate well with the presence of optic nerve dysfunction. Cardiac abnormalities were most common in the family with the highest frequency of optic neuropathy.

Uemura et al. conducted histochemical and electron microscopic studies of muscle biopsies in two patients with Leber's hereditary optic neuropathy who had no clinical evidence of a muscle abnormality.[46] They found mild but distinct myopathic changes, and considered this evidence of multisystem involvement. There were abnormal oxidative enzyme activities, aggregates of enlarged mitochondria in the subsarcolemmal regions, and disruptions of myofilaments. These changes were similar to those seen in the ragged red fibers of such diseases as the Kearns-Sayre syndrome. Limited biochemical analyses of the mitochondria did not show abnormalities. The authors reminded us that Nikoskelainen et al. had not found decreased activity of rhodanese (the cyanide detoxifying mitochondrial enzyme) in muscle biopsy specimens from patients with Leber's hereditary optic neuropathy, although this had been reported in liver samples.[47]

Lopez and Smith emphasized the diagnostic value of finding telangiectatic microangiopathy in either a symptomatic or asymptomatic family member.[48] They reported the cases of two families in which the first affected member had insufficient fundus changes for a diagnosis of Leber's hereditary optic neuropathy. The first patient was a 45-year-old woman. Her 23-year-old son subsequently presented with visual loss; he had striking circumpapillary microangiopathy. The paucity of telangiectatic microangiopathy in the initially affected family members with loss of vision led the authors to argue that peripapillary telangiectasia is a genetic marker but may not always be a pathogenetic determinant of Leber's disease.

Rizzo et al. described three patients with familial dysautonomia in whom there was slowly-progressive impairment of vision associated with bilateral optic atrophy.[49] In all cases this apparently began after the first decade. The usually short life spans of these patients and the presence of ophthalmic abnormalities such as corneal scarring that might otherwise explain visual loss or impair funduscopy were offered as explanations for the apparent rarity of optic atrophy in this disease. One case had been reported previously.[50] The authors speculated that the late onset of the optic atrophy may correlate with the later involvement of large myelinated sensory nerve fibers in this disease. They predicted that it would be more commonly recognized, and Diamond et al. confirmed this in a study of 12 patients with clear corneas from their extensive study group.[51] They found some degree of disk pallor in all of them and abnormal VEPs in 19 eyes. Visual acuities, which ranged from 20/20 to 20/100, correlated with degree of VEP abnormality.

PAPILLEDEMA

Papilledema was reported in a mildly obese patient with obstructive sleep apnea syndrome.[52] The swelling cleared after tracheostomy. The opening pressure was normal on his lumbar puncture, but was presumed to have been elevated other times, probably in relation to hypercapnia and hypoxia. The papilledema was asymmetric and correlated with the appearance of *unilateral* optic nerve swelling on CT scan.

Pollack reported the case of an obese trumpet player with benign intracranial hypertension.[53] He developed acute papilledema and lost central vision with macular edema and the fundus picture of venous stasis retinopathy. The possibility of a repeated Valsalva's maneuver playing a role in the pathogenesis was raised.

Progressive optic neuropathy is, of course, the more usual basis for loss of vision in papilledema. Wall and George studied 20 patients with idiopathic intracranial hypertension by careful perimetry using specific strategies both with static threshold and Goldmann kinetic techniques.[54] They found dysfunction in 75%. They emphasize the importance of carefully studying the visual fields and following patients very closely, as in treatment for glaucoma. As Corbett emphasized, early recognition of progressive visual field loss is the key to successful management of patients with idiopathic intracranial hypertension.[55]

Sorensen et al. studied anterior and posterior pituitary function in 15 patients with benign intracranial hypertension.[56] These included 12 women, 8 of whom were obese. This frequent association suggests some hormonal factor in the etiology. However, they found no significant abnormalities other than subnormal growth response to hypoglycemia in 4 of the patients. There was no detectable estrogen in cerebrospinal fluid and no significant abnormality of serum levels.

Durcan et al. surveyed populations for the incidence of benign intracranial hypertension, a fairly common disease (0.9 per 100,000).[57] The incidence doubled among obese young women. Again, no heightened incidence was found in association with pregnancy or the use of oral contraceptives.

Digre and Corbett compared men with benign intracranial hypertension with an age-matched group of women with that disease and with normal males.[58] Males comprised 16% of all their patients with benign intracranial hypertension. They found that the signs and symptoms were similar, but that obesity was less marked than in affected women. They also found that surgical intervention was required more often in men than in women. They again suggested that optic nerve sheath fenestration is the surgical procedure of choice, and treatment with acetazolamide or furosemide (rather than corticosteroids) is their preferred means of medical management. They found that black men (particularly those with hypertension or in treatment for hypertension) were more likely to lose vision than other groups of male patients.

The potential value of oral fluorescein ophthalmoscopy and angiography in differentiating papilledema from pseudopapilledema in children was explored in a preliminary study.[59] There were appropriately negative results in pseudopapilledema, but positive findings in some—*but not all*—instances of true papilledema.

Opticociliary shunt vessels were found in association with chronic atrophic papilledema in children aged 10 and 17 who presumably developed it from neonatal hydrocephalus.[60] The shunt vessels disappeared with surgical treatment of the hydrocephalus.

Hupp et al. reviewed the subject of optic nerve sheath decompression via the medial orbital approach.[61] Their experience consisted of studying 19 eyes of 17 patients treated at the Bascom Palmer Eye Institute over an interval of 15 years. Several of them had increased intracranial pressure, but only a few had benign intracranial hypertension. Most of them had other, local, causes of progressive visual loss with accumulation of compressible fluids in the optic nerve sheaths. They confirmed the value of optic nerve sheath decompression, finding improvement in visual function within 1 month in 7 of the 19 eyes. Postoperative complications were infrequent. The most common complication was impairment of ocular motility. They emphasized the value of comparing A-scan ultrasonography in the primary position and 30 degrees of eccentric gaze in determining whether increased optic nerve diameter was compressible by tightening and stretching of the optic nerve sheaths on eccentric gaze, i.e., when due to increased intrasheath fluid[62] (see this chapter in *Current Neuro-Ophthalmology,* vol 1[63]).

Corbett et al. found that the relative enlargement of the blind spot in papilledema was largely reversible in four of five patients when he used plus lenses.[64] This suggests that there is predominantly a refractive basis for enlargement of the blind spot. This peripapillary hyperopia could have resulted from elevation of the photoreceptors by the surrounding swollen disk and subretinal fluid. They also reported in detail the case of a patient with acquired hyperopia from choroidal folds without papilledema, in whom refraction decreased the size of the enlarged blind spot. This had previously been reported by Dailey et al.[65] Dailey et al. described the cases of seven patients, mostly males. Specific etiologies of choroidal folds, such as papilledema, lesions causing exophthalmos, and posterior scleritis (as recently reviewed by Benson[66]) were absent. Some of the cases had bilateral involvement. Ultrasonography and CT scan demonstrated increased fluid in the optic nerve sheaths and flattening of the posterior portions of the globes. There was mild disk swelling without symptoms or signs considered indicative of precerebrospinal fluid pressure. However, in one patient who was tapped the spinal fluid pressure was increased.

In a fascinating report by Fletcher et al. seven patients with the syndrome of symptomatic, monocular enlargement of the blind spot (an absolute and steep scotoma) exhibited photopsia but no corresponding disk or retinal changes even on fluorescein angiography. However, focal ERG documented a retinal basis.[67] The etiology was unclear, but it has subsequently been suggested convincingly by Hamed et al.[68] that the basis may be prior involvement by the multiple evanescent white dot syndrome described by Jampol et al.[69] Hoyt wondered whether the spectrum of the disease might include the steep blind spot enlargement and temporal photopsias without a stage of evanescent white dots or macular involvement.[70]

ISCHEMIC OPTIC NEUROPATHY

The high frequency of small cup-to-disk ratios in patients with nonarteritic anterior ischemic optic neuropathy (AION) was confirmed by another study.[71] The carefully designed study included more patients (126) than the three prior studies combined. In addition to normal controls (122), comparison was made with a group of patients with arteritic AION (23). It was suggested that temporal arteritis be considered more of a possibility when a large cup is present in the fellow eye of a patient with AION, just as when the atrophy following AION is marked by cupping, as indicated at the end of this chapter in volume 1 of this series.

The authors offered an outstanding summary of the pathogenesis of nonarteritic AION. They reminded us that, in addition to the evidence of predisposing crowded structure of the optic nerve head, there is evidence that ischemia plays a role:

1. Patients are usually middle-aged or older (and often hypertensive), likely with sclerosis and impairment of autoregulation in the optic nerve circulation.
2. Visual loss is usually sudden and most often noted on awakening (likely significant in view of the shorter hours of sleep in the elderly).
3. Fluorescein angiography often shows filling defects or delay in the peripapillary choroid, although without posterior ciliary artery occlusion, documented in temporal arteritis.

To these points might be added the association of AION with many disorders characterized by hypoperfusion, vasospasm and vaso-obliteration, including arteritis. Ischemia presumably leads to axoplasm flow stasis, known to be responsible for the disk swelling. Swollen axons in the restricted space within the scleral canal lead to a cascading effect by compression of fine vessels among the nerve fiber bundles.

Posthemorrhagic amaurosis was reviewed by Hayreh.[72] He included four of his own cases. The basis for the amaurosis is AION, and although his own cases did not show this, the disorder was most often bilateral. It can occur at any age, and there is typically a delay after the hemorrhage. Arterial hypotension need not occur. He suggested that blood loss causes an increased release of renin and endogenous vasoconstrictor agents by sympathoadrenergic activation. He pointed out that circulating vasoconstrictor agents could diffuse from the freely permeable peripapillary choroid. Failure of autoregulation and increased platelet aggregability were also considered possible factors. Fluorescein angiography showed delayed peripapillary filling of the choroid with poor perfusion of the disk with staining. He indicated that hemoglobin levels are often low in these patients, but not necessarily at the time of visual loss. Transfusion appeared to have little effect on the visual loss. Hayreh speculated that the release of endogenous vasoconstrictor agents may also play a role in idiopathic, nonarteritic AION.

Larkin and others had suggested a similar mechanism for the ischemic optic neuropathy that they encountered in 7 of 7,685 patients who underwent coronary artery bypass procedure.[73, 74] This had been previously reported by Sweeney et al.[75] and following general surgery by Jaben et al.[76] Jaben et al. considered low hemoglobin to be a factor, but as Hayreh had suggested in the amaurosis of blood loss, Larkin et al. suggested that an increase in circulating vasoconstrictors such as angiotensin in the setting of systemic hypotension and particularly in the face of elevated intraocular pressure may be more important.

Interestingly, in the paper by Jaben et al. the other surgical procedure that was mentioned in association with AION was a parathyroidectomy in a 16-year-old on hemodialysis.[76] Hypotension was not documented. An additional report by Servilla and Groggel involved a patient with AION who developed it during hemodialysis.[77] He had chronic hypotension (a common complication of dialysis), which may have been an etiologic factor. Servilla and Groggel pointed out that increased intraocular pressure may also cause a further impairment of perfusion of the optic nerve head. Previous studies have documented elevation of intraocular pressure during dialysis.[78, 79]

Hayreh in his paper on posthemorrhagic AION mentioned that such visual loss can occur with a normal rather than edematous disk appearance.[72] Johnson et al. reported the clinical and pathologic study of just such a case.[80] The patient was a 59-year-old woman with repeated gastrointestinal bleeding and hypotension, who developed only mild disk edema but who had enlargement of the optic nerves on CT scan. There was pathologic documentation of posterior, elongated, hemorrhagic infarctions of the orbital portions of the optic nerves. As they pointed out, this was reminiscent of the findings in Sharpe and co-workers' report of methanol optic neuropathy.[81] Johnson et al. considered the anemia an important contributing factor in some cases of posterior ischemic optic neuropathy consequent to bleeding.[80] This is at variance with Hayreh's formulation, and it should be noted that the patient's intraoperative and postoperative hypotension was treated with vaso-constrictors as well as transfusion. They suggested that in younger patients without arteriosclerosis (and presumably with effective autoregulatory mechanisms) the optic nerve head and immediate retrolaminar region may be less vulnerable to the effects of hypotension and anemia. This may result in a less striking disk edema and with hypoxic swelling of the orbital portion of the optic nerves, which in turn gradually compresses the fine centripetal pial vessels.[82] The result would be axial infarction.

Two cases of posterior ischemic optic neuropathy were documented by Rizzo and Lessell.[82] They described two patients in whom visual impairment was found immediately after general anesthesia. There was no delay in these cases. In one instance the patient had undergone replacement of an infected hip prosthesis. In the other the patient had undergone coronary artery bypass surgery. In both cases the optic neuropathy was bilateral and initially without any abnormality in the optic nerves. Primary optic atrophy developed later. In both patients anemia was present. The first patient, who was 62, had periods of hypotension. The other patient had arteriosclerosis and hypertension. Improvement was noted in one of these cases, which the authors considered unusual, although in some cases of posterior ischemic optic neuropathy — as the authors indicated and we have noted — surprising improvement is occasionally encountered. Late-onset optic neuritis remains an unexcluded alternative. Perhaps this will be clarified with the newer neuroimaging techniques.[2-4]

In reply to correspondence about their case, Rizzo and Lessell stated that while temporal arteritis is an important cause of posterior ischemic optic neuropathy, the erythrocyte sedimentation rate may be nonspecifically increased in the postoperative period.[83] We have seen this in the range of 90 mm/hour in two patients who suffered AION following coronary artery bypass surgery. Neither patient had other evidence of giant cell arteritis, and this did not develop later.

Another basis for posterior ischemic optic neuropathy was documented: internal carotid artery occulsion, otherwise asymptomatic.[84] In another report internal carotid artery occlusion was found in a patient with 2 years of amaurosis fugax who developed superior and then inferior branch retinal arteriolar occlusions in close sequence.[85] There was mild blurring of the disk and a dense altitudinal visual field defect. This was interpreted, perhaps correctly, as suggesting that there was AION. In this instance all the findings were attributed to thrombotic events associated with the presence of a lupus anticoagulant. The authors indicated that this should be suspected in patients who suffer thrombotic events that appear consequent to a hypercoaguable state (whether or not they have systemic lupus erythematosis), when the partial thromboplastin time is prolonged and not corrected by 1:1 dilution of the patient's plasma with normal plasma. This entity is generally confirmed by tissue thromboplastin inhibition tests and platelet neutralization procedures. It is an antibody that reacts with phospholipid antigens located on platelet membranes, clotting factors, and vascular endothelium. It may have an anticardiolipin effect, which may explain false-positive Venereal Disease Research Laboratory (VDRL) tests in some patients. The authors remind us that such false-positive serological tests were present in one of the patients with systemic lupus erythematosis and optic neuropathy reported by Jabs et al.[86] Suggested screening for the lupus anticoagulant includes a partial thromboplastin time, VDRL, platelet count, and anticardiolipin antibody test.

Jay and Williamson studied magnetic resonance images in 9 patients with AION and found small, subcortical hypertense white matter foci in 5 of the patients.[87] There were an average of 3.2 lesions per patient. Of course, these abnormalities on MRI are present in a high percentage (20% to 30%) of asymptomatic elderly patients. They may correspond to foci of atrophic perivascular demyelination, presumedly on an ischemic basis. The authors found an average of 0.9 lesions on the MRI of 5 of 11 controls. The differences were not significant. Guyer et al suggested in correspondence that if the sample size were four times as large, the same sample distribution would be significant.[88] Therefore, a larger study might confirm the prior finding in a larger series reported by Guyer et al. that there was a correlation of AION with cerebrovascular disease. Interestingly, in the second patient described by Rizzo and Lessell, who suffered posterior ischemic optic neuropathy following coronary artery bypass surgery, CT scans showed the postoperative development of a focal, hypodense cerebral lesion.[82] This is compatible with the occurrence of intraoperative cerebral infarction.

Prolonged disk swelling with little if any visual loss was reported as asymptomatic AION.[89] One of the patients was a diabetic who had frank AION in his other eye (see Beri et al.[90]). The other patient was diabetic and hypertensive and had bilateral involvement. Diabetes and hypertension are known to be associated with asymptomatic and presumed ischemic disk swelling. We have seen this as an occasional cause of the big blind spot syndrome—chronic unilateral disk edema without visual defect, often eventually resolving.

Kline emphasized that some patients with AION may have progression of their visual deficit during the period before disk swelling resolves.[91] He noted that this is well known but has not been sufficiently emphasized. He indicated that none of the AION cases with progression had giant cell arteritis. Lipton et al. have reported a fascinating case of progressive visual loss in temporal arteritis without disk swelling.[92] This presumed posterior ischemic optic neuropathy improved with corticosteroid therapy.

Interestingly, in the prospective study begun in 1974 on bilaterality in AION, Beri et al. found that less than 12% of cases of AION in their series of 438 patients were consequent to arteritis.[90] The median duration of follow-up for cases of nonarteritic AION was 28.6 months, too short to determine the ultimate percent of bilaterality since the incidence was continuing to rise almost linearly. Several points of special interest were mentioned in the paper: The prevalence of AION in the general population is not known. True simultaneous onset is rare; it is most commonly the result of unawareness of the first eye being involved until the second is affected. The authors reported that two dozen of the patients had symptomless optic disk edema. In addition, they indicated that their current practice (like ours) consists of using megadose intravenous steroids in patients suspected of temporal arteritis who present with AION in one eye, if there is any evidence of involvement of the second eye. They continue with 100 to 120 mg of prednisone by mouth in the early stages of treatment. Oral prednisone (80 to 120 mg a day) alone is used if involvement is unilateral.

Rosenfeld et al. reported an instructive case that supports their use of more aggressive therapy than just outlined.[93] A 78-year-old woman with several months of systemic symptoms of giant cell arteritis presented with 3 days of monocular vision loss and a sedimentation rate of 115 mm/hour. Her biopsy was positive. On 60 mg of prednisone/day her sedimentation rate had become normal (11 mm/hour) over a period of 2½ weeks, but vision then decreased from hand motions to no perception of light. One month later, visual observations occurred in her other eye with decrease of visual acuity from 20/20 to 20/50 with multiple cotton-wool spots even though her sedimentation rate was only 5 mm/hour. After intravenous methylprednisolone (500 mg every 12 hours for five doses) her acuity improved to 20/25. However, despite 80 mg of prednisone/day she noticed a decrease in vision 2 weeks later although her erythrocyte sedimentation rate was still 5 mm/hour. Repeat temporal artery biopsy was still positive, and she was again given intravenous methylprednisolone, 1 g every 12 hours for 5 days. Her vision improved again and her visual field defect resolved. Thereafter, she remained stable on 200 mg of prednisone/day, which was then tapered.

The authors observed that, at least in this case, intravenous megadose corticosteroids reversed visual loss that had developed while on oral prednisone treatment in doses considered adequate. One can also infer the "adequacy" by the absence of systemic symptoms and the lowering of the erythrocyte sedimentation rate. They suggested the use of intravenous megadose corticosteroids for visual loss in the first eye if the patient is seen within 36 hours of onset, in the hopes of both reversing the visual loss and protecting the second eye. They cited a case in which reversal of visual loss was reported, as well as several reports of progressive visual loss despite presumed adequate oral doses of prednisone. As they pointed out, this case shows the inadequacy of the erythrocyte sedimentation rate as a measure of activity of giant cell arteritis. The authors suggest close attention to symptoms, a point reinforced by Jacobson and Slamovits.[94]

Further discussion in correspondence of the optimal technique for measuring the erythrocyte sedimentation rate in giant cell arteritis prompts us to suggest the continued use of the Westergren method.[95] This method is simple to perform: Draw blood early in the office visit and allow it to stand 1 hour in a glass straw standing in a piece of clay; the amount of settling can then be measured.

A report by Lipton et al. reminds us that giant cell arteritis may produce transient ischemic symptoms related to the posterior circulation, and that these may respond to corticosteroid treatment.[96] There was also a review from the Mayo Clinic by Caselli et al. of the neurologic findings in 166 consecutive patients with biopsy-proven giant cell arteritis.[97] These findings were present in 51 of the patients. There were neuropathies in 23 patients (reported separately),[98] transient ischemic attacks and strokes in 12, neuro-otologic syndromes in 11, tremor in 6, neuropsychiatric syndromes in 5, tongue numbness in 3, and myelopathy in 1. Neuro-ophthalmologic problems occurred in 35 of the patients. These included transient visual loss in 17, permanent visual loss in 14, scintillating scotomas in 8; and diplopia in 3. Abnormalities in large arteries occurred in 52 patients, including bruits and diminished pulses. The carotid artery was involved in 31 patients. Thirty-five percent of patients with carotid disease had transient ischemic attacks or strokes or transient or permanent visual loss.

McDonnell et al. reviewed 237 consecutive patients with temporal artery biopsies (250 biopsies) at the Wilmer Institute over a period of 15 years and found that skip areas were infrequent.[99] They recommended cutting the vessel into short segments oriented to obtain cross-sections after taking stepped sections at 0.25 or 0.50 mm intervals. They felt there was no definite advantage to bilateral biopsy in the 13 instances where this was carried out. They allowed that it can be of some value occasionally, as has been reported and as we believe. Active arteritis was found on biopsy up to 45 days after initiation of steroid therapy, suggesting that biopsy be performed in the initial weeks, a liberalization of the time generally considered allowable. They strongly recommended biopsy for patients with relative contraindications to long-term steroid therapy, which is usually necessary once temporal arteritis is diagnosed. Complications of the procedures are rare and there were none in this series. The authors also indicated that in some patients the diagnosis of temporal arteritis can be based on clinical symptoms and signs and the response to a trial of steroids. These are probably the most important criteria, other than positive biopsies. Their findings suggested that biopsy might be avoided in some patients in whom the diagnosis is clinically suspected, although not strongly, but in whom the constitutional symptoms and headache do not resolve promptly and the erythrocyte sedimentation rate does not normalize within 1 week. In patients with giant cell arteritis on corticosteroid therapy in adequate doses, the erythrocyte sedimentation rate almost always normalizes within 1 week.

Knox et al. described the cases of six patients with uremia and anemia who developed progressive visual loss over several days.[100] Five of the patients had disk swelling, some of them with extension of edema into the retina. Four of the patients improved with hemodialysis and another with the addition of corticosteroid therapy. These therapeutic measures were suggested promptly in addition to antihypertensives. This entity is perhaps at least in part ischemic, but was thought to be more likely toxic (uremic) in part because of the reversibility. The main value of this report lies in the potential reversibility of visual loss, which has not yet been clarified from a pathogenetic point of view.

Gittinger and Asdourian reported that 2 of 150 patients on amiodarone (usually used for treatment of cardiac arrhythmias) developed papillopathy (three eyes).[101] The mechanism for the papillopathy is presumed to be ischemic, but there is relatively little visual loss and the process is reversible. Additional reports of papillopathy include 13 studied by Younge's group[102] (they found a larger than expected cup size in these patients and also that the incidence of papillopathy was higher among amiodarone patients than of AION among age-matched untreated controls) and two single case reports, the cases often resembling AION.[103, 104] One case had the typical disk swelling with acute hemorrhage and a residual visual defect.[103] Nevertheless, a toxic basis probably explained at least some of these cases. A hypothesis offered by Garrett et al. is interesting in that it postulates the possibility that glial swelling may be the primary abnormality, and axonal compression in the region of the optic nerve had a secondary effect.[104]

REFERENCES

1. Repka MX, Miller NR: Optic atrophy in children. *Am J Ophthalmol* 1988; 106:191–193.
2. Johnson G, Miller DH, MacManus D, et al: STIR sequences in NMR imaging of the optic nerve. *Neuroradiology* 1987; 29:238–245.
3. Miller DH, Newton MR, van ver Poel JC, et al: Magnetic resonance imaging of the optic nerve in optic neuritis. *Neurology* 1988; 38:175–179.
4. Eidelberg D, Newton MR, Johnson G: Chronic unilateral optic neuropathy: A magnetic resonance study. *Ann Neurol* 1988; 24:3–11.
5. Peli E, Hedges TR III, McGinnes T, et al: Nerve fiber layer photography: A comparative study. *Acta Ophthalmol* 1987; 65:71–80.
6. Newman NM, Stevens RA, Heckenlively JR: Nerve fiber layer loss in diseases of the outer retinal layer. *Br J Ophthalmol* 1987; 71:21–26.
7. Holder GE: Significance of abnormal pattern electroretinography in anterior visual pathway dysfunction. *Br J Ophthalmol* 1987; 71:166–171.
8. Celesia GG, Kaufman D, Cone SB: Simultaneous recording of pattern electroretinography and visual evoked potentials in multiple sclerosis: A method of separating demyelination from axonal damage to the optic nerve. *Arch Neurol* 1986; 43:1247–1252.
9. Weinstein GW, Arden GB, Hitchings RA, et al: The pattern electroretinogram (PERG) in ocular hypertension and glaucoma. *Arch Ophthalmol* 1988; 106:923–928.
10. Drucker MD, Savino PJ, Sergott RC, et al: Low-contrast letter charts to detect subtle neuropathies. *Am J Ophthalmol* 1988; 105:141–145.
11. Browning DJ, Buckley EG: Reliability of brightness comparison testing in predicting afferent pupillary defects. *Arch Ophthalmol* 1988; 106:341–343.
12. Sadun AA: Neuroanatomy of the human visual system: Part I. Retinal projections to the LGN and pretectum as demonstrated with a new method. *Neuro-Ophthalmol* 1986; 6:353–361.
13. Sadun AA, Johnson BM, Smith LEH: Neuroanatomy of the human visual system: Part II. Retinal projections to the superior colliculus and pulvinar. *Neuro-Ophthalmol* 1986; 6:363–370.
14. Sadun AA, Johnson BM, Schaechter J: Neuroanatomy of the human visual system: Part III. Three retinal projections to the hypothalamus. *Neuro-Ophthalmol* 1986; 6:371–379.
15. Lambert S, Hoyt CS, Narahara MH: Optic nerve hypoplasia. *Surv Ophthalmol* 1987; 32:1–9.
16. Provis JM, Van Driel D, Billson FA, et al: Human fetal optic nerve: Overproduction and elimination of retinal axons during development. *J Comp Neurol* 1985; 238:92–100.
17. Novakovic P, Taylor DSI, Hoyt WF: Localising patterns of optic nerve hypoplasia—Retina to occipital lobe. *Br J Ophthalmol* 1988; 72:176–182.
18. Stromland K: Ocular involvement in the fetal alcohol syndrome. *Surv Ophthalmol* 1986; 31:277–284.
19. Cook CS, Nowotny AZ, Sulik KK: Fetal alcohol syndrome. Eye malformations in a mouse model. *Arch Ophthalmol* 1987; 105:1576–1581.

20. Katz B, Wiley CA, Lee VW: Optic nerve hypoplasia and the syndrome of nevus sebaceous of Jadassohn. A new association. *Ophthalmology* 1987; 94:1570–1576.

21. Lincoff H, Lopez R, Kreissig I, et al: Retinoschisis associated with optic nerve pits. *Arch Ophthalmol* 1988; 106:61–67.

22. Annesley W, Brown G, Bollowing J, et al: Treatment of retinal detachment with congenital optic pit by krypton laser photocoagulation. *Graefes Arch Clin Exp Ophthalmol* 1987; 225:311.

23. Schatz H, McDonald R: Treatment of sensory retinal detachment associated with optic nerve pit or coloboma. *Ophthalmology* 1988; 95:178–186.

24. Cox MS, Witherspoon CD, Morris RE, et al: Evolving techniques in the treatment of macular detachment caused by optic nerve pits. *Ophthalmology* 1988; 95:889–896.

25. Singh J, Ghose S: Isolated coloboma of the optic nerve head: An echographic evaluation. *Ann Ophthalmol* 1987; 19:184–186.

26. Gardner T, Zaparackas ZG, Naidich TP: Congenital optic nerve colobomas: CT demonstration. *J Comp Assist Tomogr* 1984; 8:95–102.

27. Adam P, Bec P, Mathis A, et al: Morning glory syndrome: CT findings. *J Comp Assist Tomogr* 1984; 8:134–136.

28. Feist RM, Kline LB, Morris RE, et al: Recovery of vision after presumed direct optic nerve injury. *Ophthalmology* 1987; 94:1567–1569.

29. Purvin V: Evidence of orbital deformation in indirect optic nerve injury: Weight lifter's optic neuropathy. *J Clin Neuro-Ophthalmol* 1988; 8:9–11.

30. Anderson RL, Panje WR, Gross CE: Optic nerve blindness following blunt forehead trauma. *Ophthalmology* 1982; 89:445–455.

31. Chang M, Eifrig DE: Optic nerve avulsion. *Arch Ophthalmol* 1987; 105:322–323.

32. Manor RS, Cohen S, Svetliza E, et al: Papilledema in traumatic lesion of the optic nerve with amaurosis. *J Clin Neuro-Ophthalmol* 1986; 6:100–105.

33. Quigley HA, Davis EB, Anderson DER: Descending optic nerve degeneration in primates. *Invest Ophthalmol Vis Sci* 1977; 16:1841.

34. Carter KD, Nerad JA: Fluctuating visual loss secondary to orbital emphysema. *Am J Ophthalmol* 1987; 104:664–665.

35. Gross JG, Doxanas MT: Traumatic optic atrophy caused by compressed air. *Ann Ophthalmol* 1987; 19:69–74.

36. Al-Mefty O, Fox JL, Al-Rodhan, et al: Optic nerve decompression in osteopetrosis. *J Neurosurg* 1988; 68:80.

37. Leone CR Jr, Wissinger JP: Surgical approaches to diseases of the orbital apex. *Ophthalmology* 1988; 95:391–397.

38. Maroon JC, Kennerdell JS: Surgical approaches to the orbit: Indications and techniques. *J Neurosurg* 1984; 60:1226–1235.

39. Housepian EM: Intraorbital tumors, in Schmidek HH, Sweet WH (eds): *Operative Neurosurgical Techniques: Indications, Methods, and Results,* vol 1. New York, Grune & Stratton, 1982, p 153.

40. Housepian EM, Trokel SL, Jakobiec FA, et al: Tumors of the orbit, in Youmans JR (ed): *Neurological Surgery: A Comprehensive Reference Guide to the Diagnosis and Management of Neurosurgical Problems,* ed 2, vol 5. Philadelphia, WB Saunders, 1982, pp 3045–3046.

41. Hayasaka S, Yamaguchi K, Mizuno K, et al: Ocular findings in childhood lactic acidosis. *Arch Ophthalmol* 1986; 104:1656–1658.

42. Spaide RF, Diamond G, D'Amico R, et al: Ocular findings in cystic fibrosis. *Am J Ophthal* 1987; 103:204–210.

43. Snebold NG, Rizzo JF III, Lessell S, et al: Transient visual loss in ornithine transcarbamoylase. *Am J Ophthal* 1987; 104:407–412.

44. Small KW, Pollack S, Scheinman J: Optic atrophy in primary oxalosis. *Am J Ophthalmol* 1988; 106:96–97.

45. Nikoskelainen EK, Savontaus ML, Wanne OP, et al: Leber's hereditary optic neuroretinopathy, a maternally inherited disease. A genealogic study in four pedigrees. *Arch Ophthalmol* 1987; 105:665–671.

46. Uemura A, Osame M, Nakagawa M, et al: Leber's hereditary optic neuropathy: Mitochondrial and biochemical studies on muscle biopsies. *Br J Ophthalmol* 1987; 71:531–536.

47. Nikoskelainen E, Paljarvi L, Lang H, et al: Leber's hereditary optic neuropathy: A mitochondrial disease? *Acta Neurol Scand* 1984; 69:172–173.

48. Lopez PF, Smith JL: Leber's optic neuropathy. New observations. *J Clin Neuro-Ophthalmol* 1986; 6:144–152.

49. Rizzo JF III, Lessell S, Liebman SD: Optic atrophy in familial dysautonomia. *Am J Ophthalmol* 1986; 102:463–467.

50. Axelrod FB, D'Amico R: in Fraunfelder FT, Roy FH (eds): *Current Ocular Therapy,* ed 2. Philadelphia, WB Saunders, 1985, pp 260–261.

51. Diamond GA, D'Amico RA, Axelrod FB: Optic nerve dysfunction in familial dysautonomia. *Am J Ophthalmol* 1987; 104:645–648.

52. Bucci FA Jr, Krohel GB: Optic nerve swelling secondary to the obstructive sleep apnea syndrome. *Am J Ophthalmol* 1988; 105:428–430.

53. Pollack SC: Acute papilledema and visual loss in a patient with pseudotumor cerebri. *Arch Ophthalmol* 1987; 105:752–753.

54. Wall M, George D: Visual loss in pseudotumor cerebri: Incidence and defects related to visual field strategy. *Arch Neurol* 1987; 44:170–175.

55. Corbett JJ: Comment [on reference 3]. *Surv Ophthalmol* 1987; 32:217.

56. Sorensen PS, Gjerris F, Svenstrup B: Endocrine studies in patients with pseudotumor cerebri. Estrogen levels in blood and cerebrospinal fluid. *Arch Neurol* 1986; 43:902–906.

57. Durcan FJ, Corbett JJ, Wall M: The incidence of pseudotumor cerebri: Population studies in Iowa and Louisiana. *Arch Neurol* 1988; 45:875–877.

58. Digre KB, Corbett JJ: Pseudotumor cerebri in men. *Arch Neurol* 1988; 45:866–872.

59. Ghose S, Nayak BK: Role of oral fluorescein in the diagnosis of early papilloedema in children. *Br J Ophthalmol* 1987; 71:910–915.

60. Dowhan TP, Muci-Mendoza R, Aitken PA: Disappearing optociliary shunt vessels and neonatal hydrocephalus. *J Clin Neuro-Ophthalmol* 1988; 8:1–8.

61. Hupp SL, Glaser JS, Byrne SF: Optic nerve sheath decompression. Review of 17 cases. *Arch Ophthalmol* 1987; 105:386–389.

62. Gans MS, Byrne SF, Glaser JS: Standardized A-scan echography in optic nerve disease. *Arch Ophthalmol* 1987; 105:1232–1236.

63. Hupp SL, Buckley EG, Frazier-Byrne S, et al: Posttraumatic venous obstructive retinopathy associated with enlarged optic nerve sheath. *Arch Ophthalmol* 1984; 102:254–256.

64. Corbett JJ, Jacobson DM, Mauer RC, et al: Enlargement of the blind spot caused by papilledema. *Am J Ophthalmol* 1988; 105:261–265.

65. Dailey RA, Mills RP, Stimac GK, et al: The natural history and CT appearance of acquired hyperopia with choroidal folds. *Ophthalmology* 1986; 93:1336–1342.

66. Benson WE: Posterior scleritis. *Surv Ophthalmol* 1988; 32:297.

67. Fletcher WA, Imes RK, Goodman D, et al: Acute idiopathic blind spot enlargement. A big blind spot syndrome without optic disc edema. *Arch Ophthalmol* 1988; 106:44–49.

68. Hamed LA, Schatz NJ, Glaser JS, et al: Acute idiopathic blind spot enlargement without optic disc edema. *Arch Ophthalmol* 1988; 106:1029–1030.

69. Jampol LM, Sieving PA, Pugh D, et al: Multiple evanescent white dot syndrome. I. Clinical findings. *Arch Ophthalmol* 1984; 102:671–674.

70. Hoyt WF: Reply. *Arch Ophthalmol* 1988; 106:1031.

71. Beck RW, Servais GE, Hayreh SS: Anterior ischemic optic neuropathy: IX. Cup-to disc ratio and its role in pathogenesis. *Ophthalmology* 1987; 94:1503–1508.

72. Hayreh SS: Anterior ischemic optic neuropathy: VIII. Clinical features and pathogenesis of posthemorrhagic amaurosis. *Ophthalmology* 1987; 94:1488–1502.

73. Larkin DFP, Connolly P, Magner JB, et al: Intraocular pressure during cardiopulmonary bypass. *Br J Ophthalmol* 1987; 71:177–180.

74. Larkin DFP, Wood AE, Neligan M, et al: Ischaemic optic neuropathy complicating cardiopulmonary bypass. *Br J Ophthalmol* 1987; 71:344–347.

75. Sweeney PJ, Breuer AC, Selhorst JB, et al: Ischemic optic neuropathy: A complication of cardiopulmonary bypass surgery. *Neurology* 1982; 32:560–562.

76. Jaben SL, Glaser JS, Daily M: Ischemic optic neuropathy following general surgical procedures. *J Clin Neuro-Ophthalmol* 1983; 3:239–244.

77. Servilla KS, Groggel GC: Anterior ischemic optic neuropathy as a complication of hemodialysis. *Am J Kidney Dis* 1986; 8:61–63.

78. Sitprya V, Holmes JH, Ellis PP: Intraocular pressure changes during artificial kidney therapy. *Arch Ophthalmol* 1964; 72:626–631.

79. Watson AG, Greenwood WR: Studies on the intraocular pressure during hemodialysis. *Can J Ophthalmol* 1966; 1:301–307.

80. Johnson MW, Kincaid MC, Trobe JD: Bilateral retrobulbar optic nerve infarctions after blood loss and hypotension: A clinical pathologic case study. *Ophthalmology* 1987; 94:1577–1584.

81. Sharpe JA, Hostovsky M, Bilbao JM, et al: Methanol optic neuropathy: A histopathological study. *Neurology* 1982; 32:1093–1100.

82. Rizzo JF, Lessell S: Posterior ischemic optic neuropathy during general surgery. *Am J Ophthalmol* 1987; 103:808–811.

83. Rizzo JF, Lessell S: Reply. *Am J Ophthalmol* 1987; 104:556.

84. Sawle GV, Sarkies NJC: Posterior ischaemic optic neuropathy due to internal carotid artery occlusion. *Neuro-Ophthalmol* 1987; 7:349–353.

85. Levine SR, Crofts JW, Lesser GR, et al: Visual symptoms associated with the presence of a lupus anticoagulant. *Ophthalmology* 1988; 95:686–692.

86. Jabs DA, Miller NR, Newman SA, et al: Optic neuropathy in systemic lupus erythematosus. *Arch Ophthalmol* 1986; 104:564–568.

87. Jay WM, Williamson MR: Incidence of subcortical lesions not increased in nonarteritic ischemic optic neuropathy on magnetic resonance imaging. *Am J Ophthalmol* 1987; 104:398–400.

88. Guyer DR, Miller NR, Enger CL, et al: Correspondence. *Am J Ophthalmol* 1988; 105:324–325.

89. Slavin ML: Chronic asymptomatic ischemic optic neuropathy: A report of two cases in adults with diabetes mellitus. *J Clin Neuro-Ophthalmol* 1987; 7:198–201.

90. Beri M, Klugman MR, Kohler JA, et al: Anterior ischemic optic neuropathy: VII. Incidence of bilaterality and various influencing factors. *Ophthalmology* 1987; 94:1020–1028.

91. Kline NL: Progression of visual defects in ischemic optic neuropathy. *Am J Ophthalmol* 1988; 106:199–203.

92. Lipton RB, Solomon S, Wertenbaker C: Gradual loss and recovery of vision in temporal arteritis. *Arch Intern Med* 1985; 145:2252–2253.

93. Rosenfeld SI, Kosmorsky GS, Klingele TG, et al: Treatment of temporal arteritis with ocular involvement. *Am J Med* 1986; 80:143–145.

94. Jacobson DM, Slamovits TL: Erythrocyte sedimentation rate and its relationship to hematocrit in giant cell arteritis. *Arch Ophthalmol* 1987: 105:965–967.

95. Love DC, Berler DK, O'Dowd GJ, et al: Erythrocyte sedimentation rate and its relationship to hematocrit giant cell arteritis. *Arch Ophthalmol* 1988; 106:309–310.

96. Lipton RB, Rosenbaum D, Mehler MF: Giant cell arteritis causes recurrent posterior circulation transient ischemic attacks which respond to corticosteroid. *Eur Neurol* 1987; 27:97–100.

97. Caselli RJ, Hunder GG, Whisnant JP: Neurologic disease in biopsy proven giant cell (temporal) arteritis. *Neurology* 1988; 38:352–359.

98. Caselli RJ, Daube JR, Hunder GG, et al: Peripheral neuropathic syndromes in giant cell (temporal) arteritis. *Neurology* 1988; 38:685–689.

99. McDonnell PJ, Moore GW, Miller NR, et al: Temporal arteritis: Clinicopathologic. *Ophthalmology* 1986; 93:518–530.

100. Knox DL, Hanneken AM, Hollos FC, et al: Uremic optic neuropathy. *Arch Ophthalmol* 1988; 106:50–54.

101. Gittinger JW Jr, Asdourian GK: Papillopathy caused by amiodarone. *Arch Ophthalmol* 1987; 105:349–351.

102. Feiner LA, Younge BR, Kazmier FJ, et al: Optic neuropathy and amiodarone therapy. *Mayo Clin Proc* 1987; 62:702–717.

103. Nazarian SM, Jay WM: Bilateral optic neuropathy associated with amiodarone therapy. *J Clin Neuro-Ophthalmol* 1988; 8:25–28.

104. Garrett SN, Kearney JJ, Schiffman JS: Amiodarone optic neuropathy. *J Clin Neuro-Ophthalmol* 1988; 8:105–110.

CHAPTER 4

The Optic Chiasm

Joel S. Glaser, M.D.

Professor, Ophthalmology and Neurologic Surgery, Bascom Palmer Eye Institute, Department of Ophthalmology, University of Miami, Miami, Florida

This chapter consists of a review of selected literature on the optic chiasm and closely related structures. The great weight of publications dealing with computed tomography (CT) and magnetic resonance imaging (MRI) is clearly discernable. In fact, more than one third of the papers reviewed deal with CT and MRI.

ANATOMY

The anatomy of the Optic Chiasm has been an intriguing subject since the time of Galen, who in the second century likened the structure to the Greek letter *chi*, with subsequent additions and emendations by Leonardo da Vinci (1504), William Briggs (1676), Thomas Willis (1681), Descartes (1686), Isaac Newton (1704), and Ramon y Cajal (1898), among others. In "A Nineteenth Century View of the Optic Commissure", Reynolds reminds us that it was W. H. Wollaston, in 1824, who realized the significance of hemiretinal semidecussation (during his own migraine attacks), and that two Philadelphia ophthalmologists, W. W. Keen and W. Thomson, were the first to discover the vertical demarcation of the retina at the fovea, prompted by a detailed visual field examination of Pvt. Patrick Hughes.[1] Injured at Antietam in 1862, Hughes sustained a musketball injury to the left occipital region, with a residual right homonymous hemianopia. Rucker does not mention the two Philadelphians in his masterly historic review of the concept of

© 1990, Year Book Medical Publishers, Inc.
0893–0147/89/02-043-056-$04.00

chiasmal semidecussation, but neither does Reynolds cite Rucker's delightful essay.[2]

The question of nasotemporal division of different classes of retinal ganglion cells in the primate retina has been investigated in both New World and Old World monkeys, utilizing horseradish peroxidase (HRP) injection in the lateral geniculate nucleus and superior colliculus.[3] Results indicate that ipsilaterally projecting cells around the fovea can generate 2 to 3 degrees of bilateral representation in the geniculocalcarine pathways, because they are intermingled with contralaterally projecting cells on the nasal side of the foveal pit. Also, contralaterally projecting retinal ganglion cells in temporal retina cannot generate bilateral representation in the central visual pathways because there is no intermingling of ipsilaterally and contralaterally projecting cells on the temporal side of the foveal pit. Thus, a neural basis for "macular sparing" and "splitting" is suggested.

Also in the monkey, physiologic and anatomic criteria were used to clearly establish the *existence of a pretectal relay of visual information to the ipsilateral inferior olive in the macaque monkey.*[4] After injection of HRP into the inferior olivary nucleus, retrogradely labeled neurons were found in the nucleus of the optic tract (NOT) and the dorsal terminal nucleus of the accessory optic tract (DTN). The labeled cells were distributed in a sparse band arching below the margin of the brachium of the superior colliculus between the dorsal and lateral borders of the brain stem, at the caudal edge of the pulvinar. NOT-DTN neurons in the same region were also found to respond with short latencies to electrical stimulation of both the inferior olive and the optic chiasm. All neurons in the NOT-DTN that were antidromically activated from the inferior olive were also found to have direction-specific binocular visual responses. Such neurons were excited by ipsiversive motion and suppressed by contraversive motion, regardless of whether large-area random-dot stimuli moved across the visual field or small single dots moved across the fovea. Direct retinal input to these neurons was via slowly conducting fibers (3 to 9 m/sec) from the monkey's optic tract conduction velocity spectrum. As shown previously for nonprimates, NOT-DTN cells in the monkey may also carry a signal representing the velocity error between stimulus and retina (retinal slip), and relay this signal into the circuitry mediating the optokinetic reflex.[4]

The human hypothalamus can be divided into a chiasmatic region, a tuberal region, and a mammillary region.[5] The chiasmatic region comprises the magnocellular neurosecretory nuclei, several nuclei that are mainly formed of small nerve cells, and an ill-defined nerve cell assembly referred to as the chiasmatic gray. Small- to medium-sized bipolar nerve cells predominate in the chiasmatic gray. With the use of Nissl preparations counterstained for demonstration of lipofuscin pigment, four types of neurons have been distinguished. Pigmentoarchitectonic analysis of the chiasmatic region reveals the presence of eight nuclei embedded in, or partially surrounded by, the chiasmatic gray. The intermediate nucleus is a small, compact accumulation of nonpigmented nerve cells located at the level of the optic chiasm halfway between the paraventricular nucleus and the supraoptic nucleus. The supraoptic nucleus is formed of only two types of nerve cells. The cuneiform nucleus extends from the supraoptic nucleus to the ependymal lining of the third ventricle, separating the suprachiasmatic nucleus from the retrochiasmatic nucleus. The suprachiasmatic nucleus contains the smallest neurons of the region. Cells of this nucleus are devoid of lipofuscin pigment. The retrochiasmatic nucleus is formed of a heterogenous population of small and unusually large nerve cells. Numerous melanin-containing nerve cells and accumulations of nerve cells belonging to the lateral tuberal nucleus can be encountered within the boundaries of this nucleus, as well. The technique and data presented provide a basis for investigations of the aged and the diseased human brain.

NEOPLASMS

Pituitary Adenoma

A total of 255 consecutive transsphenoidal procedures for pituitary adenomas performed at the Massachusetts General Hospital were reviewed.[6] Of these pituitary tumors, 44.3% were tumors with suprasellar extension, 15.2% were intrasellar macroadenomas, and 40.4% were microadenomas. No deaths occurred during surgery. Cerebrospinal fluid rhinorrhea was the most common complication, occurring in 2.7% of cases; diabetes insipidus was next, lasting less than 1 year in 1.6% of patients and more than 1 year in 0.4%. Sinusitis occurred in 1.2% of patients, and delayed epistaxis occurred in 0.8%. Postoperative hematomas, meningitis, hydrocephalus, and deep venous thrombosis each occurred in 0.4% of cases.

Four hundred fifteen cases of suspected pituitary tumors were examined by CT and MRI.[7] Forty-one microadenomas and 26 large sellar-suprasellar pituitary tumors were diagnosed and surgically removed (61 cases), or treated with bromocriptine (6 cases). This study demonstrated that:

1. In cases of microadenomas, MRI was more accurate than CT in 3 cases and as accurate as CT in 33 cases; but MRI missed 6 cases diagnosed on CT when MRI was suboptimal (thicker than 5 mm).
2. When the sellar-suprasellar mass was markedly constricted at the diaphragma sellae on MRI sagittal slices (16 cases), transsphenoidal surgical approach was not only insufficient for total removal, but could be dangerous because the remaining suprasellar portion may rapidly increase in size following surgery, from postoperative hemorrhage and/or acute edema with severe obstructive hydrocephalus (3 cases) and/or acute blindness (2 cases).
3. Hemorrhage in pituitary tumors was easily seen on MRI and missed on CT.
4. Coronal MRI slices visualized the carotid siphon, obviating the need for angiography to rule out intrasellar aneurysm, which can mimic pituitary tumor on contrast CT.

5. Postoperative MRI was needed before considering radiotherapy to visualize accurately the relation of the optic chiasm to the residual tumor and to follow up any gradual change in tumor size.

6. In cases treated with bromocriptine, MRI was more accurate than CT in following the gradual decrease of pituitary tumor.

The CT appearances of pituitary masses after transsphenoidal surgery were obtained in 12 patients with pituitary adenomas.[8] The heights of pituitary masses on coronal CT sections were measured, and it was found that, despite complete tumor removal, the superior limits did not return to normal immediately, but gradually regressed in 3 to 4 months. The reasons for this phenomenon could be blood clot in the sella, packing material (muscle or fat) in the sella, adhesions between the diaphragma sellae or tumor and brain tissue above. Therefore, CT in the immediate postoperative period may be misleading, and baseline evaluation should be delayed for 3 to 4 months.

A thyroxine-sensitive adenoma presented in a 60-year-old woman with deteriorating vision.[9] CT scan showed pituitary enlargement with chiasmal compression. Serum prolactin levels were normal, but assessment of thyroid function showed a serum thyroxine level of 25 nmol/L (normal range 76 to 160 nmol/L) and a thyroid-stimulating hormone (TSH) level of 60 mU/L (normal range 0.5 to 5.0 mU/L). After 8 weeks of thryoxine replacement therapy (0.05 mg daily increasing to 0.1 mg daily after 3 weeks) the visual defects had resolved, serum TSH had fallen to 0.7 mU/L, and the CT scan showed pronounced reduction in the size of the pituitary gland. Therefore, measurement of TSH as well as prolactin is essential in all patients with pituitary enlargement, to avoid unnecessary pituitary surgery.

The MRI and CT scans of three proven cases of pituitary apoplexy were presented.[10] MRI scans obtained at least 5 days after the onset of symptoms suggested pituitary hemorrhage in all three cases, while CT scanning indicated pituitary hemorrhage in only one case. Increased signal on the T_1-weighted image was the hallmark of MRI scans in all three cases. These findings suggest that MRI scanning may be superior to CT scanning in identifying pituitary apoplexy, at least in the subacute phase.

The ability of high-resolution MRI (1.5 Tesla) to detect invasion of the cavernous sinuses by pituitary adenoma was determined through a retrospective review of 74 patients.[11] Patients were divided into three groups: 25 normal, 24 with invasive pituitary adenomas, and 25 with noninvasive pituitary adenomas. A fourth group of 30 patients who subsequently underwent surgery for pituitary adenoma was evaluated prospectively by MRI for the presence or absence of cavernous sinus invasion. Several features were analyzed: (1) the detectability of the medial and lateral dural margins of the cavernous sinus, (2) the size and variation in intensity of compartments within the cavernous sinus, (3) the relationship of endocrine function to the surgical and MRI appearance of the cavernous sinus, and (4) carotid artery displacement or encasement by tumor. The normal cavernous sinuses were usually symmetric, but their sizes varied. The lateral dural margin of the cavernous sinus was always recognized on MRI as a linear, discrete, low-intensity area. The medial dural margin (pituitary capsule) was seen on MR in only 2 of the 25 normal patients. In all 24 patients with cavernous sinus invasion, involvement was unilateral and was most common with laterally positioned prolactin or adrenocorticotropic hormone secretory adenomas. Invasion of the cavernous sinus was suspected by MRI in only 2 of the 13 invasive microadenomas, and was questionable in 3. In 10 of the 11 macroadenomas with surgically proven dural invasion, MR demonstrated an asymmetric increase in size and intensity of the superior and inferior cavernous sinus compartments. Noninvasive macroadenomas compressed and displaced the cavernous sinus bilaterally. The prospective MRI evaluation of 30 patients undergoing surgery for pituitary tumor revealed a sensitivity for predicting cavernous sinus invasion of 55%, a specificity of 85.7%, a positive predictive value of 62.5%, and a negative predictive value of 81.8%. No feature permitted certain distinction between invasive and noninvasive microadenomas, as the medial dural wall of the cavernous sinus could not be reliably identified. The most specific sign of cavernous sinus invasion was carotid artery encasement.

Optic Glioma

Alvord and Lofton in a literature review uncovered 623 cases of optic gliomas with sufficient information to permit actuarial (life-table) analysis concerning the prognosis of this disease by patient age, tumor site, treatment, and presence of concomitant neurofibromatosis or extension into the hypothalamus or ventricle.[12] The development of mathematical models led to the conclusion that these tumors, generally regarded histologically as low-grade astrocytomas, actually have a very wide but continuous range of growth rates. Some grow rapidly enough to be explained by simple exponential doubling at a constant rate, but most behave as though their growth decelerates. Decelerating growth rates make comparisons of various groups of patients difficult. No support is found for the classical hypothesis that some may be hamartomas. Inadequately treated gliomas of the optic nerve or chiasm bear an equally poor prognosis. However, tumors of the optic nerve (intracranial as well as intraorbital) have an excellent prognosis following complete surgical excision, and only a slightly poorer prognosis following irradiation. About 5% of optic nerve gliomas "recur" in the chiasm following "complete" intraorbital excision. Patients with neurofibromatosis have about twice the recurrence rate following complete excision of an intraorbital glioma. Optic chiasmal gliomas appear to respond to irradiation with doses above 4,500 rads. Patients with neurofibromatosis have about the same prognosis as patients without neurofibromatosis following irradiation of a chiasmal glioma.

Thirty-eight cases of optic glioma seen at the University of California were reviewed.[13] Two patients died in the postoperative period and were excluded from the follow-up analysis. Twenty-nine cases (76%) involved the optic chiasm, and 9 (24%) cases were confined to one optic nerve. Most tumors were slow-growing and progressive, although there were 3 cases of adult chiasmal gliomas that exhibited unusually aggressive behavior. These 3 cases are presented in detail. After a mean follow-up period of 9.4 years, the 10-year overall actuarial survival was 87%. Relapse-free survival was 55% at 10 years. Chiasmal tumors had poorer prognoses compared with optic nerve tumors, with 56% of chiasmal tumors recurring and 22% of optic nerve tumors recurring. Radiotherapy was beneficial in chiasmal gliomas, initially improving vision in 35% (6 of 17) and decreasing recurrence from 86% (6 of 7) without radiation therapy to 45% (9 of 20) with radiation therapy. The authors feel that optic gliomas are not benign, self-limiting lesions that require treatment, and that radiotherapy is effective in chiasmal gliomas and should be used early. No advantage to radiotherapy could be demonstrated for optic nerve gliomas, although the number of cases analyzed was small.

Thirty-six patients at the University of Pittsburgh were evaluated between 1965 and 1983 for glioma of the optic nerve and/or chiasm.[14] Median follow-up was 10.2 years. Pathologic verification was obtained in 32 patients. Tumor initially confined to the optic nerve recurred in 1 of 5 patients after complete resection. The actuarial survivals for 25 patients irradiated for biopsy-proven glioma of the optic chiasm were 96%, 90%, and 90% at 5, 10, and 15 years, respectively, and the progression-free survival was 87% at 5, 10, and 15 years. Vision stabilized or improved in 86% of patients after radiotherapy. Patients irradiated to doses greater than nominal standard dose of 1,385 radiation equivalent therapy had significantly improved progression-free survival ($P = 0.015$). One serious complication occurred after a dose of 1,533 radiation equivalent therapy. The recommended radiation dose for optic glioma is 45 to 50 Gy with 1.8 Gy fractions.

From the Hospital Infantil La Paz, Madrid, monozygotic twin sisters with optic glioma "in mirror image" (one without involvement of the left optic nerve and the other without involvement of the right optic nerve) and hydrocephalus secondary to progressive stenosis of the aqueduct were found in a series of 128 cases below 14 years of age with neurofibromatoses (NFB).[15] The optic glioma was diagnosed in the twins at 2 years of age. In one twin the tumor involved only the optic nerve, and in the other twin the glioma affected the optic nerve and homolateral optic chiasm. First symptoms of hydrocephalus appeared at 8 and 11 years of age, respectively. Ventriculoperitoneal shunting procedures were performed to relieve intracranial hypertension at 11 years and 15 years of age, respectively.

Coppeto et al. recorded an interesting case of "exophytic" suprasellar glioma that appeared to arise from the hypothalamus, insinuate forward beneath the chiasm, and produce visual loss by external compression. Surgical resection resulted in virtual complete visual recovery.[16]

MRI of the visual pathways in patients with neurofibromatosis was the subject of a study by Pomeranz et al. at the Mt. Sinai Hospital of Miami.[17] The authors found that the orbital and intracanalicular portions of the nerves were seen to best advantage with T_1-weighted sequence (TR 300 msec; TE 35 msec), axially and coronally; the chiasm was best seen with the intermediate T_2-weighted (TR 1,500; TE 35 msec) coronal sequence; and retrochiasmal structures were optimally evaluated with T_2-weighted (TR 1,500 msec; TE 70 msec) spin-echo sequence. CT was less helpful than MRI in ascertaining gliomatous involvement of hypothalamic structures.

Cranial MRI of 53 NFB patients at Indiana University were reviewed to determine the nature, extent, and number of intracranial abnormalities.[18] Twenty-three were scanned for evaluation of known central nervous system or cranial nerve involvement; the remainder were neurologically asymptomatic patients without suspected lesions referred for screening. Single lesions were noted in 32 patients, multiple lesions were identified in 14 patients, and 7 patients had normal scans. In 23 patients, small focal areas of increased signal on T_2-weighted scans within the brain were thought to represent heterotopias. Eight patients had chiasmal gliomas and 2 had optic nerve gliomas. Nine patients had parenchymal gliomas, 2 had ischemic change, and 1 had a colloid cyst. Extra-axial lesions included acoustic neuromas (5), meningiomas (4), trigeminal neurofibromas (1), and dysplasia of a sphenoid wing (2). Of the 30 asymptomatic patients referred for screening, lesions were found in 23. A screening MRI study is, therefore, recommended in patients with neurofibromatosis.

Other MRI-based studies have been conducted in the high-risk NFB population. Twenty-one patients with documented NFB were examined at Baylor College in Houston.[19] In 5 cases the indication was a known or suspected optic glioma, and two patients were examined because of a history of seizures. The remainder were examined as part of a baseline evaluation. Eighteen patients showed evidence of signal hyperintensity on T_2-weighted images. Lesions involved the optic nerve, optic chiasm, optic tract, lateral geniculate body, optic radiation, basal ganglia, periventricular white matter, cerebellar white matter, and dentate nucleus of the cerebellum. Comparison between MRI and concurrent CT scans showed MRI to be superior in demonstrating the posterior extent of optic-pathway gliomas. In addition, MRI showed focal areas of hyperintensity in the basal ganglia, internal capsule, cerebellum, and/or white matter that were not detected on CT. At the National Institutes of Health, 11 patients with gliomas of the optic chiasm were studied using a 0.5 Tesla superconducting system and third-generation CT scanners.[20] All tumors were identified with both modalities, but in the majority of cases the posterior extensions of the tumors and their relationship to adjacent brain, important to both prognosis and management, were shown better by MRI.

Craniopharyngioma

With regard to craniopharyngiomas, CT scanning still retains relevance. MRI and CT examinations were performed in nine patients with surgically proven craniopharyngioma.[21] CT was found to be superior to MRI in detection of calcification and cyst formation, but extent of involvement of adjacent structures (e.g., optic chiasm, third ventricle, and intracavernous carotid artery) was more clearly delineated by MRI. Craniopharyngioma fluid collections were found to be uniformly bright on T_2-weighted sequences. However, on T_1-weighted sequences, the signal intensity of the fluid ranged from hypointense to hyperintense, reflecting the heterogenous contents of cysts in these tumors. Since calcification and cyst formation are hallmarks of craniopharyngiomas, CT is more specific than MRI in diagnosis of craniopharyngiomas. An extraordinary case is documented, that of a young man who presented with a central scotoma in one eye and a temporal hemianopsia in the other.[22] MRI showed distinctive bilobate thickening of the chiasm and a "potbelly" expansion of the contiguous optic nerves. The distal portions of the intracranial optic nerves appeared normal. At craniotomy, incision of the lamina terminalis exposed intraventricular craniopharyngioma with anterior extension into the chiasm and proximal optic nerves. Partial resection of the tumor restored normal vision.

Leukemia

Other processes rarely infiltrate the chiasm as in the patient reported with infiltration of the optic chiasm as the primary presentation of chronic lymphocytic leukemia without lymphoreticular involvement.[23] The authors believe this to be the first report of a chiasmal syndrome due to this lymphoproliferative disorder.

DIAGNOSTIC MODALITIES

True precocious puberty occurs as a result of the premature release of luteinizing hormone–releasing hormone from the hypothalamus, which stimulates secretion of the pituitary gonadotropins, which in turn stimulate the gonadal sex steroids. The differential diagnosis of true precocious puberty includes cerebral and idiopathic categories. This distinction, which cannot be made endocrinologically due to similarities in pituitary gonadotropin and sex steroid levels, may be facilitated by high-resolution CT.

A CT study of 90 children (73 girls and 17 boys) with true precocious puberty was performed at the National Institutes of Health to detect cerebral causes of their precocious puberty.[24] Thirty-four cerebral abnormalities were demonstrated in 32 children (16 boys and 16 girls). These included hypothalamic hamartomas (17), hypothalamic astrocytoma (1), optic chiasm lesions (6), ventricular abnormalities (8), arachnoid cyst (1), and teratoma (1). The CT appearance of these cerebral abnormalities is discussed and related to the endocrinologic findings and natural history of true precocious puberty. A practical neuroradiologic approach to the evaluation of children with precocious puberty is presented.

Twenty-five patients with suspected pituitary adenoma were evaluated prospectively with CT and MRI.[25] Nine patients underwent transsphenoidal surgery, and three of these showed a documented decrease in size of mass on bromocriptine therapy. CT was more sensitive than MRI for detecting focal lesions (7 vs. 3) and sellar-floor erosion (12 vs. 6). MRI was superior to CT in identifying infundibular abnormalities (7 vs. 6), focal abnormalities of the diaphragma sellae (10 vs. 7), cavernous sinus invasion (4 vs. 2), and optic chiasm compression (6 vs. 0). Thus, MRI may be the procedure of choice for optimal identification and localization of macroadenoma. For patients with suspected microadenoma, this preliminary series indicates that CT remains the radiographic procedure of choice.

Seven patients with tumors arising in the face or paranasal sinuses, and with invasion of the anterior skull base, were evaluated with MRI and high-resolution CT.[26] MRI was superior in: (1) evaluating tumor encasement of the carotid artery and invasion of the cavernous sinus; (2) assessing the relationship of the tumor to the anterior brain, optic nerves, and optic chiasm; (3) providing coronal images free from dental artifact; and (4) determining tumor extent within the infratemporal fossa. Bone destruction was more easily observed on CT than MRI.

High-resolution MRI with a 1.5-Tesla Signa system was used to study nine patients with a previous CT diagnosis of juxtasellar meningioma.[27] In four patients, previous surgery confirmed meningiomas before MRI evaluation, which was utilized for postoperative assessment or as a baseline study for future comparisons; these patients had undergone preoperative CT and angiography. No gadolinium enhancement was used. CT was considered equal to MRI for demonstrating extra-axial configuration, superior to MRI for calcification or bony changes, but inferior to MRI for assessing suprasellar or intrasellar extension, postsurgical changes, and vascular encasement or displacement.

Two reviews in the July 1987 issue of *Radiologic Clinics of North America* are worth noting. Naheedy et al. provide an overview of the techniques of CT and MRI as applied to delineating the various pathologic processes of the sellar and parasellar regions.[28] In the second review, Rubenfeld and Wirtschafter examine current techniques for elucidating diseases in the orbit, cavernous sinus, optic chiasm, posterior visual pathways, brain stem, posterior fossa, and spinal cord.[29]

Inflammations

A most interesting case is presented by Weinstein et al.; that of a 42-year-old man with a 15-year history of rheumatoid arthritis, a 5-year history of headaches with nausea and vomiting, and progressive bilateral visual loss to hand-movement RE and 20/25 LE, with principally central scotomas.[30] Fundi showed right optic atrophy with drusen of the disk. CT demonstrated bilateral masses in the areas of the optic nerves and both cavernous sinuses. Craniotomy with biopsy disclosed "mononuclear inflammatory response with basophilic degeneration and necrosis." Plasma cells were prominent. A similar case of "rheumatoid meningitis" has been recorded by Spurlock and Richman.[31] Purvin et al (1988) reported chiasmal neuritis as a complication of Epstein-Barr virus infection.[32] A 13-year-old boy developed visual loss in association with an upper respiratory syndrome, with acuity of 20/40 RE and 20/15 LE. Visual fields showed a subtle bitemporal depression, with normal CT, MRI, and cerebrospinal fluid examination. Serologic studies were consistent with current Epstein-Barr viremia, with subsequent decline in antiviral capsid antigen. No signs or symptoms of Guillain-Barré syndrome were present.

Vascular Disease

A 25-year-old woman with two episodes of temporal hemianopic, transient loss of vision in the left eye, and complete blindness in the right, was found to have a typical circoid aneurysm replacing the right disk.[33] A left temporal field defect was present and CT followed by arteriography disclosed an arteriovenous malformation along the course of the right optic nerve, in the suprasellar space, and into the mesencephalon. This is believed to be only the third such case in the world literature. One case of bilateral ophthalmic artery aneurysm of traumatic origin is recorded.[34] The patient presented with progressive loss of vision, memory deficit, and expressive aphasia. A CT scan revealed enhancing lesions near the region of the optic chiasm. The diagnosis of cerebral aneurysm was confirmed by cerebral angiography. At operation, bilateral ophthalmic artery aneurysms were successfully clipped. A case of idiopathic intrachiasmal hemorrhage studied by MRI has been reported.[35]

MISCELLANEOUS

Trauma may take several forms, of which motor vehicle accidents, falls, and assaults are only the most obvious. At Montreal General Hospital, 24 patients sustained blunt head injuries that resulted in insults to the visual system.[36] Of these, 5 involved the optic chiasm, solely or in combination with optic nerve trauma, and all were subsequent to frontal head impacts; diabetes insipidus complicated only one case. This is a very useful review of traumatic visual loss. Iatrogenic trauma occurs (fortunately) infrequently, as a result of radiation therapy. Three such patients developed the sudden onset of total blindness several months after treatment with oral CCNU and low-dose whole-brain radiation.[37] The anterior visual system was included in the radiation field in all patients. Radiotherapy was given for a frontal lobe glioblastoma multiforme, for central nervous system prophylaxis in a patient with oat cell carcinoma of the lung, and for a parietal lobe glioblastoma multiforme. None of the neoplasms involved the anterior visual system. The radiation dose ranged from 3,000 to 4,650 rad and the oral CCNU dosage from 300 mg to 1,050 mg. Patients 1 and 2 also received other chemotherapeutic agents. Patient 3, who was treated only with oral CCNU and cranial irradiation, died. At autopsy the brain showed a widely infiltrating residual high-grade glioma, as well as patchy coagulative necrosis with swollen axons and dystrophic calcifications. The optic chiasm showed severe demyelination, axonal loss, and hyalinized vessels. Synergism between oral CCNU and radiation may account for the blindness produced.

Slavin reports a case of bitemporal hemianopia following placement of an intraventricular catheter, the tip of which lodged in the "suprasellar cistern."[38] Visual function improved after catheter removal.

Sellar anomalies are rare causes of chiasmal syndromes, but include intrasellar arachnoid cysts. Thirteen pathologically documented intrasellar arachnoid cysts treated by transsphenoidal cyst excision and marsupialization were analyzed.[39] Presenting symptoms included headache (7), visual loss (7), galactorrhea (4), and anterior pituitary dysfunction (2). Postoperatively, the 7 patients with visual loss and 4 with hyperprolactinemia improved. The 2 patients with anterior pituitary dysfunction did not improve, and 2 additional patients required hormonal supplements. Based on this operative experience, the pathophysiology of these cysts is discussed. The indications for transsphenoidal exploration include the following: to relieve optic chiasm, pituitary stalk, or gland compression, and to exclude the possibility of other sellar neoplasms. A patient with pituitary-sellar disproportion (sellar hypoplasia), a perichiasmal visual field defect, and no clinically demonstrable endocrinopathy is presented.[40] Radiographic and pathologic studies suggested that the pituitary-sellar disproportion was secondary to sellar hypoplasia, a previously unrecognized cause of the chiasmal syndrome. It remains to be seen whether hormonal manipulation aimed at suppression of gonodotropin- and/or prolactin-secreting cells might obviate the need for exploration in similar patients.

In an interesting review entitled "The Pregnant Woman's Eye" by Sunness, there is a sensible discussion of the problem of preexisting pituitary adenomas, field defects, and treatment with bromocriptine. The majority of women do well, treated or not.[41]

How does nature provide a neuroanatomic structure that permits fusion of overlapping visual fields with frontally placed eyes and subsequent stereopsis? The answer is: the optic chiasm. In a masterly thesis, Shipley provides an extensive overview of "solid seeing."[42] While the emphasis is on cortical integration and gestalt psychology, implications for neuro-ophthalmology are obvious.

REFERENCES

1. Reynolds TM: A nineteenth century view of the optic commissure. *Surv Ophthalmol* 1987; 32:214–216.
2. Rucker CW: The concept of a semidecussation of the optic nerves. *Arch Ophthalmol* 1958; 59:159–171.

3. Leventhal AG, Ault SJ, Vitek DJ: The nasotemporal division in primate retina: The neural bases of macular sparing and splitting. *Science* 1988; 240:66–67.

4. Hoffman KP, Distler C, Erickson RG, et al: Physiological and anatomical identification of the nucleus of the optic tract and dorsal terminal nucleus of the accessory optic tract in monkeys. *Exp Brain Res* 1988; 69:635–644.

5. Braak H, Braak E: The hypothalamus of the human adult: Chiasmatic region. *Anat Embryol (Berl)* 1987; 175:315–330.

6. Black PM, Zervas NT, Candia GL: Incidence and management of complications of transsphenoidal operation for pituitary adenomas. *Neurosurgery* 1987; 20:920–924.

7. Mikhael MA, Ciric IS: MR imaging of pituitary tumors before and after surgical and/or medical treatment. *J Comput Assist Tomogr* 1988; 12:441–445.

8. Teng MMH, Huang CI, Chang T: The pituitary mass after transsphenoidal hypophysectomy. *AJNR* 1988; 9:23–26.

9. Lecky BR, Williams TD, Lightman SL, et al: Myxoedema presenting with chiasmal compression: Resolution after thyroxine replacement. *Lancet* 1987; 1:1347–1350.

10. Lacomis D, Johnson LN, Mamourian AC: Magnetic resonance imaging in pituitary apoplexy. *Arch Ophthalmol* 1988; 106:207–209.

11. Scotti G, Yu CY, Dillon WP, et al: MR imaging of cavernous sinus involvement by pituitary adenomas. *AJNR* 9:657–664.

12. Alvord EC Jr, Lofton S: Gliomas of the optic nerve or chiasm. Outcome by patient's age, tumor site, and treatment (Review). *J Neurosurg* 1988; 68:85–98.

13. Wong JY, Uhl V, Wara WM, et al: Optic gliomas. A reanalysis of the University of California, San Francisco experience. *Cancer* 1987; 60:1847–1855.

14. Flickinger JC, Torres C, Deutsch M: Management of low-grade gliomas of the optic nerve and chiasm. *Cancer* 1988; 61:635–642.

15. Pascual-Castroviejo I, Verdu A, Roman M, et al: Optic glioma with progressive occlusion of the aqueduct of Sylvius in monozygotic twins with neurofibromatosis. *Brain Dev* 1988; 10:24–29.

16. Coppeto JR, Monteiro ML, Uphoff DF: Exophytic suprasellar gliomas: a rare cause of chiasmatic compression. Case report. *Arch Ophthalmol* 1987; 105:28.

17. Pomeranz SJ, Shelton JJ, Tobias J, et al: MR of visual pathways in patients with neurofibromatosis. *AJNR* 1987; 8:831–836.

18. Bognanno JR, Edwards MK, Lee TA, et al: Cranial MR imaging in neurofibromatosis. *AJNR* 1988; 9:461–468.

19. Brown EW, Riccardi VM, Mawad M, et al: MR imaging of optic pathways in patients with neurofibromatosis. *AJNR* 1987; 8:1031–1036.

20. Patronas NJ, Dwyer A, Papathanasiou M, et al: Contributions of magnetic resonance imaging in the evaluation of optic gliomas. *Surg Neurol* 1987; 28:367–371.

21. Freeman MP, Kessler RM, Allen JH, et al: Craniopharyngioma: CT and MR imaging in nine cases. *J Comput Assist Tomogr* 1987; 11:810–814.

22. Brodsky MC, Hoyt WF, Barnwell SL, et al: Intrachiasmatic craniopharyngioma: A rare cause of chiasmal thickening. Case report. *J Neurosurg* 1988; 68:300–302.

23. Howard RS, Duncombe AS, Owens C, et al: Compression of the optic chiasm due to a lymphoreticular malignancy. *Postgrad Med J* 1987; 63:1091–1093.

24. Rieth KG, Comite F, Dwyer AJ, et al: CT of cerebral abnormalities in precocious puberty. *AJR* 1987; 148:1231–1238.

25. Davis PC, Hoffman JC Jr, Spencer T, et al: MR imaging of pituitary adenoma: CT, clinical and surgical correlation. *AJR* 1987; 148:797–802.

26. Paling RM, Black WC, Levine PA, et al: Tumor invasion of the anterior skull base: A comparison of MR and CT studies. *J Comput Assist Tomogr* 1987; 11:824–830.

27. Yeakley JW, Kulkarni MV, McArdle CB, et al: High-resolution MR imaging of juxtasellar meningiomas with CT and angiographic correlation. *AJNR* 1988; 9:279–285.

28. Naheedy MH, Haag JR, Azar KB, et al: MRI and CT of sellar and parasellar disorders. *Radiol Clin North Am* 1987; 25:819–847.

29. Rubenfeld M, Wirtschafter JD: The role of medical imaging in the practice of neuro-ophthalmology. *Radiol Clin North Am* 1987; 25:863–876.

30. Weinstein GW, Powell SR, Thrush WP: Chiasmal neuropathy secondary to rheumatoid pachymeningitis. *Am J Ophthalmol* 1987; 104:439–440.

31. Spurlock RG, Richman AV: Rheumatoid meningitis. A case report and review of the literature. *Arch Pathol Lab Med* 1983; 107:129.

32. Purvin V, Herr GJ, De Myer W: Chiasmal neuritis as a complication of Epstein-Barr virus infection. *Arch Neurol* 1988; 45:458–460.

33. Defauchy M: Optochiasmatic aneurysm and Blanc Bonnet Dechaume disease: The 3rd case in the world with x-ray computed tomographic and arteriographic test. *Bull Soc Ophtalmol Fr* 1987; 87:995–1000.

34. Hahn YS, McLone DG: Traumatic bilateral ophthalmic artery aneurysms: A case report. *Neurosurgery* 1987; 21:86–89.

35. Moffit B, Diffy K, Lufkin R, et al: MR imaging of intrachiasmatic hemorrhage. *J Comput Assist Tomogr* 1988; 12:535–536.

36. Elisevich KV, Ford RM, Anderson DP, et al: Visual abnormalities with multiple trauma. *Surg Neurol* 1984; 22:565–575.

37. Wilson WB, Perez GM, Kleinschmidt-Demasters BK: Sudden onset of blindness in patients treated with oral CCNU and low-dose cranial irradiation. *Cancer* 1987; 59:901–907.

38. Slavin ML, Rosenthal AD: Chiasmal compression caused by a catheter in the suprasellar cistern. *Am J Ophthalmol* 1988; 105:560–561.

39. Meyer FB, Carpenter SM, Laws ER Jr: Intrasellar arachnoid cysts. *Surg Neurol* 1987; 28:105–110.

40. Elias Z, Powers SK, Grimson BS, et al: Chiasmal syndrome caused by pituitary-sellar disproportion. *Surg Neurol* 1987; 28:395–400.

41. Sunness JS: The pregnant woman's eye. *Surv Ophthalmol* 1988; 32:219–238.

42. Shipley T: Field processes in stereovision. A description of stereopsis appropriate to ophthalmology and visual perception. *Doc Ophthalmol* 1987; 66:95–170.

CHAPTER 5

The Retrochiasmal Visual Pathways

Carl Ellenberger, Jr., M.D.

Good Samaritan Hospital, Lebanon, Pennsylvania

Once again, in view of the multitude of visual "retrochiasmal" pathways in the brain, all subject to a vast range of diseases, I selected the contents of this chapter arbitrarily. The articles reviewed are predominantly clinical; I resisted attempts to cover more advances in understanding of the visual process, a complex field that is hardly manageable for an office physician. There is overlap with topics covered in neighboring chapters—stroke, migraine, higher cortical function, and others—when articles on these subjects relate to the cerebral visual pathways.

A new program for IBM-compatible personal computers (PCs) was invaluable in the preparation of this review. I recommend it highly, even to those readers who have daily access to the National Library of Medicine's (NLM) MEDLARS service. For about $30, "Grateful Med" can be purchased from the MEDLARS Management Section of the NLM. Installed on a PC, it allows one to "browse" through all the medical subject headings in *Index Medicus,* guides the formulation of a literature search, and then communicates with most of the MEDLARS data bases at the NLM. A search can be instantaneously reformulated according to information received back from the NLM; I usually did not "download" all of the citations I was interested in until I had made several alterations in the subject headings, an option not always practical when left to a librarian. About 70% of the citations are accompanied by abstracts. A search using the single heading "hemianopia" yielded 88 articles published in all languages during the past 2 years.

Curr Neuro Ophthalmol 2:57–74, 1990
© 1990, Year Book Medical Publishers, Inc.
0893–0147/89/02-057-074-$04.00

PHYSIOLOGY

Visual deprivation and amblyopia

Positron emission tomography (PET) is beginning to show promise as a useful tool for the elucidation of mechanisms of normal and abnormal visual processing. Using labeled 2-deoxyglucose, Demer et al. showed that glucose metabolism as an indication of neuronal activity in the primary and accessory visual cortex in humans is less activated by visual stimulation of an amblyopic eye (20/200) with a "dramatic entertainment video motion picture."[1] In addition, glucose metabolism was consistently higher in the frontal and temporal lobes contralateral to the viewing eye in some of both the normal and amblyopic subjects. Blood flow to the visual cortex was also less, measured by the tracer $H_2^{15}O$ after stroboscopic stimulation of the amblyopic eye. Given the duration (35 minutes) and apparent intensity of the visual stimuli, the differences in the resulting scans, demonstrated on a false color scheme, seem relatively slight to the naive observer; they apparently relate to the duration of stimulation. PET study of cerebral neuronal activity offers greater spatial resolution than do visually evoked potentials (VEP).

For the present, however, VEP would seem to hold the most practical potential for the *detection* of amblyopia. The "masked observer" of Friendly et al. correctly identified 22 of 27 children with anisometropic amblyopia by visual inspection of P100 amplitude of pattern-reversal VEPs, but also pronounced amblyopic 1 of 4 children with normal vision.[2] Perhaps computer-assisted analysis of the VEP waveforms will yield more specific, as well as more sensitive, results.

Rogers et al. found a linear relationship between contrast sensitivity and visual acuity in subjects with strabismic and anisometropic amblyopia. As acuity decreased, contrast sensitivity decreased along the contrast sensitivity axis, and peak sensitivity shifted to lower frequencies.[3] Although occlusion therapy brought visual acuity to 20/20, differences remained between contrast sensitivity functions of normal and amblyopic eyes. The authors attribute the apparent contradictory findings of previous investigators to measurement errors. It was disturbing to note that patching of the normal eye reduced both its acuity and contrast sensitivity.

In an attempt to restore good *binocular* vision (as well as to improve vision of the deprived eye) in monocularly deprived kittens, Murphy and Mitchell discovered another complication of occlusion therapy.[4] They examined the effects of a short but physiologically optimal period of reverse occlusion, followed by a period of binocular vision beginning at 7.5 weeks of age. Surprisingly, despite the early introduction of binocular vision, the kittens had severe *bilateral* amblyopia. Even so, cortical ocular dominance appeared similar to that of normal cats. They unexpectedly became the first to cause severe bilateral amblyopia by consecutive periods of monocular occlusion.

Two children also developed profound visual loss in a normal eye patched full time because of strabismic amblyopia in the fellow eye.[5] The first child had been patched for 13 days at age 18 months. Vision returned to normal by the 40th day of reverse occlusion. The second child had worn a patch for 1 month at age 9 months. After 3 months without treatment the initially amblyopic eye was patched for 3 years, but both eyes continue to be mildly amblyopic. Although rare, occlusion amblyopia can result from full-time patching of normal eyes of young children. The authors now avoid full-time occlusion and monitor patients at intervals of at least 1 week per 1 year of age.

In general, good response to occlusion therapy of amblyopia is thought to diminish with increasing age. But Oliver et al. challenged that conventional wisdom after assessing not only the results of patching, but also the *compliance* in different age groups.[6] Younger children were more compliant, but vision of children over age 8 years who did comply improved almost as much. The authors conclude that noncompliance—not an inflexible visual cortex—is the major reason for treatment failure in older children. Most improvement occurred in the first 3 months.

A 34-year-old man who had experienced 30 years of visual deprivation due to congenital cataracts was not so fortunate.[7] After cataract removal, despite extensive rehabilitative efforts that included training in eye-hand coordination, object recognition, mobility training, etc., he never began to use vision in daily life. The authors wonder if his failure was due to lack of motivation related to his desire to retain special status as a blind person. But this patient's visual deprivation may have been more profound than their previous patient with retinopathy of prematurity, who responded more favorably to their rehabilitative efforts.

Visual Neurotransmitters

In contrast to other projection pathways in the brain, the range of neurotransmitters in the visual system has not been conclusively determined. Although visual disturbance is not a prominent feature of Parkinson's disease, several investigators have detected both electrophysiologic and contrast sensitivity abnormalities. Bulens et al. hypothesized that if dopamine is a functional neurotransmitter in the visual system, contrast sensitivity would improve after administration of levodopa.[8] Indeed it did, in a well-designed study. Tieman et al., using a highly specific antiserum and histochemical methods, have detected the neuropeptide N-acetylaspartylglutamate in the retina, geniculate nucleus, and visual cortex of the monkey. This dipeptide activates neural receptors implicated in the action of dissociative anesthetics and hallucinogens, in long-term potentiation of synaptic efficacy in associative learning, in seizures, and in ischemic neurotoxicity.[9]

Neuroimaging

The right cerebral hemisphere may be specialized for visual processing, according to PET studies of Kushner et al.[10] Using (^{18}F)-fluorodeoxyglucose (FDG), they studied the impact of visual stimulation on cerebral metabolism in normal young men. Not surprisingly, reversing check-patterned visual stimulation of the macular regions of either visual hemifield caused significant increases in the metabolism of the contralateral posterior striate cortex. Of more interest, the stimulation induced highly significant asymmetries in the metabolism of the prefrontal and inferior parietal cortices, and also in the peristriate region. Regardless of the hemifield stimulated, metabolic activation on the right predominated. This study confirms in humans previous observations in animals that areas of cortex that process the visual stimulus extend far beyond the borders of the striate cortex. Using monocular full-field stimulation by their "dramatic video motion picture," Demer et al. also found activation of nonoccipital cortical areas in four normal subjects, and asymmetry.[1] However, with their method, activation of the hemisphere contralateral to the stimulated eye predominated. Fishbein et al. found no asymmetries in their normal, unstimulated patients (see below).[11]

To assess the effect of extraoccipital lesions on local cerebral glucose utilization in primary and associative visual cortex, Fishbein et al. studied 29 patients with hemianopic defects and 11 control subjects by PET, using FDG without visual stimulation.[11] They found reduction in the local cerebral metabolic rate for glucose in the affected hemispheres proportional to the extent of homonymous defects, but no asymmetries in normal subjects or those with bitemporal defects.

A PET study of Bosley et al. used FDG to study serial changes in the local cerebral metabolic rate of glucose in five patients with homonymous hemianopia caused by ischemic lesions of the geniculocalcarine pathways.[12] All five patients had striking impairment of glucose metabolism in the striate cortex shortly after the infarction. Increase in glucose metabolism paralleled improvement of vision in two patients with nonoccipital lesions; neither glucose metabolism nor vision improved in the remaining three with occipital lesions. PET with FDG can help distinguish between radiation necrosis and residual or recurrent tumor by showing hypometabolism in the presence of the former and hypermetabolism with the latter.[13]

Magnetic resonance imaging is not only a very sensitive way to confirm the diagnosis of multiple sclerosis, but has proved that MS may indeed involve the optic tracts.[14]

VASCULAR DISEASE

Mechanisms of Occipital Infarction

The mechanisms of cerebral infarction in the territory of the posterior cerebral artery (PCA) are being determined. Much of the credit goes to Pessin et al, whose initial work was cited incorrectly in volume 1 of *Current Neuro-Ophthalmology*.[15] Infarction in PCA territory can be caused by several mechanisms, including (1) embolism from a distant site, (2) embolism from vertebral or basilar arteries, and (3) PCA stenosis. Embolism seems to be by far the most common.[15]

Koroshetz and Ropper estimated that 20% of occipital strokes are caused by artery-to-artery embolism, i.e., from vertebral to posterior cerebral arteries.[16] This estimate is consistent with that of other observers, including Pessin et al.[15] Among 58 patients with PCA stroke, Koroshetz and Ropper identified 12 patients with vertebral artery stenosis or occlusion. They could divide their patients into two syndromes: one with prominent and multiple brain stem symptoms, the other with minor and transient brain stem symptoms. However, there were no differences on the arteriograms of the two groups that would explain these differences in clinical presentation.

Stenosis of the PCA is an uncommon vascular lesion. Pessin et al. reviewed angiograms and identified 15 patients with atheromatous PCA stenosis. Of these, 6 had related symptoms.[17] During the same period they found 80 patients with presumed embolism to the PCA. In contrast to those with PCA embolism, the patients with PCA stenosis had more transient ischemic attacks (TIAs) and fewer infarcts (only 2 patients). Preponderance of visual and sensory TIAs distinguish this vascular lesion from stenosis of the middle cerebral artery. Prognosis was good during follow-up (4 months to 4 years) on warfarin therapy.

Occipital infarction seems to be a surprisingly rare complication of dissection of the vertebral arteries, the consequences of which seem to concentrate in the brain stem after presentation with sudden occipital headache.[18, 19] Middle-aged hypertensive women seem to be especially vulnerable. The prognosis for recovery is good. Similarly, the retrochiasmal pathways are not vulnerable to ischemia in the presence of the "subclavian steal" phenomenon.[20] Most patients (64%) with reversal of blood flow in the extracranial vertebral system had no symptoms; those who did were likely to have additional stenoses in the carotid system. Instead of a predictor of stroke, subclavian steal, like carotid stenosis, is a marker for atherosclerotic vascular disease in general and risk of all its complications, including myocardial infarction.

Kosmorsky et al. reported the Cleveland Clinic experience with complications of cardiac catheterizations.[21] In a retrospective search, the authors found only 10 patients who had neuro-ophthalmic complications during a 5-year period when 30,000 catheterizations were performed. Posterior circulation events predominated, perhaps because carotid-territory embolism was less symptomatic or because the origin of the vertebral artery is at the apex of the aortic loop; eight complications were attributed to embolism and two to migraine. Among patients with complications, five had persisting visual or neurologic complications and one was lost to follow-up.

Patients do not fare so well after coronary arterial bypass (CAB) surgery: 312 such patients were compared with 50 patients who underwent major vascular surgery with cardiopulmonary bypass. Almost 5% of the CAB group experienced stroke, 25% had visual abnormalities, and 79% showed significant deterioration in ten tests of psychometric function. The authors attribute the significant differences to the contribution from cardiopulmonary bypass of emboli of air, particulate matter, platelets, valve debris, fibrin, or particles of silicone or polyvinylchloride tubing.[22]

In sickle cell disease, brain infarctions that occur in 8% to 17% of patients are focal rather than widely disseminated. They are associated with stenotic mural or occlusive transluminal thrombi involving the large arteries of the anterior circulation at the base of the brain and in the neck.[23] Rothman et al. found that the PCA territory was spared; the infarcts occurred mainly in the territory supplied by distal branches of the internal carotid artery, especially in the anterior-middle cerebral artery boundary zone.[23] They suggest that the pathogenesis of infarction involves perfusion failure or intra-arterial embolization, in addition to intravascular sickling.

Stroke Syndromes

The most recent review of "cortical blindness" was contributed by Aldrich et al., who studied 25 patients, including 15 of his own cases.[24] Cerebral vascular disease was the most common cause, but complications of surgery, particularly cardiac, and angiography also made the list. After analysis, the authors reached predictable conclusions:

1. Prognosis is poor when spontaneous stroke is the cause (and less favorable than I would have expected when iatrogenic).
2. Electroencephalograms (showing absent alpha rhythm in all patients) are more useful than VEPs for diagnosis.
3. Bioccipital computed tomography (CT) abnormalities indicate poor prognosis for recovery of vision.

An interesting feature of the article is Table 1, which correlates the CT abnormalities of 16 patients with the visual abnormalities.

Lambert et al. found that the age of onset and CT findings predicted the outcome of hypoxic cortical blindness during childhood.[25] Twenty-two of 30 infants and children regained partial vision. Poor visual outcome correlated with early age of the hypoxia and severity of CT lesions in optic radiations, but not in striate or parastriate cortex. CT would seem to have more prognostic potential than visually evoked potentials in this situation.

The combination of hemiplegia and hemianesthesia with hemianopia should alert the clinician to the possibility of infarction in the territory of the anterior choroidal artery, a rare occurrence according to Decroix et al., who report on 16 cases.[26] The syndrome can be confirmed by a CT finding of reduced density in the posterior limb of the internal capsule, sparing the thalamus medially and encroaching upon the tip of the globus pallidus laterally. Incomplete forms of the syndrome are more frequent. Left-sided spatial neglect may accompany right-sided lesions, as may slight disorders of speech in left-sided lesions.

In addition to hemianopia, PCA infarction may cause confusion, one of the most common disorders of higher function encountered by neurologists. This association has been reported before, particularly when infarctions are bilateral; however, Devinsky et al. provide the interesting observation that infarction in left PCA territory is far more likely to cause confusion than the opposite.[27] Of 19 personal or reviewed cases of PCA infarction with confusion, 18 had involvement of the left side, usually interrupting occipitotemporal connections. Thus, right homonymous hemianopia may be the clue that a confused patient has had an infarction rather than toxic-metabolic encephalopathy. The authors suggest that such infarctions disconnect the neocortex from the limbic system.

A patient of Steiner et al. was not confused when he experienced several episodes of 180-degree reversal of vision.[28] Because the duration was only minutes and the patient also had vertigo, tinnitus and nausea, the authors thought he had had basilar TIAs.

A patient developed "opticosensory ataxia" and alien hand syndrome after occlusion of the right PCA at the anterolateral midbrain, causing an extensive infarction involving the calcarine cortex, right basal temporo-occipital region, and sensory thalamic nuclei.[29] She was not aware of her left homonymous hemianopia, and her wildly ataxic left arm, which she often did not recognize as her own, felt "like a dead fish." There was no sensation to any modality in the left arm, which often moved on its own, requiring her to restrain it with her right hand. The ataxia of the contralateral arm was not diminished by visual guidance, as it is in cases of pure sensory ataxia, presumably because all visual input to the brain necessary for visual control of the left arm was to the left hemisphere, thus disconnected by infarction of the callosal connections from the right hemispheric control of the arm. Eventual improvement was "slight."

Forty percent of patients with thalamic hemorrhage had homonymous hemianopia.[30] Among the 50 patients, 84% had hypertension, 38% with larger hemorrhages died, and 5 patients with small hemorrhages experienced transient episodes of focal signs that could be mistaken for TIA. This review by Weisberg covers all the manifestations of this clinical entity and updates earlier pathologic reviews written before the advantage of CT.

A similar review by Bogousslavsky et al. defines four syndromes among 40 patients caused by PCA-territory infarctions confined to the thalamus.[31] Lacunar and embolic infarctions accounted for two thirds of the cases, in equal proportions. Only 3 patients in the category of "posterior choroidal artery infarction" had hemianopia, probably consequent to involvement of the lateral geniculate nucleus. The other categories were more common:

1. Inferolateral, characterized by contralateral sensory loss.
2. Tuberopthalmic, characterized by neuropsychologic dysfunction.

3. Paramedian, characterized by transient loss of consciousness followed by confusion, amnesia, and ocular motility disorders.

"Moyamoya disease" is a colossal misnomer, referring to the effects of a variety of causes of occlusion of the carotid arteries at the level of the siphon. It meets few of the criteria that should define a disease. Not unexpectedly, two patients had homonymous hemianopia related to occipital infarction caused by occlusion of the posterior cerebral arteries.[32]

Migraine

Olsen et al. detected reduction of regional cerebral blood flow averaging 52% in 7 of 11 patients who were unfortunate enough to suffer a migraine during measurement of blood flow by an intracarotid xenon technique.[33] In many cases the test was done because patients had suffered an earlier permanent deficit after a migraine. Although triggered by the testing procedure, the migraines, many accompanied by focal symptoms, were thought to be similar to the spontaneously occurring headaches that the patients were accustomed to having. The symptoms appeared 5 to 15 minutes after the flow reductions and resolved hours before the hypoperfusion subsided, but the authors argue that the ischemia caused the symptoms during the aura.[34] In contrast, Welch's comprehensive theory views migraine as a central nervous system dysautonomia, of which vascular phenomena are only a part.[35]

Later, Olsen's group, using single-photon emission CT found that after the initial hypoperfusion, hyperperfusion followed for 1 to as long as 24 hours, and was thought to be reactive.[36] However, because the transition from hypoperfusion to hyperperfusion came considerably *after* onset of the headache, it seems unlikely that the headache was caused by hyperperfusion, as Wolff postulated.

Regardless of the mechanism of migraine, it can definitely cause a lasting neurologic deficit in rare cases. Broderick and Swanson identified 20 patients who had had migraine-associated brain infarctions before age 50 years.[37] (Incidence was 12 cases during 176,887 person-years of observation.) Sixteen of the 20 patients were women, only 3 of whom were using oral contraceptives at the onset of the stroke. Consistent with most prior reports, the infarcts were mainly in the territory of the posterior cerebral artery. Most caused relatively mild functional impairment. Two patients had a second infarction during follow-up periods averaging 7 years.

Other authors prospectively evaluated 22 patients after migraine-related stroke, who shared no other risk factors for stroke.[38] Various scanning procedures detected infarction in 55% and cerebral arteriography showed stenosis, spasm, beading, or occlusion in 42%—and caused coma in a patient with vertebral arterial spasm. Over a mean of 22 months, one patient had another stroke. The authors postulate multiple mechanisms for migraine-related strokes, not including prolapsed mitral valves or arterial dissection.

Bogousslavsky et al. also found a preponderance of women (17 of 22) in a series of patients with classic migraine who had suffered an ischemic stroke during an attack of migraine.[39] They did not discover any nonmigrainous risk factors, including oral contraceptives, that could have caused the stroke. In contrast to the study of Rothrock et al.,[38] all arteriograms were normal and uncomplicated, so the authors minimize vasospasm as a mechanism. The infarcts were usually in the territory involved during attacks. The authors hypothesized that prolongation of the migrainous process beyond usual limits may explain most migrainous strokes.

Shuaib and Hachinski concluded, after reviewing charts of 142 patients with migraine who had 149 angiograms, that history of migraine does not increase the risk of complications caused by angiography, and that angiography during headache is a safe procedure, even though transient focal neurologic symptoms are not infrequent.[40]

On the next occasion that you confidently assure a patient that scintillating scotomas are virtually diagnostic of the benign condition called classic migraine, recall the following case: Five months after the onset of episodes of scintillating scotomas, massive cerebral hemorrhage occurred in a large right occipital lobe tumor that had not been seen on initial CT scans of a 43-year-old woman.[41] Granted, the "small areas of occipital infarction" that had been seen certainly were not characteristic of classic migraine, but most of us would not have been prepared for the malignant melanoma confirmed by autopsy. The authors believe that the visual symptoms may have related to tumor embolization. Which patients with recent onset of apparent classic migraine should have neuroimaging?

MELAS Syndrome

Another cause for alarm in the presence of apparent migraine is when the headache becomes severe, frequently recurrent, and prolonged in young patients. In that case, partial seizures and occipital infarctions leading to cortical blindness may ensue. The patient may have the MELAS syndrome (mitochondrial encephalopathy, lactic acidosis, and strokelike episodes).[42] Muscle biopsy shows the "ragged red" abnormality indicating mitochondrial myopathy. The condition is a genetically determined metabolic disorder transmitted maternally, much like Leber optic neuropathy, which appears at about the same age.[43] Mutation in the DNA of one of 13 known mitochondrial genes may affect an enzyme involved in adenosine triphosphate (ATP) manufacture. Prognosis is poor.

Another family illustrated the variability of expression of MELAS.[44] The proband became symptomatic at age 24 and followed a relentless course similar to that described by Montagna et al.[42] But his mother had been well until hearing loss began at age 35, and then fatigability at age 50. At age 61, biopsy showed evidence of a mitochondrial myopathy.

Most investigators agree that epileptic seizures without MELAS cause irreversible brain damage, but the mechanism remains elusive. A patient had prolonged unilateral status epilepticus.[45] Severe brain damage was confined to one hemisphere, related not to a vascular territory, but to the location of the epileptic discharge. This observation suggested that the damage resulted from the long-lasting epileptic activity.

Vasculitis

Younger et al. reported the clinical and pathologic findings of four patients who all died from isolated granulomatous angiitis of the brain (GAB) to illustrate their contention that GAB is a nonspecific reaction, not a disease.[46] And, because of heterogeneity of clinical and pathologic findings, they maintained that the diagnosis must rest upon pathologic criteria: inflammation of cerebral vessels by giant cells or epithelioid cells. After reviewing 74 cases of GAB reported in the literature, the authors concluded that basing diagnosis on arteriographic criteria is hazardous. They could discern no clear clinical presentation that would mandate brain biopsy, and reserved this procedure, with its 0.5% to 2.0% risk of serious morbidity, to cases for which no alternative cause emerges to explain encephalopathy evolving over days or weeks, especially if it is associated with focal cerebral signs and abnormal cerebrospinal fluid. Signs of encephalopathy were dominant in 61 of the 74 cases they reviewed. They called for a multicenter controlled therapeutic trial after the diagnosis is established by biopsy.

Additional clinical reports, similar to those reviewed in vol 1 of *Current Neuro-ophthalmology*, continue to support the conclusions of Younger et al. The patient reported by Wilson et al. was the fifth reported, but only the first with pathologic confirmation of cerebral vasculitis associated with acute posterior multifocal placoid pigment epitheliopathy (APMPPE).[47] Because headache commonly accompanies APMPPE, cerebral vasculitis may be more common in that condition than realized.

Wessel et al. reported a patient with the rare association of herpes simplex encephalitis and presumed herpes simplex retinitis.[48] They argued that the appearance of the retinitis after the encephalitis indicates that the former was infectious and not immunologic in origin, and that the retinal infection resulted either from neuron-to-neuron transmission of viruses along the optic nerve or from recurrent viral infection. In this single case, treatment with acyclovir seemed to cause improvement.

As reported in vol 1 of *Current Neuro-ophthalmology*, focal cerebral vasculitis is presumed to be the cause of the contralateral hemiparesis that uncommonly follows herpes zoster ophthalmicus (HZO), despite absence of abundant pathologic confirmation. A 17-month-old boy developed HZO and delayed contralateral hemiparesis after intrauterine varicella exposure.[49] Angiography disclosed occlusion of the lenticulostriate arteries. Recovery was "excellent."

Biopsy documented necrotizing cerebral vasculitis in a young man with ulcerative colitis.[50] The cerebral signs seemed to respond promptly to prednisone and cyclophosphamide. A 38-year-old man developed circulating immune complexes (CIC) secondary to bacterial endocarditis.[51] Superimposed on presumed subclinical radiation vasculitis, they were thought to be the cause of cerebral vasculitis (by arteriographic criteria only) in a region of the brain that had received radiation for treatment of a glioma 18 months before. CIC have not been implicated in the pathogenesis of cerebral vasculitis, but are suspected of participating in the disease process in systemic lupus erythematosis (SLE). This patient's symptoms improved after administration of dexamethasone.

Devinsky et al. have provided a good review of the clinical and neurologic findings in SLE.[52] Reviewing the medical records and autopsy reports of 50 patients, they found that cardiac emboli from Libman-Sacks endocarditis and thrombocytopenic purpura were common pathogenetic features of central nervous system (CNS) disease in SLE, but CNS vasculitis was rare.

Cerebral blood flow was found to correlate closely with CNS symptoms in patients with SLE; depressed cerebral blood flow was a sensitive indicator of active CNS disease.[53] The authors suggest that the depression could result from either a primary microvasculopathy or secondarily following the deposition of antineuronal antibody with subsequent neuronal deactivation.

Kase et al. described two patients who suffered intracerebral hemorrhage immediately after first-time use of the ubiquitous over-the-counter appetite suppressant and decongestant, phenylpropanolamine (PPA).[54] They reviewed previous similar reported cases and suggest an association of hemorrhagic stroke with PPA, probably by the mechanism of vasculitis. The circumstances in these cases were similar to those reported with amphetamine use. The chance of hemorrhage may be increased when PPA is combined with other compounds, such as caffeine, ephedrine, beta-blockers, monamine oxidase inhibitors, methyldopa, indomethacin, and oral contraceptives. Maher contributed the case of another patient, a long-time user of PPA, who experienced symptoms of cerebral vasculitis and hemorrhage for the first time during the postpartum period.[55] Cocaine may have caused cerebral vasculitis in a 22-year-old man. He experienced headache, fever, hemiparesis, and hemianesthesia, and had a CT radiolucency in the right frontotemporal region, as well as arteriographic changes compatible with vasculitis.[56]

Pregnancy

Blindness, either retinal or cortical, occurs in 3% to 5% of patients with eclampsia, and, like a variety of other toxemia-related neurologic deficits, usually resolves within a few days postpartum. Two patients with toxemia during pregnancy had hypodensities in the occipital regions by CT.[57] Vision returned and the CT abnormalities disappeared gradually after caesarean deliveries. A 35-year-old woman developed permanent homonymous hemianopia just after labor that ended a pregnancy with toxemia; two others returned to normal neurologic status after a variety of toxemia-related neurologic signs.[58] Widespread vasoconstriction was detected on cerebral angiograms of all. Another patient had TIAs in the last days of a normal pregnancy.[59] They resolved, as did a partial obstruction of the middle cerebral artery, after delivery. The authors postulate that reversible intimal hyperplasia was brought on by reproductive steroids.

HEMIANOPIA

The preservation of 5 to 10 degrees of central vision in a hemianopic defect, called "macular sparing," is generally acknowledged to result from the fact that collateral blood flow may preserve the occipital poles in PCA-territory infarction. Based mainly on anatomic studies in cats and monkeys, "foveal sparing," 2 to 3 degrees in diameter, has been attributed to bilateral representation of the maculas in the calcarine cortex. However, definite clinical examples of foveal "splitting" remained unaccounted for if human maculas were bilaterally represented. Leventhal et al. may have solved this dilemma by using refined horseradish peroxidase (HRP) methods in both Old World and New World monkeys.[60] After HRP injections into one lateral geniculate nucleus, they found that the foveal pit extended farther into temporal retina, but also that a ring of densely packed ipsilaterally-projecting cells circled the nasal side of the foveal pit. These latter cells could provide 2 to 3 degrees of bilateral representation. So, a lesion in the retrochiasmal pathways should cause homonymous hemianopia with foveal sparing in the field of the eye ipsilateral to the lesion, and splitting in the opposite field.[60]

Patients with homonymous hemianopia are quite differently handicapped in daily life. While variations in residual visual function in the blind hemifield, including sparing, can be responsible for such differences, the choice of compensatory oculomotor mechanisms or the presence of additional visual hemineglect may also play a role. In order to find objects in a blind hemifield, patients employ one of three oculomotor searching strategies: a "staircase" strategy, an "overshoot" strategy, or a "predictive" strategy. Patients with additional visual hemineglect, however, do not use the predictive strategy, nor can they learn an overshoot strategy. Meienberg developed and then applied infrared oculographic criteria to distinguish patients with hemineglect from those without, among 19 patients with hemianopia.[61, 62] The practical importance of such a delimitation is that patients with hemineglect are much more handicapped, and ignore or underestimate their handicap.

Using an eye camera, Ishiai et al. found that hemianopic patients without unilateral spatial neglect compensated by looking at the affected side of an image longer; those with neglect did not.[63]

Analysis of the CT scans of 41 cases showed that patients who are partially or fully aware of the hemianopia have purely occipital lesions.[64] The patients who were not aware of the visual defect had larger and more anterior lesions. Koehler et al. considered parietal lesions or lesions interrupting the associative pathway to the primary or secondary visual association cortex to be responsible for the lack of awareness of the defect.[64]

Poeppel et al. looked for plasticity in the visual system similar to that already found in the oculomotor system.[65] A patient with congenital left lateral rectus paresis and esotropia developed right homonymous hemianopia after a stroke at age 61. The hemianopic border of the left eye field defect was not oriented with respect to the functional vertical meridian (i.e., in line with the pseudofovea), but rather to the anatomic vertical meridian. They concluded that the striate cortex is "rigidly prewired" with reference to the anatomic vertical meridian and had not been altered by the esotropia. In contrast, plasticity in the oculomotor system enabled the patient to use a functional visual axis that did not correspond to the anatomic fovea.

Unusual Causes of Hemianopia

A patient of Barbas et al. suffered a fatal intracerebral hemorrhage after dental manipulation, perhaps by the mechanism of acute arterial hypertension caused by stimulation of trigeminal fibers.[66] Versavel et al. reversed isolated homonymous hemianopia by clipping a giant aneurysm of the anterior cerebral artery that had compressed the lateral surface of the posterior portion of the optic chiasm.[67] Chang et al. described ten patients with aneurysms of the PCA. Surgical repair of these aneurysms seemed likely to cause postoperative deficits, including hemianopia.[68]

Gans and Glaser described a patient who developed a dense homonymous hemianopia 4 days after an electrical injury, and reviewed the pathophysiology and clinical spectrum of such injuries to the CNS.[69] Soza et al. reported the unusual association between hemianopia and subdural hematoma.[70] The patient had bilateral homonymous hemianopia with preservation of central vision, spatial disorientation, and memory deficits after tentorial herniation and compression of both PCAs. Cyclosporine therapy for immunosuppression in liver transplantation caused severe CNS toxicity, including confusion, cortical blindness, quadriplegia, seizures, and coma.[71] Gittinger traced the history of our understanding of functional hemianopia.[72]

Blindsight

Shefrin recorded long-latency visually evoked potentials in four patients with homonymous hemianopia.[73] Random words appeared at a constant angle on either side of a vertical meridian. The specified target word elicited a well-formed P3 response in all intact hemifields; however, a response was seen in the hemianopic field only in the single subject in whom W. F. Hoyt had demonstrated evidence of "blindsight" at the tangent screen. Because the P3 response has been associated with cognitive aspects of sensory processing, the authors concluded that cognitive processing can take place independently of the geniculostriate pathway, even when subjective awareness of visual stimuli is absent.

Marzi et al. tested 20 patients with homonymous hemianopias for spatial summation of pairs of flashes presented simultaneously either to the same hemifield or to opposite hemifields across the vertical meridian.[74] In such experiments, normal subjects have shown summation, i.e., a shorter reaction time to key-pressing, after a pair of stimuli than after a single stimulus, regardless of whether the flashes were separated by the vertical meridian. Predictably, hemianopic subjects did not show summation across the vertical meridian, even though, like normal subjects, they showed summation within one hemifield. However, one patient did show summation across the vertical meridian; the authors interpreted this finding as evidence of blindsight. They did not demonstrate that this patient had other evidence of blindsight.

Stoerig used receiver-operating characteristic curves and tachistoscopic targets to demonstrate that five patients with clinical evidence of blindsight were able to detect only a peripheral target, not a more central one.[75]

Evoked Potentials

Ghilardi et al. examined the hemispheric distribution of the pattern visually evoked potential (PVEP) in three cynomolgus monkeys before and after right optic tractotomy or left occipital lobectomy.[76] The stimuli were vertical gratings of four spatial frequencies, counterphase and on-off modulated at 1 and 8 Hz. After experimental hemianopia, PVEPs over the midline and the intact hemisphere were normal, but partially polarity-inverted PVEPs of smaller amplitude were recorded over the deafferented hemisphere. The interhemispheric phase difference became more prominent as the spatial frequency of the stimulus was increased.

Maccolini et al. assessed the reliability of hemifield pattern-reversal VEPs in evaluating homonymous visual field defects in 13 patients with various lesions of the retrochiasmal pathways.[77] They concluded that amplitude asymmetry over 4 μV (between responses evoked by right and left hemifield stimulation, recorded ipsilaterally to the stimulated hemifield) is a reliable indicator of hemianopia. Lesions of the occipital cortex caused more pronounced bioelectrical abnormalities than those due to lesions affecting only the visual pathways, sparing the visual cortex. Experienced clinicians know, however, that confrontation methods are the most universally practical, adaptable, and sensitive methods, at least for daily, nonexperimental use.

Although intraoperative monitoring of VEPs has some theoretic and practical appeal, so far the main advantage of the technique has been to advance the careers of those who write and speak about it. After recording 35 cases, Cedzich et al. found an ". . .unacceptably high number of cases with significant VEP alteration. . .without concomitant visual function change, [and] no correlation between intraoperative VEP changes and. . .postoperative changes in visual function."[78]

REFERENCES

1. Demer JL, von Noorden GK, Volkow ND, et al: Imaging of cerebral blood flow and metabolism in amblyopia by positron emission tomography. *Am J Ophthalmol* 1988; 105:337–347.

2. Friendly DS, Weiss IP, Barnet AB, et al: Pattern-reversal visual-evoked potentials in the diagnosis of amblyopia in children. *Am J Ophthalmol* 1986; 102:329–339.

3. Rogers GL, Bremer DL, Leguire LE: The contrast sensitivity function and childhood amblyopia. *Am J Ophthalmol* 1987; 104:64–68.

4. Murphy KM, Mitchell DE: Bilateral amblyopia after a short period of reverse occlusion in kittens. *Nature* 1986; 323:536–538.

5. Simon JW, Parks MM, Price EC: Severe visual loss resulting from occlusion therapy for amblyopia. *Strabismus* 1987; 24:244–246.

6. Oliver M, Neumann R, Chaimovitch Y, et al: Compliance and results of treatment for amblyopia in children more than 8 years old. *Am J Ophthalmol* 1986; 102:340–345.

7. Carlson S, Hyvarinen L, Raininen A: Persistent behavioral blindness after early visual deprivation and active rehabilitation: A case report. *Br J Ophthalmol* 1986; 70:607–611.

8. Bulens C, Meerwaldt JD, Van der Wildt GJ, et al: Effect of Levodopa treatment on contrast sensitivity in Parkinson's disease. *Ann Neurol* 1987; 22:365–369.

9. Tieman SB, Hamilton CR, Vermeire BA, et al: N-acetylaspartylglutamate immunoreactivity in neurons of the monkey's visual pathway. *Soc Neurosci Abstr* 1987; 13:992.

10. Kushner MJ, Rosenquist A, Alavi A, et al: Cerebral metabolism and patterned visual stimulation: A positron emission tomographic study of the human visual cortex. *Neurology* 1988; 38:88–95.

11. Fishbein DS, Chrousos GA, Di Chiro G: Glucose utilization of visual cortex following extra-occipital interruptions of the visual pathways by tumor. A positron emission tomography study. *J Clin Neuro-Ophthalmol* 1987; 7:63–68.

12. Bosley TM, Dann R, Silver FL, et al: Recovery of vision after ischemic lesions: Positron emission tomography. *Ann Neurol* 1987; 21:444–450.

13. DiChiro G, Oldfield E, Wright DC, et al: Cerebral necrosis after radiotherapy and/or intraarterial chemotherapy for brain tumors. *Am J Radiol* 1988; 150:189–197.

14. Rosenblatt MA, Behrens MM, Zweifach PH, et al: Magnetic resonance imaging of optic tract involvement in multiple sclerosis. *Am J Ophthalmol* 1987; 104:74–79.

15. Pessin M, Lathi ES, Cohen MB, et al: Clinical features and mechanism of occipital infarction in the posterior cerebral artery territory. *Ann Neurol* 1987; 21:290–299.

16. Koroshetz WJ, Ropper AH: Artery-to-artery embolism causing stroke in the posterior circulation. *Neurology* 1987; 37:292–295.

17. Pessin MS, Kwan ES, DeWitt LD, et al: Posterior cerebral artery stenosis. *Ann Neurol* 1987; 21:85–89.

18. Caplan LR, Baquis GD, Pessin MS, et al: Dissection of the vertebral artery. *Neurology* 1988; 38:868–877.

19. Mokri B, Houser OW, Sandok BA, et al: Spontaneous dissections of the vertebral arteries. *Neurology* 1988; 38:880–885.

20. Hennerici M, Klemm C, Rautenberg W: The subclavian steal phenomenon: A common vascular disorder with rate neurologic deficits. *Neurology* 1988; 38:669–673.

21. Kosmorsky G, Hanson MR, Tomsak RL: Neuro-ophthalmic complications of cardiac catheterization. *Neurology* 1988; 38:483–485.

22. Shaw PJ, Bates D, Cartlidge NE, et al: Neurologic and neuropsychological morbidity following major surgery: Comparison of coronary artery bypass and peripheral vascular surgery. *Stroke* 1987; 18:700–707.

23. Rothman SM, Fulling KH, Nelson JS: Sickle cell anemia and central nervous system infarction: A neuropathological study. *Ann Neurol* 1986; 20:684–690.

24. Aldrich MS, Alessi AG, Beck RW, et al: Cortical blindness: Etiology, diagnosis and prognosis. *Ann Neurol* 1987; 21:149–158.

25. Lambert SR, Hoyt CS, Jan JE, et al: Visual recovery from cortical blindness during childhood. Computed tomographic and magnetic resonance imaging predictors. *Arch Ophthalmol* 1987; 105:1371–1377.

26. Decroix JP, Graveleau P, Masson M, et al: Infarction in the territory of the anterior choroidal artery. A clinical and computerized tomographic study of 16 cases. *Brain* 1986; 109:1071–1085.

27. Devinsky O, Bear D, Volpe BT: Confusional states following posterior cerebral artery infarction. *Arch Neurol* 1988; 45:160–163.

28. Steiner I, Shahin R, Melamed E: Acute "upside down" reversal of vision in transient vertebrobasilar ischemia. *Neurology* 1987; 37:1685–1686.

29. Levine DN, Rinn WE: Optico-sensory ataxia and alien hand syndrome after posterior cerebral artery territory infarction. *Neurology* 1986; 36:1094–1097.

30. Weisberg L: Thalamic hemorrhage: Clinical-CT correlations. *Neurology* 1986; 36:1382–1386.

31. Bogousslavsky F, Regli F, Uske A: Thalamic infarcts: Clinical syndromes, etiology, and prognosis. *Neurology* 1988; 38:837–848.

32. Noda S, Hayasaka S, Setogawa T, et al: Ocular symptoms of Moyamoya disease. *Am J Ophthalmol* 1987; 103:812–816.

33. Olsen TS, Friberg L, Lassen NA: Ischemia may be the primary cause of the neurologic deficits in classic migraine. *Arch Neurol* 1987; 44:156–161.

34. Olesen J: The ischemic hypotheses of migraine. *Arch Neurol* 1987; 44:321–322.

35. Welch KMA: Migraine: A biobehavioral disorder. *Arch Neurol* 1987; 44:323–327.

36. Anderson AR, Friberg L, Olsen TS, et al: Delayed hyperemia following hypoperfusion in classic migraine: Single photon emission computed tomographic demonstration. *Arch Neurol* 1988; 45:154–159.

37. Broderick JP, Swanson JW: Migraine-related strokes. *Arch Neurol* 1987; 44:868–871.

38. Rothrock JF, Walicke P, Swenson MR, et al: Migrainous stroke. *Arch Neurol* 1988; 45:63–67.

39. Bogousslavsky J, Regli F, Van Melle G: Migraine stroke. *Neurology* 1988; 38:223–227.

40. Shuaib A, Hachinski VC: Migraine and the risks from angiography. *Arch Neurol* 1988; 45:911–912.

41. Weinstein JM, Appen RE, Houston L, et al: Recurrent scintillating scotoma and homonymous hemianopia due to metastatic melanoma. *J Clin Neuro-Ophthalmol* 1987; 7:155–160.

42. Montagna P, Gallassi R, Medori R, et al: MELAS syndrome: Characteristic migrainous and epileptic features and maternal transmission. *Neurology* 1988; 38:751–754.

43. Novotny EJ, Singh G, Wallace DC, et al: Leber's disease and dystonia: A mitochondrial disease. *Neurology* 1986; 36:1053–1060.

44. Driscoll PF, Larsen PD, Gruber AB: MELAS syndrome involving a mother and two children. *Arch Neurol* 1987; 44:971–973.

45. Soffer D, Melamed E, Assaf Y: Hemispheric brain damage in unilateral status epilepticus. *Arch Neurol* 1986; 20:737–740.

46. Younger DS, Hays AP, Brust JM, et al: Granulomatous angiitis of the brain. An inflammatory reaction of diverse etiology. *Arch Neurol* 45:514–518.

47. Wilson CA, Choromokos EA, Sheppard R: Acute posterior multifocal placoid pigment epitheliopathy and cerebral vasculitis. *Arch Ophthalmol* 1988; 106:796–800.

48. Wessel K, Wiethoelter H, Weidle EG: Herpes simplex encephalitis with herpes simplex retinitis. *Nervenarzt* 1987; 58:317–321.

49. Leis AA, Butler IJ: Infantile herpes zoster ophthalmicus and acute hemiparesis following intrauterine chicken pox. *Neurology* 1987; 37:1537–1538.

50. Nelson J, Barron MM, Riggs JE, et al: Cerebral vasculitis and ulcerative colitis. *Neurology* 1987; 36:719–721.

51. Groothuis DR, Mikhael MA: Focal cerebral vasculitis associated with circulating immune complexes and brain irradiation. *Ann Neurol* 1986; 19:590–592.

52. Devinsky O, Petito CK, Alonso DR: Clinical and neuropathological findings in systemic lupus erythematosus: The role of vasculitis, heart emboli, and thrombotic thrombocytopenic purpura. *Arch Neurol* 1988; 23:380–384.

53. Kushner MJ, Chawluk J, Fazekas F, et al: Cerebral blood flow in systemic lupus erythematosus with or without cerebral complications. *Neurology* 1987; 37:1596–1598.

54. Kase CS, Foster TE, Reed JE, et al: Intracerebral hemorrhage and phenylpropanolamine use. *Neurology* 1987; 37:399–404.

55. Maher LM: Postpartum intracranial hemorrhage and phenylpropanolamine use. *Neurology* 1987; 37:1686.

56. Kaye BR, Fainstat M: Cerebral vasculitis associated with cocaine abuse. *JAMA* 1987; 258:2104–2106.

57. Lau SP, Chan FL, Yu UL, et al: Cortical blindness in toxaemia of pregnancy: Findings on computed tomography. *Br J Radiol* 1987; 60:347–349.

58. Will AD, Lewis KL, Hinshaw DB, et al: Cerebral vasoconstriction in toxemia. *Neurology* 1987; 37:1555–1557.

59. Brick JF: Vanishing cerebrovascular disease of pregnancy. *Neurology* 1988; 38:804–806.

60. Leventhal AG, Ault SJ, Vitek DJ: The nasotemporal division in primate retina: the neural bases of macular sparing and splitting. *Science* 1988; 240:66–67.

61. Meienberg O, Harrer M, Wehren C: Oculographic diagnosis of hemineglect in patients with homonymous hemianopia. *J Neurol* 1986; 233:97–101.

62. Meienberg O: Eye movement patterns in homonymous hemianopsia and visual hemineglect. Criteria of oculographic delineation based on 19 cases and their diagnostic significance. *Klin Monatsbl Augenheilkd* 1988; 192:108–112.

63. Ishiai S, Furukawa T, Tsukagoshi H: Eye-fixation patterns in homonymous hemianopia and unilateral spatial neglect. *Neuropsychologia* 1987; 25:675–679.

64. Koehler PJ, Endtz LJ, Te Velde J, et al: Aware or non-aware. On the significance of awareness for the localization of the lesion responsible for homonymous hemianopia. *J Neurol Sci* 1986; 75:255–262.

65. Poeppel E, Stoerig P, Logothetis N, et al: Plasticity and rigidity in the representation of the human visual field. *Exp Brain Res* 1987; 68:445–448.

66. Barbas N, Caplan L, Baquis G, et al: Dental chair intracerebral hemorrhage. *Neurology* 1987; 37:511–512.

67. Versavel M, Witmer JP, Matricali B: Giant aneurysm arising from the anterior cerebral artery and causing an isolated homonymous hemianopsia. *Neurosurgery* 1988; 22:560–563.

68. Chang HS, Fukushima T, Takakura K: Aneurysms of the posterior cerebral artery: report of ten cases. *Neurosurgery* 1986; 19:1006–1011.

69. Gans M, Glaser JS: Homonymous hemianopia following electrical injury. *J Clin Neuro-Ophthalmol* 1986; 6:218–223.

70. Soza M, Tagle P, Kirkham T, et al: Bilateral homonymous hemianopia with sparing of central vision after subdural hematoma. *Can J Neurol Sci* 1987; 14:153–155.

71. deGroen PC, Aksamit AJ, Rakela J, et al: Central nervous system toxicity after liver transplantation. *N Engl J Med* 1987; 317:861–866.

72. Gittinger JW: Functional hemianopsia: A historical perspective. *Surv Ophthalmol* 1988; 32:427–432.

73. Shefrin SL, Goodin DS, Aminoff MJ: Visual evoked potentials in the investigation of "blindsight." *Neurology* 1988; 38:104–109.

74. Marzi CA, Tassinari G, Aglioti S: Spatial summation across the vertical meridian in hemianopics: A test of blindsight. *Neuropsychologia* 1986; 24:749–758.

75. Stoerig P, Poeppel E: Eccentricity-dependent residual target detection in visual field defects. *Exp Brain Res* 1986; 64:469–475.

76. Ghilardi MF, Marx MS, Onofrj MC, et al: Scalp distribution of pattern visual evoked potentials in normal and hemianopic monkeys. *Physiol Behav* 1987; 41:297–302.

77. Maccolini E, Andreoli A, Valde G, et al: Hemifield pattern-reversal visual evoked potentials (VEPs) in retrochiasmal lesions with homonymous visual field defect. *Ital J Neurol Sci* 1986; 7:437–442.

78. Cedzich C, Schramm J, Fahlbusch R: Are flash-evoked visual potentials useful for intraoperative monitoring of visual pathway function? *Neurosurgery* 1987; 21:709–715.

CHAPTER 6

Higher Visual Functions

Jeffrey L. Cummings, M.D.

Dementia Research Program, Department of Neurology, Department of Psychiatry and Biobehavioral Sciences, UCLA School of Medicine; Neurobehavior Unit, West Los Angeles Veterans Administration Medical Center (Brentwood Division), Los Angeles, California.

In the recent past there has been a rapid accumulation of information in several areas pertinent to considerations of higher visual function. The main themes to be developed in this chapter include neuro-ophthalmologic aspects of dementia of the Alzheimer type, studies of visuospatial neglect, investigations of the role of subcortical structures in visuospatial abilities, new information regarding agnosia syndromes, investigations of alexia, and studies of the contributions of the left and right hemispheres to visuospatial skills.

NEURO-OPHTHALMOLOGIC ASPECTS OF DEMENTIA OF THE ALZHEIMER TYPE

Dementia of the Alzheimer type (DAT) is rapidly becoming one of the greatest challenges to the health care of elderly citizens. The disease currently affects approximately 2 million Americans and is the fourth most common cause of death in the United States. DAT becomes increasingly prevalent among individuals beyond the seventh decade of life through a combination of rising incidence in the elderly and the long survival of the victims. There have been recent advances in both the clinical characterization of DAT and the understanding of its neurobiologic foundations. Clinically, DAT features an insidious onset and gradual progression of memory disturbances, aphasia, visuospatial deficits, personality changes, and impairment of abstraction and judgment capabilities.[1] Motor function is retained until the final stages of the illness. The clinical sydrome is sufficiently characteristic that, with careful application of diagnostic criteria, the accuracy rate of premorbid diagnosis is now approximately 90%.[2] Pathologically: (1) neurons in affected regions of the brain contain neurofibrillary tangles, (2) there are numerous cortical neuritic plaques, and (3) a majority of patients have an amyloid angiopathy affecting the cerebral blood vessels. The principal neurochemical deficits include acetylcholine and somatostatin.[3] Despite vigorous efforts, successful treatment remains an unachieved goal.

The explosion of information concerning DAT has included relatively little data concerning the neuro-ophthalmologic aspects of the disease. There have been, however, a few recent studies of the visuomotor and visuoperceptual aspects of DAT. Pursuit movements were investigated by Fletcher and Sharpe.[4] They found that among 13 patients with DAT, smooth pursuit was uniformly decreased in speed and large catch-up saccades were needed to maintain foveation. The abnormality was particularly marked when, after a period of constant velocity, there was a small acceleration of target speed. In addition, there were large-amplitude saccadic intrusions that frequently disrupted pursuit movements. No relationship was found between the severity of the pursuit abnormalities and the magnitude of the mental status changes as measured by a standard mental status questionnaire. The authors attributed the abnormalities to bilateral parietal lobe dysfunction in DAT. Hutton and colleagues also studied pursuit abnormalities in DAT with slightly contrasting findings.[5] Like Fletcher and Sharpe, they found that DAT patients required significantly more catch-up saccades to maintain eye tracking than did controls. In the investigation of Hutton et al., however, there was a good correlation between pursuit abnormalities and degree of dementia ($r = 0.74$, $p < 0.005$). The latter findings suggested that eye tracking abnormalities potentially could be used as an index of severity of the neuropathologic changes.

In a second study, Fletcher and Sharpe studied saccadic eye movement dysfunction in DAT.[6] Thirteen patients were compared with 11 age-matched control subjects. They found that when targets had predictable amplitudes, the DAT patients manifested hypometric saccades, and when the target motion was unpredictable, they had prolonged saccadic latencies and reduced peak velocities. Impersistence of gaze was evidenced by large-amplitude saccadic intrusions away from the intended position of gaze. In addition, the authors observed reflexive saccades toward the target even when the patients were instructed to look away. They attributed the latter abnormality to a visual grasp reflex. A significant negative correlation was found between peak saccadic velocities and estimated change in intelligence quotients (IQs) of the patients (slower velocities were found in patients with the largest changes in IQ). Most of the saccadic abnormalities observed were attributed to frontal lobe dysfunction. Hershey et al. had previously documented increases in saccadic latency in DAT and observed similar abnormalities in patients with other types of dementia (multi-infarct dementia, brain tumors, alcohol-related dementia), suggesting that this finding does not have differential diagnostic value.[7] The potential differentiating value of the other eye movement abnormalities has not been investigated.

The sensory aspects of visual function have also been assessed recently. Hinton and co-workers studied the optic nerves of ten DAT patients and found that eight of them exhibited marked abnormalities.[8] Compared with age-matched controls, DAT patients exhibited a 15% to 80% depletion of optic nerve axons, diminished axon diameter, and an increase in glial cells. Retinas from three of the DAT patients were also examined, and were found to have a loss of retinal granule cells. The remaining cells showed degenerative changes such as atrophy or swelling with vacuolization. Studies revealed no neurofibrillary tangles, neuritic plaques, or amyloid angiopathy. The meaning of these findings is not clear. They do not occur in all DAT patients and therefore cannot be regarded as a necessary or inevitable part of the disease; however, these findings occurred more commonly in DAT patients than in normal controls, suggesting an important relationship to some aspect of DAT. Elementary visual perceptual abilities remain intact throughout most of the course of DAT, suggesting that the observed changes rarely produce functional disability.

The integrity of recognition abilities in DAT has been a source of controversy. Agnosia has often been described as part of the early symptomatology of DAT and the naming disturbances observed have sometimes been attributed to recognition disturbances. Using reading abilities as a model of visual recognition abilities, however, Cummings and colleagues were able to demonstrate that these functions were remarkably robust in DAT.[9] They demonstrated that the ability to correctly read words, numbers, and letters was preserved until relatively late in the course of the disease. Patients who scored only 1 or 2 points on an elementary 30-point mental status questionnaire were frequently able to read aloud accurately. Reading comprehension was impaired much earlier, so that despite preservation of the ability to verbally encode the written symbol, the patients were not able to decode its meaning. These findings imply that visual agnosia is a late finding in DAT and that the reading comprehension disturbances observed are more likely attributable to the language deficits that commonly accompany DAT.

HEMISPATIAL NEGLECT

A major theme of inquiry in the recent study of neglect has been the investigation of the role of subcortical structures in mediating spatial attention. Ferro and co-workers investigated 15 patients with right-sided subcortical infarctions localized by computerized tomography (CT) or magnetic resonance imaging (MRI).[10] Lesions were distributed in the anterior internal capsule, caudate nucleus, lenticular nucleus, posterior internal capsule, or periventricular white matter. Twelve of

14 patients tested soon after onset of the infarction evidenced hemispatial neglect. Except for a tendency for patients with large posterior internal capsule lesions to make more errors on a line-crossing test, no specific correlations emerged between type of neglect (visual, auditory, tactile) and lesion site. The authors concluded that disruption of a cortico-striatal-nigral-collicular pathway accounts for the failure to explore the contralesional hemispace.

Bogousslavsky et al. studied two patients with anterior choroidal artery territory infarctions who manifested severe unilateral neglect.[11] Single-photon emission tomography (SPECT) studies demonstrated decreased cerebral hemispheric blood flow in the ipsilateral parietal and frontal cortex as well as in subcortical structures. This observation suggests that the neglect was a product of cortical dysfunction, even though the lesion leading to the compromise of cortical metabolism was subcortical in location. Similar findings have been reported in the studies of "subcortical aphasias," where cerebral cortical metabolism is decreased in patients with a subcortical lesion and an accompanying aphasia and is preserved in those without language dysfunction. These reports indicate the potential information to be gained by adding the study of cerebral metabolism or blood flow to the traditional structural studies of brain lesions.

A single case report relevant to the role of subcortical structures in neglect was submitted by House and Hodges.[12] They observed a patient with an infarction of the right internal capsule, globus pallidus, and putamen. The lesion was documented by CT and later confirmed at autopsy. Despite preserved intellect and no evidence of hemispatial neglect, the patient exhibited marked anosognosia with complete denial of her left-sided weakness. Anosognosia and hemispatial neglect frequently occur simultaneously. This case demonstrates that the two can be dissociated and that anosognosia as well as neglect can be produced by lesions involving the basal ganglia.

The role of the thalamus in visual hemiattention was also studied. Rafal and Posner[13] investigated three patients with unilateral thalamic hemorrhages soon after onset, and again 6 months later. Only one patient exhibited neglect, and this resolved during the observation period. However, all patients exhibited slow reaction times for stimuli presented contralateral to the lesion both at the time of onset of the disorder and after 6 months of recovery. The authors concluded that even in the absence of an overt neglect syndrome, there is frequently an impairment in timely exploration of the contralateral hemispace following thalamic injury.

These observations expand the understanding of the role of subcortical structures in intellectual and visuospatial function. Left-sided subcortical lesions produce aphasia and right-sided lesions cause hemispatial neglect. The precise role of the subcortical lesions, however, remains to be determined. Neuropsychologic deficits are more common with hemorrhagic lesions than with infarctions, and the association between lesions and deficits is more variable than with cortical injury. Moreover, as noted above, metabolic and cerebral blood flow studies show cortical defects in patients with symptomatic subcortical lesions and none in those without symptoms. Together, the studies suggest that the symptomatic syndromes reflect co-occurring cortical and subcortical dysfunctions. This conclusion is consistent with studies of subcortical dementias (e.g., Huntington's disease) where constructional disturbances and mild naming deficits occur, but more marked aphasic and attentional abnormalities are not observed. Unresolved questions in this area include: What is the cause of the cortical hypometabolism associated with subcortical lesions? What is the role of the white matter involvement often associated with subcortical lesions?

In addition to the role of subcortical lesions in producing hemispatial neglect, several other aspects of the neglect syndrome were explored, including altitudinal neglect, ipsilateral neglect with right hemisphere lesions, and hemispatial neglect of recalled memories. Rapcsak and co-workers studied a single patient with Balint's syndrome associated with bilateral parietal-occipital infarctions.[14] In addition to the elements of Balint's syndrome (psychic paralysis of gaze, simultanagnosia, optic ataxia), the patient exhibited an altitudinal pattern of visual neglect. She consistently extinguished stimuli in the inferior quadrants despite near normal visual fields, while perceiving stimuli in the upper quadrants. In addition, she failed to perceive the inferior halves of fixated objects. The authors concluded from these provocative observations that attention may be distributed along vertical as well as horizontal axes.

Weintraub and Mesulam compared patients with left-sided and right-sided lesions and found that neglect was more severe with right brain dysfunction.[15] They also observed that patients with right brain pathology were more likely to make ipsilateral attentional errors than patients with left brain lesions. This observation supports the evolving hypothesis that the right hemisphere mediates spatial attention for both sides of space, whereas the left hemisphere mediates contralateral spatial attention only. Thus, right brain lesions produce attentional errors in both hemiuniverses, while left-sided lesions lead to contralateral hemispatial neglect only. In a study of related importance, Rapcsak et al. found that patients with right-sided lesions may extinguish one of two stimuli presented simultaneously within the same visual hemifield.[16] They interpreted this finding as suggesting that the limited attentional resources remaining after a right brain lesion are insufficient to accommodate distribution to two spatial locations.

Meador and colleagues studied three patients with right hemisphere lesions and asked them to recall a visual scene well known to the patients. They found that the patients failed to recall significantly more left-sided items, and that the amount of recall could be improved by having the patients turn their heads in the neglected direction. This investigation adds further data to support the theory that the neglect syndrome extends to the mental representation of hemispatial items in memory as well as affecting ongoing perceptual events.

Voeller and Heilman investigated the novel hypothesis that children with attention deficit disorder (ADD) may share features with patients manifesting hemispatial neglect.[18] They found that seven boys with ADD made more errors on the left side of a letter cancellation task than five normal controls. They concluded that ADD may result from an early injury to the right hemisphere and that spatial inattention is demonstrable as part of the ADD syndrome. This suggestion gains further support from experimental studies showing that right but not left hemisphere lesions produce motor hyperactivity in rats. Thus, several aspects of the ADD syndrome are potentially ascribable to right hemispheric dysfunction.

Mark and colleagues proposed the hypothesis that unilateral neglect may result not only from inattention to one field of vision, but from failure to disengage from stimuli in the ipsilateral field.[19] They attempted to test the idea by having patients with evidence of unilateral neglect mark lines on a piece of paper (condition 1) or erase similar lines on a piece of paper (condition 2). There was significantly more neglect with the marking task than the erasure task. The results were interpreted as suggesting that the continued presence of stimuli in the non-neglected space increases the severity of neglect in the contralateral hemispace. The findings might also suggest that the engagement of the patient (greater in the erasure task) reduces the relative degree of neglect in both hemifields.

The most promising advance with regard to hemispatial neglect concerned the experimental application of pharmacotherapy. Fleet et al., reasoning that ascending dopaminergic pathways were disrupted by most lesions known to induce neglect, administered bromocriptine (a dopamine receptor agonist) to two patients with hemispatial neglect.[20] In this open therapeutic trial, both patients improved during therapy and worsened after withdrawal on their performance tests of line, letter, and geometric figure cancellation. Further trials with blinded designs will be necessary to establish the efficacy of pharmacotherapy and determine the appropriate patients for treatment, but these preliminary observations suggest that pharmacologic management may be useful in this treatment-resistant syndrome.

AGNOSIA SYNDROMES

Simultanagnosia, visual object agnosia, and prosopagnosia were all objects of recent investigations. Rizzo and Hurtig studied three patients with simultanagnosia associated with bilateral superior occipital lobe lesions.[21] The patients had normal visual acuity and were without visual field defects. Electro-oculographic (EOG) recordings revealed normal fixation, pursuit velocity, ocular tracking, and saccadic function. Scanning of target objects and scenes was also intact, although verbal reports of the perceived material lacked appropriate detail. During fixation (verified by EOG) objects disappeared from vision. This study suggests that the heretofore mysterious syndrome of simultanagnosia may be due in some cases to the disappearance of objects from vision during sustained fixation. It remains to be seen if this mechanism accounts for all cases of simultanagnosia; several previously reported patients with this syndrome were described as having deficient visual search activities, and more than one mechanism may play a role in the disorder.

Two classic varieties of visual object agnosia have previously been described:

apperceptive agnosia, wherein the patient can distinguish intensity, width, and direction but not the form of objects; and associative visual agnosia, characterized by intact form perception (as demonstrated by the ability to draw the object) but an inability to recognize the perceived object. New observations suggest that these two forms of agnosia may represent but two recognizable steps in a complex process leading to object identification. These recent investigations provide new information in the understanding of this process.

A case of visual agnosia was intensively studies by Riddoch and Humphreys.[22] The patient exhibited features of the associative visual agnosia syndrome, including inability to recognize objects visually, intact tactile recognition and naming, and preserved ability to copy figures that he could not recognize. Storage and recall of visual information were also shown to be performed normally. The patient suffered from bilateral occipital lobe infarctions and had bilateral superior altitudinal visual field defects. The authors showed that the severity of the agnosia was influenced by the duration of stimulus exposure and the complexity of the object. The patient could discriminate figures when presented in isolation, but failed to identify them when overlapped with other figures. Object silhouettes were more readily identified than the objects themselves. The authors argued that although the patient had many features of associative visual agnosia, his deficits went beyond those of an impairment of semantic association with the intact perception. They suggested that recognition occurs on a continuum and that "associative agnosia" and "apperceptive agnosia" are umbrella terms embracing two multifaceted aspects of the recognition process. They suggested the term "integrative visual agnosia" for the syndrome they described.

Warrington and James reported three cases under the term "visual apperceptive agnosia."[23] Each of the patients had a large lesion of the posterior aspect of the right hemisphere. The patients had intact elementary vision and performed shape recognition tasks normally. When the visual details of the stimulus were degraded, distorted, or obscured, the patients' abilities to recognize the objects were severely impaired. The authors suggested that the cardinal failure in apperceptive agnosia is the failure to perform perceptual categorization. They also hypothesized a two-stage model of object recognition, one involving perceptual categorization that is impaired in apperceptive agnosia, and one involving visual semantic processing that is impaired in associative visual agnosia. There have been few other cases of apperceptive agnosia reported, and most previously described patients have had bilateral posterior hemispheric lesions. The study by Warrington and James suggests that lesions limited to the right hemisphere may be capable of producing the syndrome.

Prosopagnosia was the object of study by Tranel et al.[24] They investigated four patients, three with "pure" prosopagnosia (impaired ability to identify familiar faces) and one with an inability to identify faces in conjunction with a memory disorder. The authors attempted to identify which aspects of facial identification remained intact and which were disturbed in the prosopagnosia syndrome. Three of the four patients had no difficulty discriminating among different facial expressions and deducing their emotional meaning, estimating the age of the individual whose face was depicted, or recognizing the gender of the individual. All had the expected difficulty identifying the exact identity of the person pictured. The authors hypothesized that the identification of age, gender, and emotional expression depends on categorical recognition skills, whereas the identification of individual faces calls on the unique repertoire of experience of each individual to make a specific association. Examination of the lesions of the patients suggested that disruption of the anterior multimodal and limbic structures is responsible for classic prosopagnosia. If there is more posterior dysfunction involving visual association cortex, then the syndrome includes the inability to make more elementary visual discriminations, including differentiating age, gender, and emotional expression.

ALEXIA

Both alexia with agraphia and alexia without agraphia received extensive recent study. Kawahata et al. reported three cases of alexia with agraphia in which the lesion was identified radiologically (CT and positron emission tomography) to be in the posterior inferior temporal lobe of the left hemisphere, rather than in the more conventional location involving the left angular gyrus.[25] In one case the reading disability involved Kana (Japanese phonograms) more than Kanji (Japanese ideograms), whereas two cases had disproportionate difficulty with Kanji. The patient with more impaired Kana had a more dorsal lesion involving the left posterior temporal lobe and lateral occipital lobe sparing the angular gyrus; the other two patients had infarctions of the left inferior posterior temporal lobe. These cases demonstrate that interruption of reading and writing is not confined to lesions occurring in the angular gyrus, and when the pathologic changes involve the posterior inferior temporal lobe the ideographic form of Japanese may be more affected.

The typical lesions producing alexia without agraphia involve the splenium of the corpus callosum and the left occipital cortex. Silver and co-workers studied a unique case of alexia without agraphia in which the lesions involved the left lateral geniculate body and the splenium, but spared the occipital lobe.[26] The report included anatomic investigations with CT and MRI as well as metabolic studies with positron emission tomography using F-fluorodeoxyglucose. The authors surmised that this was a case with double disconnection in which the geniculate lesion interrupted information going to the left occipital cortex while the splenial lesion prevented information in the right hemisphere from reaching the "reading areas" of the left brain. Although not involved structurally, the left occipital cortex exhibited diminished metabolic activity in the acute phase of the illness and had largely recovered when the patient was rescanned 5 months later after substantial improvement. This suggests that disconnection of a cortical structure by a subcortical lesion results in reversible decrease in metabolic activity of the cortical region. An alternate explanation to be resolved by further studies is that the occipital cortex actually sustained reversible ischemic injury during the initial insult and the geniculate lesion was incidental. In either case, the report stimulates new ways of viewing the alexia without agraphia syndrome and initiates the use of new technologies to study these complex disorders.

VISUOSPATIAL AND CONSTRUCTIONAL DISORDERS

Swindell et al. approached one of the most pressing areas of research in visuospatial and constructional performance.[27] Previous observations with commissurotomy patients and patients with left or right hemisphere lesions indicated that the two hemispheres make different contributions to the constructional process. In copying and drawing tasks, for example, right hemisphere lesions tended to disrupt the external configuration and overall orientation of the figure, suggesting a primary role for the right brain in these functions. Left brain lesions, on the other hand, tended to produce more disturbances of internal detail, supporting a larger role for the left hemisphere in detail analysis. Application of this information to the study of copies made by patients, however, had not given satisfactory results in previous studies attempting to deduce the side of the lesion from the type of constructional errors. Swindell and coworkers obtained drawings of a person done at the time of discharge from the hospital and at 1, 2, and 6 months later. The patients with right-sided lesions produced scattered, fragmented, elaborately detailed drawings and frequently manifested left-sided neglect. Left brain damaged patients made simple, often incoherent, drawings that omitted details and were usually placed in the upper left quadrant of the page. The drawings of those with left-sided injuries improved more quickly and more completely than the drawings of those with right-sided lesions. Abnormalities continued to be evident in the drawings of those with right brain injury 12 months after onset at a time when the drawings of left brain injured patients had normalized. When expert neuropsychologists and a neurologist were asked to assign the drawings to a right brain damaged or left brain damaged group without knowledge of the patient's lesion site, they made only 5 errors in 48 choices. When asked to order the four drawings made by each patient during the course of the study, they were able to correctly order those of patients with left-sided damage much more adequately than those from patients with right-sided injuries. The left brain damaged patients showed a lawful progression of recovery, whereas those with right-sided lesions tended to make more random changes. This study demonstrates that visuospatial functions as assessed by drawing tests can be used to determine the side of hemispheric dysfunction. It also shows that drawing disability produced by right brain lesions is more severe and more persistent than that associated with left brain damage.

Acknowledgments

This project was supported by the Veterans Administration.
Appreciation is extended to Ms. Norene Hiekel for typing the manuscript.

REFERENCES

1. Cummings JL, Benson DF: Dementia of the Alzheimer type: An inventory of diagnostic clinical features. *J Am Geriatr Soc* 1986; 34:12–19.
2. Tierney MC, Fisher RH, Lewis AJ, et al: The NINCDS-ADRDA Work Group criteria of the clinical diagnosis of probable Alzheimer's disease: A clinicopathological study of 57 cases. *Neurology* 1988; 38:359–364.
3. Katzman R: Alzheimer's disease. *N Engl J Med* 1986; 314:964–973.
4. Fletcher WA, Sharpe JA: Smooth pursuit dysfunction in Alzheimer's disease. *Neurology* 1988; 38:272–277.
5. Hutton JT, Nagel JA, Loewenson RB: Eye tracking dysfunction in Alzheimer-type dementia. *Neurology* 1984; 34:99–102.
6. Fletcher WA, Sharpe JA: Saccadic eye movement dysfunction in Alzheimer's disease. *Ann Neurol* 1986; 20:464–471.
7. Hershey LA, Whicker L Jr, Abel LA, et al: Saccadic latency measurements in dementia. *Arch Neurol* 1983; 40:592–593.
8. Hinton DR, Sadun AA, Blanks JC, et al: Optic-nerve degeneration in Alzheimer's disease. *N Engl J Med* 1986; 315:485–487.
9. Cummings JL, Houlihan JP, Hill MA: The pattern of reading deterioration in dementia of the Alzheimer type: Observations and implications. *Brain Lang* 1986; 29:315–323.
10. Ferro JM, Kertesz A, Black SE: Subcortical neglect: Quantitation, anatomy, and recovery. *Neurology* 1987; 37:1487–1492.
11. Bogousslavsky J, Miklossy J, Regli F, et al: Subcortical neglect: Neuropsychological, SPECT, and neuropathological correlations with anterior choroidal artery territory infarction. *Ann Neurol* 1988; 23:448–452.
12. House A, Hodges J: Persistent denial of handicap after infarction of the right basal ganglia: A case study. *J Neurol Neurosurg Psychiat* 1988; 51:112–115.
13. Rafal RD, Posner MI: Deficits in human visual-spatial attention following thalamic lesions. *Proc Natl Acad Sci* 1987; 84:7349–7353.
14. Rapcsak SZ, Cimino CR, Heilman KM: Altitudinal neglect. *Neurology* 1988; 38:277–281.
15. Weintraub S, Mesulam M-M: Right cerebral dominance in spatial attention. *Arch Neurol* 1987; 44:621–625.
16. Rapcsak SZ, Watson RT, Heilman KM: Hemispace-visual field interactions in visual extinction. *J Neurol Neurosurg Psychiatry* 1987; 50:1117–1124.
17. Meador KJ, Loring DW, Bowers D, et al: Remote memory and neglect syndrome. *Neurology* 1987; 37:522–526.
18. Voeller KKS, Heilman KM: Attention deficit disorder in children: A neglect syndrome? *Neurology* 1988; 38:806–808.
19. Mark VW, Kooistra CA, Heilman KM: Hemispatial neglect affected by non-neglected stimuli. *Neurology* 1988; 38:1207–1211.
20. Fleet WS, Valenstein E, Watson RT, et al: Dopamine agonist therapy for neglect in humans. *Neurology* 1987; 37:1765–1770.

21. Rizzo M, Hurtig R: Looking but not seeing: Attention, perception, and eye movements in simultanagnosia. *Neurology* 1987; 37:1642–1648.
22. Riddoch MJ, Humphreys GW: A case of integrative visual agnosia. *Brain* 1987; 110:1431–1462.
23. Warrington EK, James M: Visual apperceptive agnosia: A clinicopathological study of three cases. *Cortex* 1988; 24:13–32.
24. Tranel D, Damasio AR, Damasio H: Intact recognition of facial expression, gender, and age in patients with impaired recognition of face identity. *Neurology* 1988; 38:690–696.
25. Kawahata N, Nagata K, Shishido F: Alexia with agraphia due to the left posterior inferior temporal lobe lesions—neuropsychological analysis and its pathogenetic mechanisms. *Brain Lang* 1988; 33:296–310.
26. Silver FL, Chawluk JB, Bosley TM, et al: Resolving metabolic abnormalities in a case of pure alexia. *Neurology* 1988; 38:730–735.
27. Swindell CS, Holland AL, Fromm D, et al: Characteristics of recovery of drawing ability in left and right brain-damage patients. *Brain Cognit* 1988; 7:16–30.

PART TWO

THE OCULAR MOTOR SYSTEM

CHAPTER 7

The Eyelid

Patrick A. Sibony, M.D.

Associate Professor of Ophthalmology, State University of New York at Stony Brook, Stony Brook, New York

FACIAL ANATOMY AND PATHOLOGY

Weakness of the lower facial muscles with preservation of upper facial movements is a well-grounded sign of upper motor neuron dysfunction. The usual explanation, that corticofacial fibers project bilaterally to the facial motor nucleus to control upper facial movement and contralaterally to control lower facial movements, is an explanation that has never been anatomically substantiated. In primates, Jenny and Saper[1] found that descending corticofacial fibers project directly to the motor neurons supplying the lower facial muscles on both sides with contralateral predominance. Upper facial movement is preserved because the facial motor neurons that innervate the upper facial muscles receive little direct cortical input.

The human orbicularis oculi contains a higher percentage of phasic contracting muscle fibers (type II) than other muscles of the face.[2] A study of the intrinsic blood supply of the feline facial nerve shows that the labyrinthine segment contains fewer blood vessels than the mastoid or tympanic segments; the geniculate ganglion has a dense vascular plexus.[3] Denervation of human facial muscles exhibits a wide spectrum of ultrastructural changes, including abnormal sarcomeres and organelles, as well as a variety of inclusion bodies.[4]

Controversies on the pathophysiologic mechanisms of facial synkinesias have been reviewed.[5] Misdirection, ephaptic transmission, and central reorganization

Curr Neuro Ophthalmol 2:89–114, 1989
© 1989, Year Book Medical Publishers, Inc.
0893–0147/89/02-089-114-$04.00

are still the main contenders. In my view, an experimental study by Thomander[6] provides additional support for the misdirection hypothesis. Using retrograde horseradish-peroxidase (HRP), the somatotopic organization of the facial motor nucleus was mapped before and after transecting the facial nerve. Normally, transport along the zygomatic or buccal rami results in discrete labeling of specific regions of the facial motor nucleus. Eleven months after reanastomosis, application of HRP to these same branches results in labeling of cells throughout the nucleus, confirming the results of similar experiments on the oculomotor[7] and sciatic nerves.[8] For traumatically acquired forms of synkinesis, misdirection appears consistent with both clinical and experimental observations. With respect to other well-recognized synkinesias, the explanation may not be quite so evident, as in the discussion below on the pathophysiology of hemifacial spasm. Also, Lyness et al.[9] studied the levator palpebrae from 12 patients with trigemino-oculomotor synkinesis and described a neurogenic pattern of atrophy. Although its genesis is still poorly understood, the presence of pathologic changes in both the affected and unaffected sides compared with normal controls would seem to support a central mechanism.

BLINKS

Eyelid Movements

Eyelid closure during spontaneous, voluntary, and reflex blinking is a product of the reciprocal activity of the levator palpebrae and the orbicularis oculi. Electromyographic (EMG) studies have shown that the open eyelid position is maintained by tonic activity of the levator; inhibition of the levator with simultaneous contraction of the orbicularis oculi results in a blink. The dynamics of upper eyelid movement during a blink consist of a smooth, high-velocity downward phase followed by a slower upward phase; moreover, the upward phase consists of an initial rapid rise followed by an exponential-like return to the elevated position. Kennard and others were the first to analyze eyelid movements systematically and quantitatively. A variety of techniques have recently been used to study eyelid kinematics including mechanical levels,[10] a photodiode limbus reflectance spectacle,[11] an infrared image sensor,[12] and the magnetic search coil.[13]

Manning and Evinger[14] have demonstrated stimulus-dependent differences in the eyelid movements of rabbits. A blink induced by an air puff is more rapidly completed and achieves a higher velocity than a light-stimulated blink of equal amplitude. The dissimilarity is due to the relative timing of levator and orbicularis oculi contraction. Analysis of the effects of stimulus duration and intensity on blink amplitude, orbicularis activity, and blink duration led them to conclude that blinks may be controlled by a "two-stage neural process": an early preprogrammed component and a late phase under stimulus control.

Holder et al.[11] correlated surface and needle EMG of the levator and orbicularis with human eyelid movements during voluntary blinks. Coinhibition was found just before orbicularis activity, and cocontraction was present during lid closure.

Becker and Fuchs,[13] using a search coil, demonstrated tight coupling between the eyelid and eye during smooth pursuits and saccadic eye movements. Upward "lid saccades" tend to be slightly smaller and slower than saccadic eye movements; a postsaccadic glissade moves the eyelid to its final position. The slight disparity between eye and lid movement was attributed to viscous drag on the levator. Analysis of the levator during upward saccades discloses a pulse-step change in EMG activity; however, there is no levator burst activity during the upward phase of a blink. Since downward saccadic eye velocities tend to be slower than upward saccades, the velocity of downward lid saccades was slower—but more closely linked to eye movements—than upward lid saccades. The downward saccadic velocities of the upper lid remain unexplained because the orbicularis oculi does not contract during a downward lid saccade. It has been suggested that mechanical factors, such as the elastic properties of the upper lid, friction drag against the eyeball, and gravity, might account for the slow downward eyelid movements observed in patients with neuropathies (Kennard and others), but the high velocities generated by a downward lid saccade would seem to require active contraction. Becker and Fuchs[13] raise the possibility that an undetected phasic contraction of a portion of the orbicularis oculi might be responsible.

Niida et al.,[12] using a noncontact imaging technique, also studied lid movements during vertical eye movements and found, in contrast to Becker and Fuchs,[13] that upward lid saccades were slower than downward lid saccades. Moreover, there was no pulse-step activity of the levator during upward saccades. The discrepancies between these two studies are difficult to explain but may relate to differences in recording techniques and testing paradigms.

Prior studies have shown that blinks can facilitate abnormal saccadic eye movements in a variety of supranuclear oculomotor disturbances. Kurlan et al.[15] found that the percentage of blink-associated saccadic eye movements increased with fatiguing saccadic tasks in a patient with coexistent Meige's syndrome and myasthenia gravis. Neuromuscular fatigue with slow drifts in eye position was corrected with blink-associated saccades. They suggest that blinks and facial contractions might represent a compensatory mechanism for myasthenic oculomotor fatigue.

Torsional eye movements were studied under a variety of oculomotor tasks including the voluntary blink.[16] As has already been shown in a prior study by the same authors, the eye is transiently displaced 1 to 3 degrees inferonasally during a blink. Torsional movements during a blink, however, were not as predictable, sometimes exhibiting incyclotorsion, excyclotorsion, or both.[16]

Blink Reflexes

Reflex blinks to sound are the earliest and most consistent response of the audiogenic startle reflex. The subject was recently studied in a number of publications,[17-19] including an excellent article by Wilkins et al.[19] that reviews the literature and discusses the EMG parameters of the normal startle reflex as distinguished from other startle syndromes.

The blink reflex is clinically studied by stimulating the supraorbital nerve, which elicits two responses in the orbicularis oculi: an early R1 and a late R2. The R1 is thought to be mediated by an ipsilateral oligosynaptic pontine pathway. The R2 is a bilateral response mediated by polysynaptic pathways in the pons and medulla.

Suprasegmental factors may facilitate or inhibit the blink reflex as shown in patients with extrapyramidal and hemispheric diseases. Presentation of a warning stimulus has a facilitatory effect on R1 and an inhibitory effect on R2.[20] Stimulation of the posterior tibial nerve (i.e., proprioceptive impulses along type Ia afferent fibers) was found to increase the amplitude of the R1 component, presumably mediated by the spinoreticular pathways.[21] Klug and Csecsei[22] presented clinical evidence that the R2 component may be altered by midbrain and pontomesencephalic lesions. Acute intracranial pressure elevation, in an animal model, shows that R2 is suppressed bilaterally with early signs of mesencephalic herniation, whereas R1 disappears just before the onset of respiratory arrest, again underscoring the importance of the mesencephalon in modulating the blink reflex.[22] Adaptive gain of the blink reflex was studied by Evinger and Manning,[23] who found that gain changes, habituation, and reflex modification selectively affect the longer-latency polysynaptic components of the blink.

Tobacco smoking transiently prolongs the R2 latency and reduces the magnitude of both R1 and R2; R1 latency was unaffected. It is unclear if this is a direct nicotine effect on pontine interneurons or a remote inhibitory process caused by nicotine-mediated dopamine release.[24]

There have been a number of studies in the past suggesting anatomic and physiologic dissimilarities between the corneal blink and the blink induced by supraorbital stimulation. For example, the corneal blink reflex has no early R1 component and does not habituate. A recent study by Cruccu et al.[25] disputes this contention by demonstrating clear signs of habituation using electrical rather than mechanical stimuli.

The blink reflex was studied in newborns and premature infants.[26, 27] There was a longer latency of both R1 and R2 among premature infants and a normal R1 latency and longer R2 latency among newborns; there were no contralateral R2 responses among either newborns or premature infants.[26] Repeated glabella taps with variable interstimulus intervals were used to study blink reflex inhibition. Reflex inhibition, not present in premature infants, occurred in newborns when the interstimulus interval was longer than that required in adults.[27] The developmental implications of these findings were discussed in both studies. The photic blink reflex was found to have "limited value" in patients with optic neuritis because latency was unaffected and changes in amplitude were noted in only 38% of those studied.[28]

Blink Rate

The blink rate is thought to reflect central dopaminergic activity; for example, blink rates are low in patients with Parkinson's disease and abnormally high in patients with schizophrenia. Goldberg et al.[29] found that patients with autism, a disorder associated with dopaminergic hyperactivity, had elevated blink rates compared with normal subjects. Similarly, Karson et al.[30] studied psychotic adolescent patients before neuroleptic treatment or psychiatric hospitalization and found an increase in the blink rate. That mentally retarded children (without parkinsonian signs) were found to have diminished blink rates suggests that factors other than dopaminergic activity are involved.[29] This point was also emphasized by Stern et al.,[31] who reviewed the cognitive factors that may alter the blink rate.

FACIAL NERVE

Those readers with broader interests in the facial nerve might also refer to a more comprehensive survey of the recent literature on facial neuropathies and Bell's palsy.[32]

In an attempt to bring about a standard method for grading facial nerve function, the American Academy of Otolaryngology–Head and Neck Surgery adopted a grading system based on work carried out by House and Brackmann.[33] The grading system consists of a six-point scale where grade I is normal and grade VI represents total, flaccid paralysis. Grades II through V are defined by the degree of weakness based on gross inspection of facial appearance, symmetry at rest, and motility of the muscles of the forehead, eye, and mouth. A more elaborate system, the Linear Measurement Index (LMI), quantitates movement during standard facial expressions using anatomic landmarks.[34] Integrated EMG (which quantitates the magnitude of a muscle contraction) has also been used in conjunction with the LMI.[35] Comparisons of these systems and others were discussed by Burres and Fisch.[36]

Bell's Palsy

There have been numerous studies suggesting that Bell's palsy might be due to a viral infection or an autoimmune disorder, although the precise cause remains unknown. The evidence consists of studies showing elevated serum viral antibodies, inflammatory changes of the nerve, widespread subclinical disturbances in the peripheral and central nervous system, clinical similarities between Bell's palsy and Guillain-Barré syndrome, abnormalities of the cerebrospinal fluid (CSF), and epidemiologic studies. In support of the immunologic hypothesis, several studies demonstrated circulating immune complexes[37] and abnormalities in the cell-mediated immune system.[38, 39] Several recent articles support the contention that Bell's palsy is a polyneuropathy by electrophysiologically demonstrating subclinical dysfunction of the ipsilateral acoustic and trigeminal nerves, the contralateral facial nerve, ulnar nerve, optic nerve, and the brain stem.[40–42]

Edstrom et al.[43] found myelin basic protein was significantly elevated among ten of 28 patients with Bell's palsy. In one of the larger studies of its kind, Weber et al.[44] performed an extensive CSF-serum analysis in adult patients with Bell's palsy and compared them with patients with Bannwarth's syndrome and herpes zoster oticus. They looked at total blood cell count, protein concentration, blood-CSF permeability, CSF-serum ratios for IgG, IgA, and IgM, and specific CSF antibodies to six viral agents (cytomegalovirus [CMV], herpes, measles, mumps, rubella, and varicella zoster) in 62 patients with Bell's palsy. Only 10% had a pathologic CSF analysis without any other identifiable cause. Among 13 patient studied for specific antibody production, only 2 exhibited evidence of intrathecal production of a viral specific antibody, one case showing mild elevation to herpes simplex and the other to CMV and measles. These findings were in striking contrast to those in patients with herpes zoster oticus and Bannwarth's syndrome, who consistently showed a variety of abnormalities. Because of the inconsistency of the CSF findings, the authors questioned whether the majority of idiopathic facial neuropathies are due to direct viral infection or that they represent a mild variant of Guillain-Barré syndrome.

A retrospective epidemiologic analysis of Bell's palsy was reported by Katusic et al.,[45] who found that the annual incidence of Bell's palsy from 1968 to 1982 was 25 cases per 100,000. In all, 208 cases were identified, and, as has been observed before, 86% recovered completely. The presence of complete facial weakness, pain (other than ear pain), and hypertension was associatd with incomplete recovery. The clinical features of 228 children with Bell's palsy over a 10-year period was studied by Prescott.[46] He found that the overall recovery rate was 96%, that females were more commonly affected than males, and that steroids had no effect on the overall outcome. McGregor et al.[47] described 7 patients with Bell's palsy acquired in late pregnancy or post partum and reviewed the literature on this questionable association.

Familial Bell's palsy has been associated with both autosomal dominant and recessive patterns of inheritance. Some of these cases may be associated with other cranial nerve palsies. Recently, Aldrich et al.[48] described a family in which the father and seven (of ten) children had a total of 20 episodes of Bell's palsy. There were multiple recurrent cranial neuropathies affecting the sixth, third, and fourth cranial nerves among five family members. Another series was notable because

Bell's palsy occurred in four female family members. That three of four developed the palsy at ages 12 to 13 led the authors to speculate that hormonal factors may play a role in genetically predisposed families.[49]

There is still no final word on the benefits of steroids in the treatment of Bell's palsy. Stankiewicz[50] critically reviewed 94 publications and concluded that the definitive study has yet to be done but there is a strong suggestion that steroids may be beneficial. Though steroids do not affect the cause of the disease or prevent partial denervation or contracture, they may prevent denervation, synkinesia, and progression and may hasten recovery.

Facial Neuropathies

Several reports have dealt with the use of computed tomography (CT) in patients with facial neuropathies[51–54] but few have dealt with magnetic resonance imaging (MRI). A review of the clinical, pathologic, and radiographic records of 42 patients with facial neuropathies disclosed that half of 24 patients with "occult" facial nerve lesions received unnecessary or inappropriate radiologic examinations. Thirteen of these patients were ultimately found to have tumors. Not surprisingly, the most common error was the ordering of a routine head scan with improper views of the region of interest. The authors proposed a detailed CT protocol for the facial nerve based on clinical localization of the lesion.[55]

In the past 2 years, there have been a number of reports describing iatrogenic facial neuropathies caused by general anesthesia induced by pressure behind the mandibles,[56] embolization for severe epistaxis,[57, 58] a modified O'Brien facial nerve block for cataract surgery,[59] dental surgery,[60] and carotid endarterectomy.[61] Both nitrofurantoin[62] and lithium[63] were alleged to have caused facial neuropathy.

Facial neuropathies have also been associated with a variety of conditions, including Kawasaki disease,[64] prostatic carcinoma,[65] parotid tumors,[66–68] glomus jugulare,[69] histiocytosis X,[70] parotitis,[71, 72] familial amyloidosis,[73] intrapetrous carotid artery aneurysm,[74] nose blowing,[75] traumatic neuromas,[76] human immunodeficiency virus infection,[77] and herpes simplex.[78] Be warned that a large wad of chewing tobacco in the mouth can mimick a facial palsy.[79]

The management of traumatic facial neuropathies remains controversial. Despite the use of high-resolution CT[51, 54] and a variety of clinical and electrodiagnostic indicators, it is not possible to predict reliably which patients will recover and which might benefit from surgical decompression. Moreover, the natural history of untreated fractures is unclear. Nonetheless, some still advocate prompt surgical decompression whereas others manage conservatively. More recently, Coker et al.[80] retrospectively reviewed their experience with 18 temporal bone fractures, 7 gunshot wounds, and 4 iatrogenic complications; all had complete facial paralysis (grade VI), 90% denervation, and elevated thresholds for stimulation. They recommended a variety of approaches depending on the nature of the injury (penetrating vs. nonpenetrating injuries) and the presence of hearing loss. Among 22 cases due to fractures and iatrogenic causes, 60% improved to grades I to III. However, without surgical intervention,[81] 44 of 45 patients with traumatic facial neuropathies improved to satisfactory levels, 65% of whom recovered completely.

Lyme Disease

Lyme disease is a systemic seasonal infection caused by a tick-borne spirochete, *Borrelia burgdorferi*. Tick-borne meningopolyneuritis (Bannwarth's syndrome), long known in the Euopean literature, is very similar if not the same disease. The clinical manifestations include constitutional symptoms, with cutaneous, cardiac, rheumatologic, and neurologic findings. The neurologic manifestations consist of a lymphocytic meningitis, painful peripheral neuritis, or cranial neuropathies. The disease can be mistaken for Guillain-Barré syndrome, multiple sclerosis, sarcoidosis, and syphilis. A monograph summarizing the Proceedings of the Second International Symposium on Lyme Disease and Related Disorders held in 1985 was recently published with numerous contributions from recognized experts in the field.[82]

Unilateral or bilateral facial neuropathies have been reported in up to 63% of cases of Bannwarth's syndrome[83] and 50% of cases of Lyme disease with neurologic manifestations.[84] Among 951 patients with Lyme disease, Clark et al.[85] found 101 cases (11%) with facial neuropathies, 23% of which were bilateral. Facial neuropathy was associated with erythema chronicum migrans (in 85%), a history of a tick bite (38%), meningoencephalitis (19%), radiculoneuritis (14%), and arthritis (49%). Three of their patients had isolated facial paralysis with normal CSF studies. With or without treatment, facial palsies had an excellent prognosis. Schmutzhard et al.[86] found that 14 of 17 patients with meningopolyneuritis had a facial paralysis (50% were bilateral). Among 37 patients with isolated seventh nerve palsies, 15 were found to have serum antibodies to *B. burgdorferi*. Though all the patients with meningopolyneuritis had intrathecal borrelial antibody, only 1 of the 15 with isolated facial palsies had CSF antibody. Jonsson et al.[87] performed Lyme enzyme-linked immunosorbent assay (ELISA) titers in 94 patients with "Bell's palsy," and 58 controls. Based on their criteria for reactivity, 15 of the 94 patients had positive Lyme titers to IgG and/or IgM, whereas only 2 of the controls had positive titers. Among the 15 with positive titers, only 6 patients had other clinical manifestations of Lyme disease.

Because of the recent flurry of case reports and commentaries describing the ophthalmic manifestations of Lyme disease,[88–99] several general points should be emphasized. There seems little doubt that Lyme disease can be associated with ocular and neuro-ophthalmic manifestations. Leaving aside Lyme facial neuropathy, the ophthalmic findings appear to be somewhat unusual, and no clear pattern of uveitis or optic neuropathy has emerged. Early in the course of the disease,

Lyme titers may be negative, and persistently seronegative, culture-positive cases have been described.[90, 91] In this setting, the diagnosis is based on a strong clinical suspicion based primarily on the characteristic rash: erythema chronicum migrans. The spirochete is fastidious, and cultures have proved to be clinically impractical because of their low yield. Moreover, histopathologic demonstration of the organism is difficult and can occasionally be quite misleading. The diagnostic problems are compounded by the fact that elevated Lyme titers alone should not be taken as positive proof of active Lyme disease, because 6% to 8% of those "positive" titers occur in asymptomatic subjects without a history of Lyme disease.[100, 101] Thus, lacking the rash, arthritis, or abnormal spinal fluid, it can be difficult to assess the significance of an isolated cranial neuropathy with a positive Lyme titer.

Since all of the spirochetes share common antigens, serologic tests may cross-react. Depending on the method, Lyme titers may be positive in approximately 20% to 60% of patients with syphilis,[102, 103] and 20% of patients with Lyme disease may have a weakly positive FTA-Abs.[104] Yet to be substantiated in large numbers of patients, some have suggested that, among patients with Lyme disease, the rapid plasma reagin (RPR) test and microhemagglutination-Treponema Pallidum (MHA-TP) are usually negative, and the FTA, if positive, is present in low titers (< 1:10) only.[104] Nonetheless, a false-positive Lyme titer or a false-positive FTA presents a diagnostic dilemma for the neuro-ophthalmologist faced with an isolated optic neuropathy, uveitis, or isolated sixth nerve palsy.[88] A recently published case report illustrates the problem.[89] Fortunately, the treatment does not differ radically in either case. Finally, it is becoming increasingly evident that, like neurosyphilis, there exists a late form of Lyme disease, characterized by diffuse or focal encephalopathy, that can resemble multiple sclerosis.[105-109]

Given these uncertainties, the clinician sometimes treats without surely knowing whether the patient, in fact, has Lyme disease. Clearly, there is much more to learn about this troublesome disease.

BLEPHAROSPASM

Jancovic and Tolosa[110] edited an excellent monograph on the facial dyskinesias that includes a number of authoritative reviews and some new material covering the spectrum of craniocervical movement disorders. The clinical features and differential diagnosis are discussed at length.[111-115] Physiology of the blink rate and the blink reflexes in a variety of pathologic states are discussed in two separate articles.[116, 117] Based on personal letters, Koster[118] of the Benign Essential Blepharospasm Research Foundation describes the devastating impact these disorders can have on the patient. Jankovic and Nutt[119] report on the incidence of the movement disorders among relatives of patients with craniocervical disorders. Among 238 patients studied, 37% had a close relative with a movement disorder. Lee's travels to and from work on the London Underground have provided him with a laboratory in which to study the normal and pathologic human face.[120] This is an observant and thoughtful description of facial stereotypes, mannerisms, and tics. The pathophysiologic and therapeutic pharmacology of the facial dyskinesias are covered in several chapters.[121–123] The monograph also discusses a variety of other subjects including torticollis, tardive dyskinesia, tremors, voice and speech disorders, chorea, and myoclonus of the facial structures as well as hemifacial spasm and apraxia of lid opening (discussed later).

A newly recognized disorder consisting of familial hypoceruloplasminemia, blepharospasm, retinal degeneration, and high-density areas in the basal ganglia by CT was described. The disorder was thought to be due to a lack of apoceruloplasmin, with iron deposition in the basal ganglia and other organs.[124]

With the recognition that botulinum provides only temporary relief, there remains continued interest in the surgical treatment of blepharospasm. Anderson and Patrinely[125] describe their experience with myectomies in which nearly all of the eyelid protractors in the upper eyelid, brow, and sometimes the lower lid are removed. They claim that improvement in functional disability averaged in the 85% to 95% range; however, the procedure can be complicated by lymphedema lasting weeks to months, drying and exposure, facial hypoesthesia, localized skin flap necrosis, loss of brow hairs, hematoma formation, and ectropion. Surgery does little for the lower facial and cervical muscle spasms. Dobie and Fisch[126] report on their experience with selective facial neurectomies in 191 patients, 74% of whom had a "satisfactory result." Complications were surprisingly few: no patient had more than mild to moderate permanent damage; only 1.5% required tarsorraphy; none had serious postoperative complications. Among 69 patients with essential blepharospasm or hemifacial spasm, 12 required reoperation because the results were unsatisfactory. Even among the strongest proponents of surgical therapy, most agree that surgery should be restricted to those patients with disabling blepharospasm that fails to respond to botulinum.

Botulinum Therapy

There seems to be general agreement about the efficacy and safety of botulinum toxin, in the treatment of essential blepharospasm, Meige's syndrome, and hemifacial spasm. Most patients experience a significant degree of improvement for about 12 weeks, and in most cases, side effects are mild and transient, consisting of ptosis, lagophthalmos, dry eye symptoms, and diplopia. Recent publications have expanded the total number of patients studied, investigated the effects of repeated injections and the side effects more systematically, and expanded its use to treat related problems.[127–130]

Based on the larger series of recently published studies,[131–134] repeated administration of botulinum appears to be safe and well tolerated. This includes one study with 14 patients receiving five or more injections,[131] another study with 37 patients undergoing four or more injections,[132] and 44 patients receiving three or more injections.[134] Though one group observed a slight increase in the duration of effect after the second and third injections,[134] the others showed no such change.[131, 133] Some have suggested that repeated injections may be less effective and shorter in their duration[135]; however, there have been no clear signs of tolerance or increased side effects.[131–134] Moreover, Biglan et al.[136] found no detectable levels of antibotulinum antibody from 28 patients who received a total of 57 doses (12 patients received two to five injections).

The rate of nonresponse, previously reported to be anywhere from 4% to 22%,[131] depends on how "nonresponse" is defined. Using a more rigorous definition, Cohen et al.[131] found a nonresponse rate of 14% of 224 injections among 32% of their 75 patients. However, nearly half of these patients responded to prior or subsequent injections. Most patients will, to some degree, respond to botulinum,[132, 134] but the Cohen et al.[131] criteria for nonresponse appear to give a more critical and realistic appraisal of the beneficial effects of botulinum.

The standard initial dose of 12.5 units per eye injected at multiple sites appears to be optimum. For those patients (approximately 18% to 21%) who fail to respond initially or exhibit a short duration of action, some have resorted to a double-dose regimen[131, 132] and, in some cases, triple and quadruple doses.[132] In one study, the double-dose injections appeared to increase the duration but reduced the degree of effect and slightly increased the number of nonresponders.[131] The use of double-dose regimens has not been associated with significant increases in side effects.[131, 137]

Some investigators have noted a prolonged duration of action among patients who have undergone prior surgical treatment for blepharospasm,[133, 138] whereas others have not.[132, 134] Those patients with hemifacial spasm may have longer durations of effect than those patients with other forms of blepharospasm,[132] although Engstrom et al.[134] found no differences in duration between Meige's syndrome and essential blepharospasm. Patients with generalized neurologic disorders do not appear to respond as well as those without.[134]

Though the occurrence of mild ptosis, lid swelling, tearing, and exposure is common, these effects tend to be mild, usually lasting days to several weeks. The occurrence of disabling complications has fortunately been rare. Patrinely et al.[135] reviewed the local side effects associated with botulinum therapy. Elston[133] reported marked ptosis and ophthalmoplegia lasting 7 weeks in three of 101 patients who were inadvertently given a tenfold overdose. Diplopia, usually lasting 3 weeks, has been noted in 1% to 6% of patients.[131–133] Avoiding the medial lower eyelid may reduce the likelihood of diplopia[135, 139] or ectropion.[132] Elston[133] described four patients who were visually disabled by a persistent Bell's phenomenon, that is, the eyes continued to deviate upward with the eyelids open.[132, 140] Notwithstanding the absence of systemic side effects, there appears to be some systemic absorption, as shown by recording abnormal single fiber activity in the arm muscles following facial injection.[141]

The frequency of ptosis following botulinum treatment for 39 patients with strabismus and four patients with blepharospasm was reported by Burns et al.[140] Mild ptosis developed in 53% of 57 injections. Visually significant ptosis, which developed in 21% of patients, resolved within 8 weeks of injection.

The use of botulinum toxin has been expanded to treat patients with spastic entropion,[137] torticollis,[130, 132] and apraxia of lid opening,[142] and to induce a protective ptosis for patients with indolent corneal ulcers, exposure, and neuroparalytic keratopathy.[143, 144]

Given the limited duration of botulinum toxin in treating blepharospasm, a pharmacologic alternative that provides longer if not permanent effects would be desirable. Baker and Wirtschafter[145] have been studying the effects of orbicularis oculi injection of doxorubicin, a drug which appears to cause permanent injury to the muscle and central motor neurons (by suicide retrograde transport). More animal studies will be needed before considering this drug for human studies.

HEMIFACIAL SPASM

Pathophysiology

There continues to be some disagreement, to say the least, about whether hemifacial spasm (HFS) is due to ephaptic transmission or central reorganization.[146–148] Recall that several years ago, Moller and Jannetta[147] proposed a central mechanism based on intraoperative electrophysiologic recordings in patients with HFS. Stimulating one branch of the facial nerve evokes contraction in a muscle supplied by a nonstimulated branch. Antidromic impulses along the stimulated branch presumably spread laterally and are then transmitted orthodromically along the unstimulated branch; all this occurs in about 10 msec (total conduction time). However, the antidromic conduction time along one branch plus the orthodromic conduction time following proximal stimulation in the other takes only 8 msec (summed conduction time).

The controversy has focused on this 2-msec disparity between the summed and total conduction times and where lateral spread occurs (i.e., within the facial motor nucleus or the root entry zone of vascular compression). Moller and Jannetta dismissed an ephaptic mechanism, arguing that there should be no difference between the summed and total conduction times. The additional 2 msec seen in the total conduction time probably represents the time required for lateral spread to occur within the facial motor nucleus before the impulse is transmitted orthodromically. In support of the ephaptic mechanism, Nielsen[148] has argued that lateral spread occurs at the site of compression where a focal area of demyelination would be expected to slow conduction and increase total conduction time. The summed conduction time is less because it only reflects the activity along undamaged fast conducting fibers. That there is slowing of conduction among some of the axons in the facial nerve has also been shown by a delay in the R1 component of the blink reflex in patients with HFS. For a more detailed summary of the data and a list of pertinent references, please refer to an exchange of letters to the editor.[146-148]

More recently, Moller[149] has shown an early orthodromic mentalis response following antidromic stimulation of the temporalis branch. This early response had a latency equal to the summed conduction times along each of the individual branches. Based on this early response, Moller suggests that ephaptic transmission can indeed occur; however, it was present in only three of 50 patients studied. Moreover, this early response was small in magnitude and could be demonstrated only after the nerve was manipulated.

Overall, there seems to be general agreement about the experimental observations, but the interpretation remains controversial. Further understanding of this problem may follow the recent development of an animal model. Sen and Moller,[150] using chronic periodic intracranial stimulation of the rat facial nerve, have recorded similar differences between total and summed conduction latencies.

Clinical Aspects

The differential diagnosis and management of HFS were recently reviewed.[150a] The great majority of cases are due to vascular compression; tumors are rare.[151] Levin and Lee[152] reported a unique case of a cerebellopontine lipoma presenting with hemifacial spasm. Nishi et al.[153] reported the second example of HFS as a false localizing sign in a patient with a contralateral acoustic neuroma.

Though microvascular decompression offers a cure for many patients, the surgical results vary with the experience of the surgeon (75% to 95% cure rates); the recurrence rate can vary between 3% and 7%; and mild to severe complications can include hearing loss, facial paresis, stroke, and death (15% to 20%).[150] Among 278 patients undergoing microvascular decompression, nine (3.2%) developed major complications, including hematomas, acute hydrocephalus, stroke, and status epilepticus; two patients died.[154] Intraoperative monitoring of the facial EMG has been used to identify the offending blood vessel and predict the likelihood of success.[155] This technique may improve the cure rate. Jho and Jannetta[156] summarized their experience with HFS and microvascular decompression in young patients under the age of 20.

Aoki and Nagao[157] described an exceptional case of HFS. At craniotomy, the patient was found to have a normal facial nerve without signs of vascular compression. The case was terminated without performing a microvascular decompression, and the patient awoke completely free of spasm. They suggest that vascular compression does not explain this case, although a series of letters following publication brought forth several other possible explanations: that the offending blood vessel was moved when the subarachnoid cistern was dissected, that the offending vessel was too small to appreciate or the nerve was not completely explored,[158] and that the HFS was due to some unidentified factor such as downward shift of the brain stem.[159] Inadvertent injury of the facial nerve during surgery would explain improvement without decompression.

Myectomy, selective facial neurectomy, and thermocoagulation[160] are surgical alternatives to microvascular decompression. Garland et al.[161] discussed the results of myectomy in 21 patients with HFS and reported "excellent or good results" in 94%. Postsurgical lymphedema was common, although the authors state that all complications tended to be "mild and transient." At present, if medications fail, botulinum toxin appears to be the most reasonable next step, recognizing that there are limitations.

SUPRANUCLEAR EYELID DISTURBANCES

"Apraxia" of eyelid opening, or more appropriately supranuclear paresis of eyelid opening, is a transient inability to initiate eyelid opening voluntarily in the absence of neuromyopathic disorders or active contraction of the orbicularis oculi. During the episode, attempted voluntary eyelid opening is accompanied by vigorous frontalis contraction.

Previously reported causes include progressive supranuclear palsy (PSP), Parkinson's disease, atypical Parkinson's (probably multiple-system atrophy), adult-onset Hallervorden-Spatz disease, Shy-Drager syndrome, Huntington's chorea, cerebral diplegia with parkinsonism, methyl-phenyl-tetrahydropyridine–induced Parkinson's disease, and frontotemporal gunshot injury. More recently, this finding has been described most commonly among patients with PSP[162, 163] and rarely in patients with right hemispheric strokes,[162] Wilson's disease,[164] Parkinson's disease,[165] and neuroacanthocytosis with PSP.[166]

Though the mechanism is unknown, it has been suggested that apraxia of eyelid opening results from an involuntary supranuclear inhibition of the levator associated with rostral brain-stem and extrapyramidal lesions. Others suggest that it is a consequence of generalized slowness and diminution of motor activity characteristic of extrapyramidal disease.[165] If apraxia of eyelid opening is not associated with orbicularis activity, it is difficult to explain why such patients should respond to botulin injection of the orbicularis oculi[132] or the frontalis[142] (although some do not respond[133]). It would be interesting to confirm by EMG the clinical impression that the orbicularis oculi and levator do not, in fact, contract during episodes of eyelid closure.

"Apraxia of eyelid closure" (supranuclear paralysis of eyelid closure) is characterized by an inability to close the eyes on command with preservation of eyelid closure to reflex stimuli. This has been previously described in patients with Creutzfeld-Jakob syndrome, hemispheric vascular disease, and amyotrophic lateral sclerosis. Lepore[162] has described four additional patients one with a static encephalopathy and the rest with PSP.

Apraxia of eyelid closure should be distinguished from eyelid impersistence in which initiation of eyelid closure is maintained but cannot be sustained. De Renzi et al.[167] found that failure to keep the eyelids closed was the most common manifestation of motor impersistence with acute brain lesions. It sometimes affected only the contralateral eyelid and was more frequent after right-sided brain damage.

Unilateral hemispheric lesions can rarely be associated with both contralateral and bilateral ptosis. Lepore[168] has recently summarized 13 cases of bilateral cerebral ptosis associated with massive right hemisphere lesions (10 infarcts, 3 hemorrhages), midline shift, gaze deviation to the right, and other signs of right hemispheric dysfunction. In a related report, Lowenstein et al.[169] described patients with long-standing unilateral ptosis and contralateral hemispheric arteriovenous malformations.

In an epileptic girl with Lennox syndrome, seizures were consistently precipitated by repetitive voluntary and reflex blinking. Eye movements and photic stimulation had no such effect.[170]

MYOKYMIA

Facial myokymia consists of involuntary, continuous, rapid undulating contractions of the face frequently involving the orbicularis. These contractions may, on rare occasion, result in monocular oscillopsia.[171] Electrophysiologically, there are brief tetanic bursts of motor unit potentials. In most instances it is a benign symptom attributed to fatigue, stress, or excess caffeine; however, it may be associated with both peripheral and central lesions due to multiple sclerosis, intrinsic brain-stem tumors, and Guillain-Barré syndrome.

Eight of 100 patients with Bell's palsy had clinical evidence of myokymia, and another 15 patients exhibited EMG findings consistent with myokymia.[172] Facial and limb myokymia was described in four patients bitten by a timber rattlesnake.[173]

In a presumptive case of multiple sclerosis, myokymia was associated with an MRI lesion in the inferolateral dorsal pons near the junction of the middle cerebellar peduncle and an abnormal brain-stem auditory evoked potential (reduced amplitude in III; absent wave IV, V).[174] Similarly, in a patient with a pontine glioma, myokymia was associated with a focal expansion of the superior cerebellar peduncle and upper pons by MRI.[175] Myokymia was a false localizing sign in a patient with obstructive hydrocephalus and resolved after shunting.[176]

PTOSIS

The occurrence of lid retraction secondary to contralateral ptosis is often explained by Hering's law of equal innervation to yoke muscles. There is still some question, however, as to whether Hering's law, which was originally intended to explain the actions of the extraocular muscles, applies to the coordinated movements of both eyelids. It appears that if Hering's law applies, it does so infrequently and may be restricted to certain groups of patients. For example, among 21 patients with ptosis from a variety of causes, only 1 (with myasthenia gravis) showed lid retraction.[177] Even among myasthenic patients, lid retraction appears to be rare: only 4 of 150 myasthenic patients had lid retraction.[178] Most of the previously reported cases have occurred with lesions at or distal to the neuromuscular junction.[177]

The explanation for the infrequent occurrence of contralateral lid retraction is unknown, but Lepore[177] suggests several possibilities. Compensatory unilateral orbicularis oculi contraction may mask the lid retraction. Thus, if the orbicularis is also weakened, as it is in myasthenia, contralateral lid retraction becomes more evident. Kansu and Subutay[178] also question the validity of Hering's law in their cases and suggest instead that the activity of a myasthenically weakened muscle is facilitated by acetylcholinesterase inhibitors.[178] A combination of both arguments (facilitation and Hering's law) was proposed to explain why two patients showed a paradoxical response to edrophonium (Tensilon), with the onset of ptosis in one eye and reversal of ptosis in the other.[179] Finally, in response to the Kansu and Subutay report, the editor suggests that if the ptotic eye is fixating, both lids will elevate, whereas if the nonptotic eye is fixating, there is no need to retract the contralateral lid.

These articles raise fundamental questions about the determinants of lid position of each eye and the relative lid position between both eyes. One other factor that needs to be considered is that lid retraction may also be influenced by the relative activity of the ipsilateral superior rectus, perhaps more so than the contralateral levator. As discussed in the section on blinks, the position of the lid is closely linked to vertical eye movements. Moreover, lid retraction can sometimes result from a paresis of upgaze, inferior rectus restriction in thyroid orbitopathy,[180] and blowout fractures. In these instances, attempted upgaze may disproportionately raise the eyelid more than the eye. More quantitative studies using the search coil may provide a more precise understanding of these observations.

Exploiting the fact that myasthenia is exacerbated by heat and improved by cold, Sethi et al.[181] showed that myasthenic ptosis can improve after applying an ice pack to the eyelid. Eight of ten myasthenic patients improved after the ice pack test; in one case the ice pack test was positive where the Tensilon test was negative.

A number of articles have described new syndromes and reviewed previously recognized syndromes in which ptosis or eyelid involvement was a prominent feature.[182–186] The report by Cornel et al.[186] is of interest because it underscores a previously recognized association between ptosis and cardiac disease (aortic coarctation).

The Marcus Gunn phenomenon was described in a patient with Waardenburg's syndrome and aganglionic megacolon.[187] Correction of ptosis alone in patients with the Marcus Gunn phenomenon will usually aggravate the aberrant lid elevation with jaw movement. Thus, the surgical approach in these cases is aimed toward eliminating levator function and elevating the lid. Two reports describe similar approaches to this problem in which the levator is transected above the tarsal plate. The distal levator-aponeurosis, which is still attached to the tarsus, is then used as a sling.[188, 189]

Pang et al.[190] described two patients with lid retraction on adduction. Four other family members in three consecutive generations were similarly affected, suggesting an autosomal dominant pattern of inheritance. Similarly, a 17-year-old woman with unilateral congenital ptosis and esotropia was found to have lid elevation on abduction and ptosis on adduction. Electro-oculographic analysis of saccades showed no limitation of eye movements.[191]

Ptosis due to levator disinsertion can complicate radial keratotomy.[192, 193] Ptosis and dermatochalasis were the presenting signs of an occult primary systemic amyloidosis.[194]

Malone and Nerad[195] summarized their experience with treatment of ptosis in oculomotor nerve palsies. The treatment of ptosis in patients with chronic progressive ophthalmoplegia was discussed in two recent publications.[196, 197] The predictability of certain parameters in aponeurotic ptosis repair under local anesthesia was reported by Linberg et al.[198] They found a linear relationship between lid position at surgery and 3 months postoperatively. Lid position at 1 week was highly predictive of the 3-month result. If the operative lid fissure was greater than 10 mm, a rise was subsequently observed; if less than 10 mm, a fall was noted. If after the aponeurotic repair the lid is still overcorrected or undercorrected, Jordan and Anderson[199] described a simple method for adjusting lid position after surgery using local anesthesia. Karesh and Putterman[200] reported on their experience in 56 eyelids undergoing levator recessions. A retrospective study of 58 patients with thyroid orbitopathy who underwent eyelid surgery stressed the importance of relieving inferior rectus restriction, the limitations of lateral tarsorrhaphy to treat lid retraction, and the usefulness of scleral grafts to treat lower lid retraction.[201]

REFERENCES

1. Jenny AB, Saper CB: Organization of the facial nucleus and corticofacial projection in the monkey: A reconsideration of the upper motor neuron facial palsy. *Neurology* 1987; 37:930–939.

2. Happak W, Burggasser G, Gruber H: Histochemical characteristics of human mimic muscles. *J Neurol Sci* 1988; 83:25–35.

3. Balkany T: The intrinsic vasculature of the cat facial nerve. *Laryngoscopy* 1986; 96:70–77.

4. Bardosi A, Goebel H, Stennert E: The ultrastructure of normal and denervated human facial muscle. *Plast Reconstr Surg* 1987; 79:171–176.

5. Monserrat L, Benito M: Facial synkinesis and aberrant regeneration of facial nerve. *Adv Neurol* 1988; 49:211–224.

6. Thomander L: Reorganization of the facial motor nucleus after peripheral nerve regeneration. *Acta Otolaryngol* 1984; 97:619–626.

7. Sibony PA, Evinger C, Lessell S: Retrograde horseradish peroxidase transport after oculomotor nerve injury. *Invest Ophthalmol Vis Sci* 1986; 27:975–980.

8. Brushert TM, Mesulum NM: Alteration in connections between muscle and anterior horn motoneurons after peripheral nerve repair. *Science* 1980; 208:603–605.

9. Lyness RW, Collin JR, Alexander RA, et al: Histological appearances of the levator palpebrae superioris muscle in the Marcus Gunn phenomenon. *Br J Ophthalmol* 1988; 72:104–109.

10. Evinger C, Shaw MD, Peck CK, et al: Blinking and associated eye movements in humans, guinea pigs, and rabbits. *J Neurophysiol* 1984; 52:323–339.

11. Holder DS, Scott A, Hannaford B, et al: High resolution electromyogram of the human eyeblink. *Electromyogr Clin Neurophysiol* 1987; 27:481–488.

12. Niida T, Mukuno K, Ishikawa S: Quantitative measurement of upper eyelid movements. *Jpn J Ophthalmol* 1987; 31:255–264.

13. Becker W, Fuchs AF: Lid-eye coordination during vertical gaze changes in man and monkey. *J Neurophysiol*, 1988; 60:1227–1252.

14. Manning KA, Evinger C: Different forms of blinks and their two-stage control. *Exp Brain Res* 1986; 64:579–588.

15. Kurlan R, Jankovic J, Rubin A, et al: Coexistent Meige's syndrome and myasthenia gravis: A relationship between blinking and extraocular muscle fatigue? *Arch Neurol* 1987; 44:1057–1060.

16. Ferman L, Collewijn H, Vandenberg AV: A direct test of Listing's law: II. Human ocular torsion measured under dynamic conditions. *Vision Res* 1987; 27:939–951.

17. Ljubin C, Knesaurek K, Ljubin T: Mathematical and graphic model of the audiomotor reflex of the musculus orbicularis oculi and the law of energy. *Electromyogr Clin Neurophysiol* 1986; 26:229–240.

18. Krauter EE: Reflex modification by the human auditory startle blink by antecedent interruption of a visual stimulus. *Percept Mot Skills* 1987; 64:727–738.

19. Wilkins DE, Hallett M, Wess MM: Audiogenic startle reflex of man and its relationship to startle syndromes: A review. *Brain* 1986; 109:561–573.

20. Beolhouwer AJ, Bruggemans E, Brunia CH: Blink reflex magnitude during the foreperiod of a warned reaction time task: Effects of precueing. *Psychophysiology* 1987; 24:625–631.

21. Raffaele R, Emery P, Palmeri A, et al: Influences on blink reflex induced by IA afferents in human subjects. *Eur Neurol* 1986; 25:373–380.

22. Klug N, Csecsei G: Electrically elicited blink reflex and early acoustic evoked potentials in circumscribed and diffuse brain stem lesions. *Acta Neurochir Suppl* 1987; 40:57–94.

23. Evinger C, Manning KA: A model system for motor learning: Adaptive gain control of the blink reflex. *Exp Brain Res* 1988; 70:527–538.

24. Evinger C, Sibony P, Manning KA, et al: A pharmacological distinction between long and short latency pathways of the human blink revealed with tobacco. *Exp Brain Res* 1988; 149:1–4.

25. Cruccu G, Inghilleri M, Fraioli B, et al: Neurophysiologic assessment of trigeminal function after surgery for trigeminal neuralgia. *Neurology* 1987; 37:631–638.

26. Khater-Boidin J, Duron B: The orbicularis oculi reflexes in healthy premature and full-term newborns. *Electroencephalogr Clin Neurophysiol* 1987; 67:479–484.

27. Hoffman HS, Cohen ME, Anday EK: Inhibition of the eyeblink reflex in the human infant. *Dev Psychobiol* 1987; 20:277–283.

28. Malin JP: Visual evoked blink reflex in optic neuritis. *J Neurol* 1987; 235:49–52.

29. Goldberg TE, Maltz A, Bow JN, et al: Blink rate abnormalities in autistic and mentally retarded children: Relationship to dopaminergic activity. *J Am Acad Child Adolesc Psychiatry* 1987; 26:336–338.

30. Karson CN, Goldberg TE, Leleszi JP: Increased blink rate in adolescent patients with psychosis. *Psychiatry Res* 1986; 17:195–198.

31. Stern JA, Walrath LC, Goldstein R: The endogenous eyeblink. *Psychophysiology* 1984; 21:22–33.

32. May M, Hughes GB: Facial nerve disorders: Update 1987. *Am J Otolaryngol* 1987; 8:167–180.

33. House JW, Brackmann DE: Facial nerve grading system. *Otolaryngol Head Neck Surg* 1985; 93:146–147.

34. Burres SA: Objective grading of facial paralysis. *Ann Otol Rhinol Laryngol* 1986; 95:238–241.

35. Burres SA: Facial biomechanics, the standards of normal. *Laryngoscopy* 1985; 95:708–714.

36. Burres SA, Fisch U: The comparison of facial grading systems. *Arch Otolaryngol Head Neck Surg* 1986; 112:755–758.

37. Jonsson L, Larsson A, Thomander L: Immune complexes and complement components in Bell's palsy. *J Otorhinolaryngol Relat Spec* 1987; 49:294–301.

38. Manos-Pujol M, Buendia E, Mestre M, et al: Cellular immunity abnormalities in patients with recurrent Bell's palsy. *Clin Otolaryngol* 1987; 12:283–287.

39. Jonsson L, Sjoberg O, Thomander L: Activated T cells and Leu-7+ cells in Bell's palsy. *Acta Otolaryngol* 1988; 105:108–113.

40. Hanner P, Anderson O, Frisen L, et al: Clinical observations of effects on central nervous system in patients with acute facial palsy. *Arch Otolaryngol Head Neck Surg* 1987; 113:516–520.

41. Nieuwmeyer PA, Visser SL, Feenstra L: Bell's palsy: A polyneuropathy. *Am J Otol* 1985; 6:250–252.

42. Uri N, Schuchman G: Vestibular abnormalities in patients with Bell's palsy. *J Laryngol Otol* 1986; 100:1125–1128.

43. Edstrom S, Hanner P, Anderson O, et al: Elevated levels of myelin basic protein in CSF in relation to auditory brainstem responses in Bell's palsy. *Acta Otolaryngol* 1987; 103:198–203.

44. Weber T, Jurgens S, Luer W: Cerebrospinal fluid immunoglobulins and virus-specific antibodies in disorders affecting the facial nerve. *J Neurol* 1987; 234:308–314.

45. Katusic SK, Beard M, Wiederholt WC, et al: Incidence, clinical features, and prognosis in Bell's palsy, Rochester, Minnesota, 1968–1982. *Ann Neurol* 1986; 20:622–627.

46. Prescott CA: Idiopathic facial nerve palsy in children and the effect of treatment with steroids. *Int J Pediatr Otorhinolaryngol* 1987; 13:257–264.

47. McGregor JA, Guberman A, Amer J, et al: Idiopathic facial nerve paralysis (Bell's palsy) in late pregnancy and the early puerperium. *Obstet Gynecol* 1987; 69:435–438.

48. Aldrich MS, Beck RW, Albers JW: Familial recurrent Bell's palsy with ocular motor palsies. *Neurology* 1987; 37:1369–1371.

49. Amit R: Familial juvenile onset of Bell's palsy. *Eur J Pediatr* 1987; 146:608–609.

50. Stankiewicz JA: A review of the published data on steroids and idiopathic facial paralysis. *Otolaryngol Head Neck Surg* 1987; 97:481–486.

51. Aguilar EA III, Yeakley JW, Ghorayeb BY, et al: High resolution CT scan of temporal bone fractures: Association of facial nerve paralysis with temporal bone fractures. *Head Neck Surg* 1987; 9:162–166.

52. Wadin K, Thomander L, Wilbrand H: The labyrinthine portion of the facial canal in patients with Bell's palsy investigated by computed tomography. *Acta Radiol* 1987; 28:25–30.

53. Inoue Y, Tabuchi T, Hakuba A, et al: Facial nerve neuromas: CT findings. *J Comput Assist Tomogr* 1987; 16:942–947.

54. Schubiger O, Valavanis A, Stuckmann G, et al: Temporal bone fractures and their complications: Examination with high resolution CT. *Neuroradiology* 1986; 28:93–99.

55. Harnsberger HR, Davis RKL, Parkin JL, et al: The tailored CT evaluation of persistent facial nerve paralysis. *Laryngoscope* 1986; 96:347–352.

56. Glauber DT: Facial paralysis after general anesthesia. *Anesthesiology* 1986; 65:516–517.

57. Prescott CA: An unusual complication of epistaxis. *J Laryngol Otol* 1988; 102:176.

58. DeVries N, Versluis RJJ, Valk J, et al: Facial nerve paralysis following embolization for severe epistaxis (a case report and a review of the literature). *J Laryngol Otol* 1986; 100:207–210.

59. Spaeth GL: Total facial nerve palsy following modified O'Brien facial nerve block. *Ophthalmic Surg* 1987; 18:518–519.

60. Burke RH, Adams JL: Immediate cranial nerve paralysis during removal of a mandibular third molar. *Oral Surg Oral Med Oral Pathol* 1987; 63:172–174.

61. Downs AR, Jessen M, Lye CR: Peripheral nerve injuries during carotid endarterectomy. *Can J Surg* 1987; 30:22–24.

62. Thomson RG, James OF: Seventh-nerve palsy and hepatitis associated with nitrofurantoin. *Hum Toxicol* 1986; 5:387–388.

63. McCall WV, Coffey CE: Transient facial palsy during lithium toxicity, letter. *J Clin Psychopharmacol* 1987; 7:280–281.

64. Hattori T, Tokugawa K, Fukushige J, et al: Facial palsy in Kawasaki disease: Report of two cases and review. *Eur J Pediatr* 1987; 146:601–602.

65. Seymore CH, Peeples WJ: Cranial nerve involvement with carcinoma of prostate. *Urology* 1988; 31:211–213.

66. Van Niekerk JL, Wobbles T, Monstrey S, et al: The management of parotid tumors: A 10-year experience. *Acta Chir Belg* 1987; 87:1–5.

67. Broderick JP, Auger RG, DeSanto LW: Facial paralysis and occult parotid cancer: A characteristic syndrome. *Arch Otolaryngol Head Neck Surg* 1988; 114:195–197.

68. Sullivan MJ, Breslin K, McClatchey KD, et al: Malignant parotid gland tumors: A retrospective study. *Otolaryngol Head Neck Surg* 1987; 97:529–533.

69. Basma NJ, Robin PE: Glomus jugulare tumor masquerading as idiopathic facial nerve palsy. *J Laryngol Otol* 1987; 101:605–606.

70. Zachariades N, Anastasea-Vlachou K, Xypolyta A, et al: Uncommon manifestations of histiocytosis X. *Int J Oral Maxillofac Surg* 1987; 16:355–362.

71. Shone GR, Stewart S: Facial paralysis in parotitis. *Br J Surg* 1985; 72:902.

72. Robertson JF, Azmy AA: Facial paralysis in acute parotisis. *Z Kinderchir* 1987; 42:312.

73. Darras BT, Adelman LS, Mora JS, et al: Familial amyloidosis with cranial neuropathy in corneal lattice dystrophy. *Neurology* 1986; 36:432–435.

74. Brandt TW, Jeulius HA, Cohen NJ: Facial paralysis as the initial presentation of an internal carotid aneurysm. *Arch Otolaryngol Head Neck Surg* 1986; 112:198–202.

75. Onundrasen DT: Acute nose blow palsy: A pneumatic variant of sudden facial paralysis. *N Engl J Med* 1987; 317:1227.

76. Snyderman C, May M, Berman MA, et al: Facial paralysis: Traumatic neuromas vs. facial nerve neoplasms. *Otolaryngol Head Neck Surg* 1988; 98:53–59.

77. Wiselka MJ, Nicholson KG, Ward SC, et al: Acute infection with human immunodeficiency virus associated with facial nerve palsy and neuralgia (letter). *J Infect* 1987; 15:189–190.

78. Smith MD, Scott GM, Rom S: Herpes simplex virus and facial palsy. *J Infect* 1987; 15: 259–261.

79. Linzer M, Miller MJ: Tobacco chewer's pseudopalsy (letter). *Lancet* 1987; 1:860.

80. Coker NJ, Kendall KA, Jenkins HA, et al: Traumatic intratemporal facial nerve injury: Management rationale for preservation of function. *Otolarygol Head Neck Surg* 1987; 97:262–269.

81. Maiman DJ, Cusick JF, Anderson AJ, et al: Nonoperative management of traumatic facial palsy. *J Trauma* 1985; 25:645–648.

82. Stanek G, Flamm H, Barbour AG, et al (eds): *Proceedings of the Second International Symposium on Lyme Disease and Related Disorders, Vienna 1985*. New York, Gustav Fischer Verlag, 1987.

83. Ackerman R, Horstrup P, Schmidt R: Tick-born meningopolyneuritis (Garin-Bujadoux, Bannwarth). *Yale J Biol Med* 1984; 57:485–490.

84. Pachner AR, Steere A: The triad of neurologic manifestations of Lyme disease: Meningitis, cranial neuritis and radioculoneuritis. *Neurology* 1985; 35:47–53.

85. Clark JR, Carlson RD, Sasaki CT, et al: Facial paralysis in Lyme disease. *Laryngoscope* 1985; 95:1341–1345.

86. Schmutzhard E, Pohl P, Stanek G: Involvement of *Borrelia burgdorferi* in cranial nerve affection. *Zentralbl Bakteriol Mikrobiol Hyg A* 1986; 263:328–333.

87. Jonsson L, Stiernstedt G, Thomander L: Tick-born *Borrelia* infection in patients with Bell's palsy. *Arch Otolaryngol Head Neck Surg* 1987; 113:303–306.

88. Sibony PA, Golub B, Halperin J, et al: Neuro-ophthalmic manifestations of Lyme disease: Pitfalls in diagnosis (abstract INOS-39). International Neuro-ophthalmology Symposium, Vancouver, BC, May 7–12, 1988.

89. Farris BK, Webb RM: Lyme disease and optic neuritis. *J Clin Neuro Ophthalmol* 1988; 8:73–78.

90. MacDonald AB: Ambiguous serologies in active Lyme borreliosis, invited editorial. *J Clin Neuro Ophthalmol* 1988; 8:79–80.

91. MacDonald AB: Lyme disease: A neuro-ophthalmologic view. *J Clin Neuro Ophthalmol* 1987; 7:185–190.

92. Bertuck AW, Rocco E, Schwartz EG: Eye findings in Lyme disease. *Conn Med* 1987; 5:151–152.

93. Wu G, Lincoff H, Ellsworth RM, et al: Optic disc edema and Lyme disease. *Ann Ophthalmol* 1986; 18:252–255.

94. Racher HS, Kaufman DM, Goldfarb J, et al: Pseudotumor cerebri and Lyme disease: A new association. *J Pediatr* 1985; 6:931–933.

95. Schechter SL: Lyme disease associated with optic neuropathy. *Am J Med* 1986; 81:143–145.

96. Baum J, Barza M, Weinstein P, et al: Bilateral keratitis as a manifestation of Lyme disease. *Am J Ophthalmol* 1988; 105:75–77.

97. Steere AC, Duray PH, Danny JH, et al: Unilateral blindness caused by infection with Lyme disease spirochete, *Borrelia burgdorferi*. *Ann Intern Med* 1985; 103:382–384.

98. Smith JL: Syphilis/Lyme/AIDS, editorial comment. *J Clin Neuro Ophthalmol* 1987; 7:196–197.

99. Bialasiewicz AA, Ruprecht KW, Naumann GOH: Bilateral diffuse choroiditis and exudative vitreal detachments with evidence of Lyme disease. *Am J Ophthalmol* 1988; 105:419–420.

100. Hanrahan JP, Benach JL, Coleman JL: Incidence and cumulative frequency of endemic Lyme disease in a community. *J Infect Dis* 1984; 150:489–496.

101. Steere AC, Taylor E, Wilson ML: Longitudinal assessment of the clinical and epidemiological features of Lyme disease in a defined population. *J Infect Dis* 1986; 154:295–300.

102. Magnarelli LA, Anderson JF, Johnson RC: Cross-reactivity in serological tests for Lyme disease and other spirochetal infections. *J Infect Dis* 1987; 156:183–188.

103. Russell H, Sampson JS, Schmidt GP, et al: Enzyme-linked immunosorbent assay and indirect immunofluorescence assay for Lyme disease. *J Infect Dis* 1984; 149:465–470.

104. Hunter EF, Russell H, Farshy CE, et al: Evaluation of sera from patients with Lyme disease in FTA-Ab test for syphilis. *Sex Transm Dis* 1986; 13:232–236.

105. Ackerman R, Rehse-Kupper B, Gollmer R: Progressive *Borrelia* encephalomeylitis. *Zentralbl Bakteriol Mikrobiol Hyg A* 1986; 263:297–300.

106. Weder B, Wiedesheim P, Matter L: Chronic progressive neurological involvement in *Borrelia burgdorferi* infection 1987. *J Neurol* 1987; 234:40–43.

107. Kollikowski HH, Schwendemann G, Schulz M, et al: Chronic *Borrelia* encephalomyeloradiculitis with severe mental disturbance. *J Neurol* 1988; 235:140–142.

108. Schmutzhard E, Pohl P, Stanek G: Lyme borreliosis and multiple sclerosis. *Lancet* 1987; 1:167–168.

109. Broderick JP, Sandok BA, Mertz LE: Focal encephalitis in a young woman 6 years after the onset of Lyme disease: Tertiary Lyme disease? *Mayo Clin Proc* 1987; 62:313–316.

110. Jancovic J, Tolosa E (eds): Facial dyskinesias. *Adv Neurol* 1988; 49.

111. Jankovic J: Etiology and differential diagnosis of blepharospasm and oromandibular dystonia. *Adv Neurol* 1988; 49:103–116.

112. Tolosa E, Marti MJ: Blepharospasm-oromandibular dystonia syndrome (Meige's syndrome): Clinical aspects. *Adv Neurol* 1988; 49:73–84.

113. Pita-Salorio D, Quintana-Conte R: Ophthalmologic causes of blepharospasm. *Adv Neurol* 1988; 49:91–102.

114. Fahn S: Blepharospasm: A form of focal dystonia. *Adv Neurol* 1988; 49:125–133.

115. Dogre K, Corbett JJ: Hemifacial spasm: Differential diagnosis, mechanism, and treatment. *Adv Neurol* 1988; 49:151–176.

116. Kimura J: Blink reflex in facial dyskinesia. *Adv Neurol* 1988; 49:39–63.

117. Karson CN: Physiology of normal and abnormal blinking. *Adv Neurol* 1988; 49:25–37.

118. Koster ML: Blepharospasm: Patient's perspective. *Adv Neurol* 1988; 49:65–72.

119. Jankovic J, Nutt JG: Blepharospasm and cranial-cervical dystonia (Meige's syndrome): Familial occurrence. *Adv Neurol* 1988; 49:117–123.

120. Lees A: Facial mannerisms and tics. *Adv Neurol* 1988; 49:255–262.

121. Klawans HL, Tanner CM: Cholinergic pharmacology of blepharospasm with oromandibular dystonia (Meige's syndrome). Adv Neurol 1988; 49:443–450.

122. Gimenez-Roldan S, Mateo D, Orbe M, et al: Acute pharmacologic tests in cranial dystonia. *Adv Neurol* 1988; 49:451–466.

123. Tolosa E, Kulisevsky J: Dopaminergic mechanisms in cranial dystonia. *Adv Neurol* 1988; 49:433–441.

124. Miyajima H, Nishimura Y, Mizoguchi K, et al: Familial apoceruloplasmin deficiency associated with blepharospasm and retinal degeneration. *Neurology* 1987; 37:761–767.

125. Anderson RL, Patrinely JR: Surgical management of blepharospasm. *Adv Neurol* 1988; 49:501–520.

126. Dobie RA, Fisch U: Primary and revision surgery (selective neurectomy) for facial hyperkinesia. *Arch Otolaryngol Head Neck Surg* 1986; 112:154–163.

127. Jankovic J: Botulinum A toxin in the treatment of blepharospasm. *Adv Neurol* 1988; 49:467–472.

128. Arthurs B, Flanders M, Codere F, et al: Treatment of blepharospasm with medication, surgery and type A botulinum toxin. *Can J Ophthalmol* 1987; 22:24–28.

129. Tolosa E, Marti MJ, Kulisevsky J: Botulinum toxin injection therapy for hemifacial spasm. *Adv Neurol* 1988; 49:479–491.

130. Jankovic J, Orman J: Botulinum A toxin for cranial-cervical dystonia: A double-blind, placebo-controlled study. *Neurology* 1987; 37:616–623.

131. Cohen DA, Savino PJ, Stern MB, et al: Botulinum injection therapy for blepharospasm: A review and report of 75 patients. *Clin Neuropharmacol* 1986; 9:415–429.

132. Mauriello JA Jr, Coniaris H, Haupt EJ: Use of botulinum toxin in the treatment of 100 patients with facial dyskinesias. *Ophthalmology* 1987; 94:976–979.

133. Elston JS: Long-term results of treatment of idiopathic blepharospasm with botulinum toxin injections. *Br J Ophthalmol* 1987; 71:664–668.

134. Engstrom PF, Arnoult JB, Mazow ML, et al: Effectiveness of botulinum toxin therapy for essential blepharospasm. *Ophthalmology* 1987; 94:971–975.

135. Patrinely JR, Whiting AS, Anderson RL: Local side effects of botulinum toxin injections. *Adv Neurol* 1988; 49:493–500.

136. Biglan AW, Gonnering R, Lockhart LB, et al: Absence of antibody production in patients treated with botulinum A toxin. *Am J Ophthalmol* 1986; 101:232–235.

137. Carruthers J, Stubbs HA: Botulinum toxin for benign essential blepharospasm, hemifacial spasm and age-related lower eyelid entropion. *Can J Neurol Sci* 1987; 14:42–45.

138. Shore JW, Leone CR, O'Conner PS, et al: Botulinum toxin for the treatment of essential blepharospasm. *Ophthalmic Surg* 1986; 17:747–753.

139. Freuh BR, Nelson CC, Kapustiak JF: The effect of omitting botulinum toxin from the lower eyelid in blepharospasm treatment. *Am J Ophthalmol* 1988; 106:45–47.

140. Burns CL, Gammon A, Gemmill MC: Ptosis associated with botulinum toxin treatment of strabismus and blepharospasm. *Ophthalmology* 1986; 93:1621–1627.

141. Sanders DB, Massey WE, Buckley EG: Botulinum toxin for blepharospasm: Single fiber EMG studies. *Neurology* 1986; 36:545–547.

142. Katz B, Rosenberg JH: Botulinum therapy for apraxia of eyelid opening. *Am J Ophthalmol* 1987; 103:718–719.

143. Kirkness CM, Gillian WA, Dilly PN, et al: Botulinum toxin A–induced protective ptosis in corneal disease. *Ophthalmology* 1988; 95:473–480.

144. Adams GG, Kirkness CM, Lee JP: Botulinum toxin A induced protective ptosis. *Eye* 1987; 1:603–608.

145. Baker L, Wirtschafter JD: Experimental doxorubicin myopathy: A permanent treatment for eyelid spasms? *Arch Ophthalmol* 1987; 105:1265–1268.

146. Ravits J, Hallet M: Pathophysiology of hemifacial spasm: Localization of the lesion in hemifacial spasm (letter). *Neurology* 1986; 36:591.

147. Moller AR, Jannetta PJ: Reply from the authors. *Neurology* 1986; 36:591.

148. Nielsen VK: Indirect and direct evidence of ephaptic transmission in hemifacial spasm, (letter). *Neurology* 1986; 36:592.

149. Moller AR: Hemifacial spasm: Ephaptic transmission or hyperexcitability of the facial motor nucleus? *Exp Neurol* 1987; 98:336–349.

150. Sen CN, Moller AR: Signs of hemifacial spasm created by chronic periodic stimulation of the facial nerve in the rat. *Exp Neurol* 1987; 98:336–349.

150a. Digre K, Corbett JJ: Hemifacial spasm: Differential diagnosis, mechanism and treatment. *Adv Neurol* 1988; 49:151–176.

151. Spirk C, Wirtschafter JD: Hemifacial spasm due to intracranial tumor: An international survey of botulinum investigators. *Ophthalmology* 1988; 95:1042–1045.

152. Levin JM, Lee JE: Hemifacial spasm due to cerebellopontine angle lipoma: Case report. *Neurology* 1987; 37:337–339.

153. Nishi T, Matsukado Y, Nagahiro S, et al: Hemifacial spasm due to contralateral acoustic neuroma: Case report. *Neurology* 1987; 37:339–342.

154. Hanakita J, Kondo A: Serious complications of microvascular decompression operations for trigeminal neuralgia and hemifacial spasm. *Neurosurgery* 1988; 22:348–352.

155. Moller AR, Jannetta PJ: Monitoring facial EMG responses during microvascular decompression operations for hemifacial spasm. *J Neurosurg* 1987; 66:681–685.

156. Jho HD, Jannetta PJ: Hemifacial spasm in young people treated with microvascular decompression of the facial nerve. *Neurosurgery* 1987; 20:767–770.

157. Aoki N, Nagao T: Resolution of hemifacial spasm after posterior fossa exploration without vascular decompression. *Neurosurgery* 1986; 18:478–479.

158. Jannetta PJ: Hemifacial spasm resolution without vascular decompression, letter. *Neurosurgery* 1987; 20:63.

159. Maroun F, Jacob J, Mangan M: Hemifacial spasm, letter. *Neurosurgery* 1987; 20:994–995.

160. Salar G, Iob I, Ori C, et al: Treatment of hemifacial spasm with percutaneous radiofrequency thermocoagulation of the facial nerve. *Acta Neurochir Suppl* 1987; 39:132–135.

161. Garland PE, Patrinely JR, Anderson RL: Hemifacial spasm: Results of unilateral myectomy. *Ophthalmology* 1987; 94:288–294.

162. Lepore FE: So-called apraxias of lid movement. *Adv Neurol* 1988; 49:85–90.

163. Golbe LI, Davis PH, Lepore FE, et al: Eyelid movement abnormalities in progressive supranuclear palsy. *Neurology* 1987; 37(suppl 1):259.

164. Keane JR: Lid-opening apraxia in Wilson's disease. *J Clin Neuro Ophthalmol* 1988; 8:31–33.

165. Brusa A, Mancardi G, Meneghini S, et al: 'Apraxia' of eye opening in idiopathic Parkinson's disease, letter. *Neurology* 1986; 36:134.

166. Bonaventura I, Matias-Guiu J, Cervera C, et al: Neuroacanthocytosis syndrome, apraxia of eyelid opening, and progressive supranuclear palsy, letter. *Neurology* 1986; 36:1276.

167. De Renzi E, Gentillini M, Bazolli C: Eyelid movement disorders and motor impersistence in acute hemisphere disease. *Neurology* 1986; 36:414–418.

168. Lepore FE: Bilateral cerebral ptosis. *Neurology* 1987; 37:1043–1046.

169. Lowenstein DH, Koch TK, Edwards MS: Cerebral ptosis with contralateral arteriovenous malformation: A report of two cases. *Ann Neurol* 1987; 21:404–407.

170. Rafal RD, Laxer KD, Janowsky JS: Seizures triggered by blinking in a non-photosensitive epileptic. *J Neurol Neurosurg Psychiatry* 1986; 49:445–447.

171. Krohel GB, Rosenberg PN: Oscillopsia associated with eyelid myokymia. *Am J Ophthalmol* 1986; 102:662–663.

172. Bettoni L, Bortone E, Ghizzoni P, et al: Myokymia in the course of Bell's palsy: An electromyographic study. *J Neurol Sci* 1988; 84:69–76.

173. Brick JF, Gutmann L, Brick J, et al: Timber rattlesnake venom–induced myokymia: Evidence for peripheral nerve origin. *Neurology* 1987; 37:1545–1546.

174. Scaioli V, Savoiardo M, Bussone G, et al: Brain-stem auditory evoked potentials (BAEPs) and magnetic resonance imaging (MRI) in a case of facial myokymia. *Electroencephalogr Clin Neurophysiol* 1988; 71:153–156.

175. Merchut MP, Biller J, Brumlik J, et al: Isolated facial myokymia and facial contracture: Computed tomography and magnetic resonance imaging correlation. *J Clin Neuro Ophthalmol* 1985; 5:120–123.

176. Sandyk R: Facial myokymia: A false localizing sign in obstructive communicating hydrocephalus: A case report. *Eur Neurol* 1985; 24:112–114.

177. Lepore FE: Unilateral ptosis and Herring's law. *Neurology* 1988; 38:319–322.

178. Kansu T, Subutay N: Lid retraction in myasthenia gravis. *J Clin Neurol Ophthalmol* 1987; 7:145–150.

179. Komiyama A, Hirayama K: Paradoxical reversal of ptosis in myasthenia gravis by edrophonium administration (letter). *J Neurol Neurosurg Psychiatry* 1988; 51:315.

180. Wesley RE, Bond JB: Upper eyelid retraction from inferior rectus restriction in dysthyroid orbit disease. *Ann Ophthalmol* 1987; 19:34–36, 40.

181. Sethi KD, Rivner MH, Swift TR: Ice pack test for myasthenia gravis. *Neurology* 1987; 37:1383–1385.

182. Naguib KK: Hypertelorism, proptosis, ptosis, polysyndactyly, hypospadias and normal height in three sibs: A new syndrome? *Am J Med Genet* 1988; 29:35–41.

183. Cohen SM, Nelson LB: Aniridia with congenital ptosis and glaucoma: A family study. *Ann Ophthalmol* 1988; 20:53–57.

184. Baraitser M, Winter RM: Iris coloboma, ptosis, hypertelorism, and mental retardation: A new syndrome. *J Med Genet* 1988; 25:41–43.

185. Oley C, Baraitser M: Blepharophimosis, ptosis, epicanthus inversus syndrome (BPES syndrome). *J Med Genet* 1988; 25:47–51.

186. Cornel G, Sharratt GP, Virmani S, et al: Familial coarctation of the aortic arch with bilateral ptosis: A new syndrome? 1987; 22:724–726.

187. Meire F, Standaert L, DeLaey JJ, et al: Waardenburg syndrome, Hirschsprung megacolon, and Marcus Gunn ptosis. *Am J Med Genet* 1987; 27:683–686.

188. Betharia SM, Kumar S: Levator sling for Marcus Gunn ptosis. *Br J Ophthalmol* 1987; 71:685–689.

189. Neuhaus RW: Eyelid suspension with a transposed levator palpebrae superioris muscle. *Am J Ophthalmol* 1985; 100:308–311.

190. Pang MP, Zweibach PH, Goodwin J: Inherited levator-medial rectus synkinesis. *Arch Ophthalmol* 1986; 104:1489–1491.

191. Rice CD, Weaver RG, Benjamin E, et al: Unilateral blepharoptosis with synkinetic movements of the eyelids on horizontal gaze. *J Pediatr Ophthalmol Strabismus* 1986; 23:201–205.

192. Bonham RD, Iliff WJ, Stark WJ, et al: Ptosis following refractive corneal surgery: Case report. *Arch Ophthalmol* 1987; 105:25.

193. Linberg JV, McDonald MB, Safir A, et al: Ptosis following radial keratotomy performed using a rigid eyelid speculum. *Ophthalmology* 1986; 93:1509–1512.

194. Gonnering RS, Sonneland PR: Ptosis and dermatochalasis as presenting signs in a case of occult primary systemic amyloidosis (AL). *Ophthalmic Surg* 1987; 18:495–497.

195. Malone TJ, Nerad JA: The surgical treatment of blepharoptosis in oculomotor nerve palsy. *Am J Ophthalmol* 1988; 105:57–64.

196. Lane CM, Collin JR: Treatment of ptosis in chronic progressive external ophthalmoplegia. *Br J Ophthalmol* 1987; 71:290–294.

197. Olenius M, Nylen B: Ocular myopathy with palpebral ptosis. *Ann Plast Surg* 1987; 19:146–153.

198. Linberg JV, Vasquez RJ, Gung-Mei C: Aponeurotic ptosis repair under local anesthesia: Prediction of results from operative lid height. *Ophthalmology* 1988; 95:1046–1052.

199. Jordan DR, Anderson RL: A simple procedure for adjusting eyelid position after aponeurotic ptosis surgery. *Arch Ophthalmol* 1987; 105:1288–1291.

200. Karesh JW, Putterman AM: Correction of postoperative eyelid retraction with a simplified levator palpebrae superioris (LPS) muscle recession: Analysis of a 10-year experience. *Ophthalmic Surg* 1987; 18:815–820.

201. Thaller VT, Kaden K, Lane CM, et al: Thyroid lid surgery. *Eye* 1987; 1:609–614.

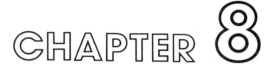

CHAPTER 8

Cerebral Control of Smooth Pursuit and Optokinetic Nystagmus

Ronald J. Tusa, M.D., Ph.D.
Department of Neurology, The Johns Hopkins University School of Medicine, Baltimore, Maryland

David S. Zee, M.D.
Departments of Neurology and Ophthalmology, The Johns Hopkins University School of Medicine, Baltimore, Maryland

Our knowledge of the cerebral control of smooth visual tracking systems has burgeoned in the last decade. In this chapter we will discuss how smooth pursuit is mediated by specific areas in the occipito-temporal and frontal cortex. We will then discuss how the visual-tracking capabilities of the subcortical optokinetic system found in subprimates have been expanded in primates via cerebral cortical mechanisms. We will also describe a newly discovered large-field short-latency (approximately 70 msec) visual-tracking system found in primates.

SMOOTH PURSUIT

Functional Description

Smooth pursuit eye movements are slow-phase tracking movements that maintain images of small moving targets on the fovea whether the head is stationary or

Curr Neuro Ophthalmol 2:115–146, 1989
© 1989, Year Book Medical Publishers, Inc.
0893–0147/89/02-115-146-$04.00

moving. The latter is called vestibulo-ocular reflex (VOR) cancellation. Three different types of signals about target motion may serve as stimuli to pursuit: retinal-position error (target position minus eye position), retinal-velocity error (target velocity minus eye velocity), and retinal-acceleration error (target acceleration minus eye acceleration). Initiation of pursuit primarily depends on a retinal-velocity and a retinal-acceleration error signal, whereas steady-state pursuit probably uses all three signals.

Figure 1 illustrates three different target trajectories that are used to assess initiation and steady-state smooth pursuit. Figure 1,A shows a Rashbass trajectory, which is the best stimulus to examine initiation of pursuit.[93] In this trajectory, the target is stepped away from the fixation point and ramped at a constant velocity back toward the fixation point such that the target crosses the fixation point within 100 to 200 msec of stimulus onset. The eye will begin to track the target smoothly without generating a saccadic eye movement. Figure 1,B shows a step-ramp tra-

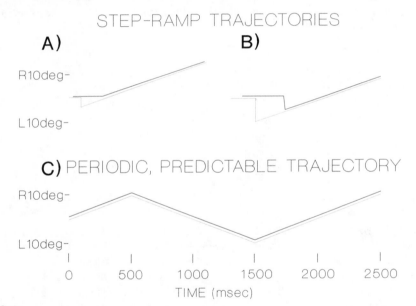

FIG 1.
Various types of target trajectories used to test smooth pursuit eye movements. Eye position is shown as a *solid line* and target position is shown as a *light dotted line*. In step-ramp trajectories **(A and B),** the target is stepped away from the fixation point and then ramped at a constant velocity. By allowing the target to cross the fixation point within 100 to 200 msec of stimulus onset, the eye will track the target smoothly without generating a saccadic eye movement **(A;** Rashbass trajectory). This is the preferred trajectory to examine initiation of pursuit. By stepping the target well into one visual hemifield before ramping it toward **(B)** or away from (not shown) the fixation point, a saccadic eye movement will be made followed by smooth pursuit. This type of trajectory is useful in testing initiation of pursuit within one visual hemifield. Periodic, predictable trajectories **(C)** should be used to examine steady-state pursuit and the use of prediction.

jectory in which the target is placed several degrees within one visual hemifield. This type of target trajectory is useful in assessing the accuracy of saccades and initiation of smooth pursuit to moving targets within one visual hemifield. Figure 1,C shows a periodic, predictable trajectory, which is useful for assessing steady-state pursuit and the ability to predict target motion. In this section the properties of initiation of pursuit and of steady-state pursuit will be described, then the role of predictability of target motion and visual attention in smooth pursuit will be discussed.

During pursuit initiation to a small target moving in an unpredictable Rashbass trajectory, the eye accelerates to a velocity that closely matches the velocity of the target. This initiation period of pursuit is primarily open loop, i.e., because of inherent delays in processing of visual information there is not enough time for any new retinal-velocity error information to be used to modify the initial eye acceleration. In both monkeys and humans, the initiation of pursuit consists of two distinct phases, an early phase and a late phase.[18, 60, 122] The early phase begins about 100 msec after the onset of target motion and continues for about 20 msec. Eye acceleration during the early phase is a constant 100 degrees/sec^2 that does not vary according to the brightness of the target or its velocity and location in the visual field. The late phase immediately follows the early phase and lasts about 80 msec. During this phase, eye acceleration ranges from 100 to 300 degrees/sec^2 and does vary according to the intensity of the target and its velocity and location in the visual field. Eye acceleration is highest for a bright target that starts within the central 6 degrees of the visual field and moves toward the center of gaze at a velocity of 90 degrees/sec. For a dim target, the optimal location in the visual field for eliciting maximum eye acceleration is the same as that for a bright target, but the preferred target speed is only 30-45 degrees/sec.

Steady-state pursuit follows the initiation period of pursuit for targets moving at a constant velocity. During steady-state pursuit, eye velocity can be altered both by retinal-position and by retinal-velocity errors.[18, 82, 90] During steady-state pursuit, eye velocity can reach values as high as 60 degrees/sec to targets moving in a nonpredictable step-ramp trajectory (unpublished results, 1988).

Steady-state pursuit can continue even when the visual target is turned off. When a subject tries to continue to pursue a target after it disappears, the eye continues to move at a velocity that is about 50% of the previous eye speed, and that value can be maintained for several seconds.[7] It has been suggested that this residual eye velocity is due to prediction of target movement. This predictive behavior in the smooth pursuit system may also relate to the generation of smooth pursuit eye movements to predictable targets without a time delay[65] and to the generation of anticipatory smooth pursuit eye movements.[9, 49] During smooth pursuit of a target moving in a periodic, predictable trajectory, eye accelerations and velocities can reach values as high as 1,250 degrees/sec^2 and 150 degrees/sec, respectively, and pursuit of the target is significantly improved compared with pursuit of targets moving in a nonpredictable trajectory.[58, 76] Peak eye velocities to a target moved

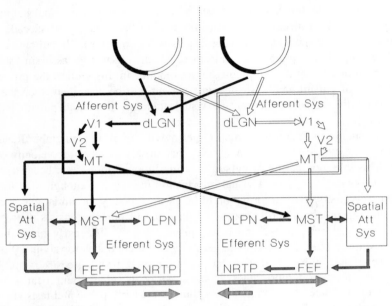

FIG 2.
Schematic diagram illustrating the cerebral systems believed to be involved in smooth pursuit eye movements in the monkey. A cortical afferent system *(Sys)* includes a projection from the dorsolateral geniculate nucleus *(dLGN)* to striate cortex *(V1)* to the middle temporal area *(MT)* directly and indirectly via prestriate cortex *(V2)*. This system processes information about target motion in the contralateral visual field. In the schematic, the regions and pathways mediating motion information from the right and left visual hemifields are outlined by thick black lines and open double lines, respectively. The cortical efferent system includes a projection from the medial superior temporal area *(MST)* to the dorsolateral pontine nucleus *(DLPN),* and probably a projection from the frontal eye field *(FEF)* to the nucleus reticularis tegmenti pontis *(NRTP)*. The bidirectional arrow below the box enclosing each cortical efferent system indicates the relative extent each hemisphere mediates smooth pursuit eye movements in the horizontal direction. The cortical efferent system in each hemisphere receives a projection from both the ipsilateral and contralateral cortical afferent systems. The spatial attention *(Att)* system includes areas within prefrontal and posterior parietal cortex. It interacts with the cortical afferent and efferent systems. See text for details. (Adapted from Tusa RJ, Ungerleider LG: Fiber pathways of cortical areas mediating smooth pursuit eye movements in monkeys. *Ann Neurol* 1988; 23:174–183.)

once across the screen at a constant velocity can reach values as high as 100 degrees/sec when the subject knows the direction and the time of onset of the upcoming target.[75]

Smooth pursuit in the laboratory is generally examined in a relatively sterile visual environment. The normal visual environment, though, is complex, with stimuli of different size, shape, color, and brightness moving in different directions at different speeds. Accordingly, a spatially selective system is needed to focus attention to one stimulus. Such a system must be able to engage or disengage the pursuit system for stimuli at any location in the visual field. Furthermore, as a consequence of generating smooth pursuit eye movements to a moving target in an otherwise stationary visual environment, there is motion on the retina of the background that occurs in the direction opposite to the pursuit eye movement. There must be a mechanism to prevent the large-field tracking systems from stabilizing the eyes, which would oppose smooth pursuit eye movements.

Pathophysiology

The cerebral cortical control of smooth pursuit eye movements can be divided into cortical afferent, efferent, and spatial attention systems. These systems are

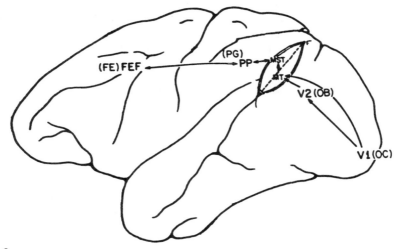

FIG 3.
Lateral view of the monkey brain illustrating the location and connections of cortical areas believed to be involved in smooth pursuit eye movements. The locations of these cortical areas are based on electrophysiologic studies. The cytoarchitectonically defined areas of Von Bonin and Bailey[127] that best correspond to these functional areas are enclosed in parentheses. A portion of the superior temporal sulcus (containing middle temporal *[MT]* and medial superior temporal *[MST]* areas) has been spread apart, and the fundus of this sulcus is represented as a dashed line. The functional divisions of monkey cortex correspond better to the Von Bonin and Bailey cytoarchitectonic areas than to the more familiar visual areas of Brodmann[13] (areas 17 through 21). *FEF* = frontal eye field; *PP* = posterior parietal; *V2* = prestriate cortex; *V1* = striate cortex. *FE, PG, OB,* and *OC* are abbreviations for German terms described by Von Economo.[128] They will assist the reader in identifying corresponding areas in the monkey brain and the human brain (see Fig 4). (Adapted from Tusa RJ: Cortical control of eye movements, in Kennard C, Clifford Rose F (eds): *Physiological Aspects of Clinical Neuro-Ophthalmology.* London, Chapman & Hall, 1988, pp 249–264.)

schematized in Figure 2, and the location of the cortical areas contained within these systems in the monkey brain is shown in Figure 3. These cortical areas include striate cortex (V1), prestriate cortex (V2), middle temporal (MT) area, medial superior temporal (MST) area, posterior parietal (PP) area, and frontal eye field (FEF). These cortical areas have been identified based primarily on neurophysiologic criteria.[67]

There is some evidence that the human brain contains areas homologous to these cortical areas in the monkey brain. First, areas V1, V2, MT, MST, PP, and FEF in the monkey brain correspond to areas defined cytoarchitectonically by Von Bonin and Bailey[127] (see Fig 3), which were originally based on the cytoarchitectonic areas in the human brain defined by Von Economo[128] (Fig 4). Second, specific regions in these cytoarchitectonic areas in the human brain have increased blood flow during the generation of smooth pursuit eye movements. These include striate cortex (corresponding to V1 in the monkey), an adjacent prestriate cortical area (V2?), a lateral area in temporo-occipital cortex (MST?), and a region in parieto-occipital cortex (PP?).[77] The area in temporo-occipital cortex is adjacent to an area selectively activated by a low-contrast set of moving dots, which is thought to be the homologue of area MT in the monkey.[78]

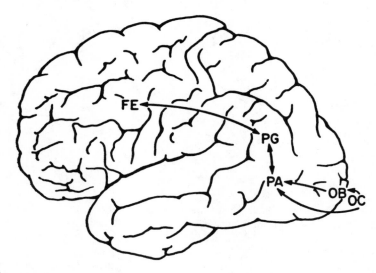

FIG 4.
Cytoarchitectonically defined cortical areas in the human brain (Von Economo[128]) that correspond to the cytoarchitectonically defined areas in the monkey brain shown in Fig 3. Based on the myelination pattern, portions of *PA* in the human brain may be the homologue to middle temporal and medial superior temporal areas in the monkey brain. The anatomic connections among the cortical areas are based on connections described in the monkey brain. (Adapted from Tusa RJ: Cortical control of eye movement, in Kennard C, Clifford Rose F (eds): *Physiological Aspects of Clinical Neuro-Ophthalmology*. London, Chapman & Hall, 1988, pp 249–264.)

Cortical Afferent System

Anatomy and Physiology.—The major afferent stimulus for smooth pursuit eye movements is the motion of an image of the target across the retina. Perception of motion is mediated by a neural pathway separate from that which mediates perception of color and shape.[24, 61, 67] The motion pathway begins with large-cell, β-retinal–ganglion neurons. These cells receive converging input from all three types of cone receptors, and so they are color nonspecific. These retinal-ganglion neurons in turn project to the magnocellular layers of the dorsal lateral geniculate nucleus (dLGN; layers 1 and 2), which in turn project to layer 4Cα in cortical area V1. Layer 4B of V1 in turn projects directly to cortical area MT and indirectly to MT via the thick cytochrome oxidase stripe regions of cortical area V2. Most of the neurons within area MT have receptive fields located within the central 10 degrees of the visual field and prefer stimulus velocities of about 30 degrees/sec (at moderate target intensities).[68] These physiologic features coincide with the location and velocity of visual targets that are optimal for initiating smooth pursuit. Neurons within V1, V2, and MT encode the direction and the velocity of targets moving within the contralateral visual field. All directions of motion are represented within these cortical areas in each hemisphere. Further processing of motion perception is mediated in cortical areas MST and PP, but the receptive fields in these two areas are extremely large and include portions of both visual hemifields.

At successive stages of the cortical pathway from V1 to PP cortex, the physiologic properties of neurons change in two major ways. First, neurons process more complex features of target motion.[23, 67] For example, cells in striate cortex only encode motion of stimuli in the frontal plane, cells in area MT encode stimulus motion in three dimensions, cells in area MST encode motion of objects rotating in space, and cells in area PP encode the visual motion encountered during movement through the environment (optic flow). Second, complex interactions occur between the receptive field center and the receptive field periphery in neurons within areas MT, MST, and PP.[2, 48, 67] For example, if within the center of a receptive field a small target is moved in one direction while within the periphery of the receptive field a large target is moved in the opposite direction—precisely the condition that occurs during smooth pursuit of a small target in a visually textured environment—the neural activity of certain neurons in areas MT, MST, and PP is either further enhanced or suppressed.

Stereopsis and visual information used to encode target location within craniotopic (head-referenced) space is also processed in the cortical pathway from V1 to PP.[24, 61, 126] In contrast, color and shape perception is processed in a cortical projection system consisting of V1, V2, V4 (prestriate cortex), and inferior temporal cortex sequentially interconnected by white matter "U" fibers.[119, 126] This anatomic segregation of different perceptual functions provides the substrate for selective deficits following focal cortical lesions.

Lesions.—*V1 Acute Deficits.*—Unilateral ablation of V1 results in a hemifield visual defect contralateral to the lesion, and all visual perceptual functions are lost within the defective portion of the visual field. This is expected since information used for all types of visual perceptual functions are first processed in V1 before being distributed to specific areas in parietal and temporal cortex. Because a unilateral lesion in V1 only causes a visual afferent defect, there is no impairment in the ability to initiate smooth pursuit eye movements as long as the target is stepped into and moved within the intact visual hemifield.[99, 113] This is best examined with step-ramp trajectories in which the target is stepped 5-10 degrees into the visual field and then ramped at about 15 degrees/sec toward or away from the fixation point (Fig 5,A and B). Once the eye moves to the target, steady-state pursuit is normal in both horizontal directions to targets moving in both step-ramp and periodic, predictable trajectories.[99, 113]

Several mechanisms may account for the preserved ability to generate normal steady-state pursuit, even with a complete hemianopia, including the use of prediction of target trajectory and the use of a region of macular sparing in the visual

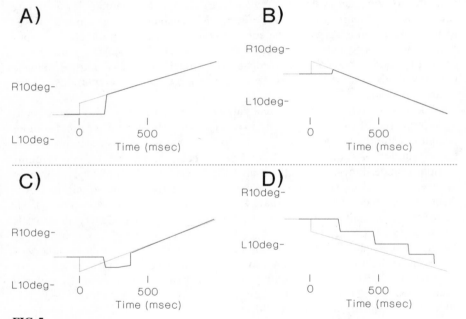

FIG 5.
Schematic of horizontal visual-tracking eye movements to a target moved in a step-ramp trajectory in a monkey several months following a unilateral right-sided striate cortex ablation. Eye position is shown as a *solid line* and target position is shown as a *light dotted line*. Targets stepped into the intact field and then ramped either to the left or right elicit accurate saccades followed by normal smooth pursuit **(A and B).** The first saccade to targets stepped into the defective field is either hypermetric or hypometric for targets moving toward or away from the fixation point, respectively **(C and D).** No smooth pursuit follows the first saccade. These findings are consistent with a retinotopic defect for initiation of pursuit for targets stepped into the defective visual field.

field to prevent the target from disappearing in the defective visual field even when small retinal-position errors occur. We have found a region of macular sparing in monkeys with complete V1 ablations and in hemidecorticate monkeys.[120] This region extends about 1.5 degrees into the defective visual field, and targets confined to this region will elicit smooth pursuit eye movements with velocities up to 60 degrees/sec. This area of macular sparing is due to the presence of retinal-ganglion cells in the nasal hemiretina of each eye that project to the ipsilateral instead of the contralateral dLGN.[15, 57] Macular sparing has also been described in human patients following occipital lobectomies,[37] but studies have not determined whether visual information from this region can be used to generate smooth pursuit eye movements.

V1 Chronic Deficits.—Following unilateral V1 lesions, monkeys recover the ability to detect target lights and generate saccades to targets in their defective visual field, but they do not appear to recover motion perception in the defective visual field.[81, 99] Consequently, stationary targets stepped into the defective visual field elicit an accurate saccadic eye movement, but targets stepped into and then moved within the defective visual field elicit an inaccurate saccade and no smooth pursuit. For targets stepped into the defective field and moved toward the fixation point, the saccade is hypermetric, and for targets stepped into the defective field and moved away from the fixation point, the saccade is hypometric (see Fig 5,C and D). Recovery of the ability to use retinal-position errors to generate accurate saccadic eye movements in destriated monkeys appears to be mediated by an extrastriate pathway to the superior colliculus, as no recovery occurs following hemidecortication, and no recovery occurs following sequential V1 and superior collicular lesions.[81, 120] We have found that hemidecorticate monkeys will often initiate low acceleration eye movements to targets stepped into and ramped within the defective field, but we believe these are predictive pursuit eye movements triggered by the offset of the fixation point and not pursuit eye movements guided by the motion of the target (unpublished observation, 1988). Eye acceleration did not depend on the velocity of the target, and the direction of pursuit initiation was the same whether the target was moving toward or away from the fixation point.

Monkeys with bilateral V1 lesions do recover smooth pursuit eye movements in contrast to monkeys with unilateral V1 lesions.[135] Within several months of a bilateral occipital lobectomy, monkeys are able to initiate and maintain smooth pursuit eye movements to small targets moved in both a step-ramp and a periodic, predictable trajectory, though many of the features of these eye movements are abnormal. Pursuit latencies during initiation are increased twofold to threefold, and there are low-frequency, sinusoidal oscillations and erratic fluctuations in eye velocity. We speculate that these animals are using an extrastriate source for motion perception that is imprecise in coding target velocity. In addition, we believe the monkeys are extensively relying on prediction of target motion. They frequently made brief smooth eye movements that were in the correct direction but with a velocity and trajectory that only roughly approximated that of the target.

Why are there such differences in the recovery of pursuit between monkeys with unilateral and those with bilateral loss of striate cortex? Perhaps the development of alternative sources of afferent information for the generation of smooth tracking is stimulated when the pursuit pathways have been completely deafferented from striate cortex. With a unilateral striate lesion, the actual time when there is any stimulus (or need) for adaptation is minimal since saccadic eye movements quickly bring the image of the target into the intact visual field.

Two preliminary reports suggest that some patients with unilateral striate cortical or optic radiation lesions can initiate smooth pursuit to targets stepped into and then moved within the defective field.[83, 123] It is not clear whether these patients are actually using target motion mediated by an extrastriate pathway to initiate pursuit or whether they are using predictive pursuit eye movements triggered by the offset of the fixation point similar to what we found in hemidecorticate monkeys. It is also controversial whether patients with visual field deficits recover any motion perception. Riddoch[95] described a group of patients with either unilateral or bilateral visual field deficits from occipital lobe trauma that were able to perceive targets and occasionally identify them if they were moving but not if they were stationary. This has become known as the Riddoch phenomenon. We have found no evidence of motion perception using the brightest and largest target of the Goldmann perimeter in a group of patients who had unilateral occipital lobectomies at least 2 years previously (unpublished findings, 1988). Perhaps the Riddoch phenomenon is due to incomplete involvement of striate cortex requiring patients to use relative movement of the object against its background to enhance figure-ground discrimination. The surround antagonism properties found in neurons within the motion perception pathway are ideal for this kind of visual discrimination.[2]

MT Acute Deficits.—A unilateral lesion in area MT in monkeys does not cause a homonymous hemianopia but does cause a selective defect in perception of motion in the contralateral visual field.[86] Unilateral MT lesions also result in visual tracking deficits resembling those following chronic unilateral V1 lesion. Accurate visually guided saccades are made to stationary targets in the contralateral visual field, but saccades to targets moving in any direction within the contralateral visual field are inaccurate because the speed of the target is not taken into account when the saccade is generated.[87] In addition, initiation of smooth pursuit is normal for targets in the intact visual field but is impaired for targets moving in any direction in the defective visual hemifield, i.e., the smooth pursuit deficit is retinotopic in nature. A similar retinotopic deficit in smooth pursuit with preservation of saccades to stationary targets has been described in patients with a unilateral occipito-temporal lobe lesion.[83, 113]

MT Chronic Deficits.—One week following unilateral MT lesions, monkeys completely recover perception of motion and their ability to pursue moving targets accurately.[86, 87] The basis for this recovery may be sparing of parts of MT that can assume the function of the ablated portion, or the use of other cortical pathways to area MST such as area V4 in prestriate cortex or area STP in the superior temporal sulcus.[67]

Cortical Efferent System

Anatomy and Physiology.—The cortical efferent system for generating smooth pursuit eye movements in the monkey includes an ipsilateral projection from the MST area to the dorsolateral pontine nucleus (DLPN), and possibly a parallel projection from the FEF to the nucleus reticularis tegmenti pontis (NRTP) (see Fig 2). Areas MST and DLPN have received the most detailed investigation. Neurons in these two areas encode both target velocity and smooth pursuit eye velocity.[47, 84, 88, 110, 112] All directions appear to be represented for both the target velocity and the smooth pursuit eye velocity signals (in area MST there may be a slight predominance of cells for the ipsilateral direction within each hemisphere for both of these signals). The smooth pursuit eye velocity signal in these two areas is not thought to be a "motor command signal" to generate smooth pursuit eye movements, as the vast majority of neurons encoding this signal discharge after the initiation of smooth pursuit. Instead, it is believed these neurons are encoding a signal representing target velocity in space by adding the retinal-velocity error signal from area MT to an eye velocity signal coming from some other source. This concept is consistent with the finding that microstimulation of areas MST and DLPN does not initiate pursuit but does change eye velocity during steady-state pursuit.[46, 70]

Less is known about areas FEF and NRTP with respect to smooth pursuit. Neurons within these two areas encode smooth pursuit eye velocity but do not encode target motion for small targets.[14, 44, 80] Microstimulation of the FEF in monkeys initiates ipsilateral smooth pursuit,[64] but further studies are needed to determine whether neurons in the FEF are encoding a "motor command signal" to generate smooth pursuit eye movements.

We have suggested that the projections from MST to DLPN, and from FEF to NRTP, form two parallel cortical efferent pursuit pathways, although there are a number of other potential cortical pathways to the pons that could mediate smooth pursuit. Area DLPN receives projections from all of the cortical areas within the motion perception system (V1, V2, MT, MST, and PP) and also receives a minor projection from the FEF.[11, 54, 69, 118, 125]

Based on physiologic and lesion studies, the remaining pursuit pathway appears to involve the flocculus and posterior vermis of the cerebellum.[43, 59, 109, 136] These cerebellar regions each receive projections from DLPN and NRTP and in turn project to the oculomotor nuclei via the vestibular nuclei.[12, 50, 51, 132]

Lesions.—*MST and FEF Acute Deficits.*—A unilateral lesion in area MST in monkeys causes a directional defect in pursuit for targets moving toward the side of the lesion regardless of the visual field in which the target was initially stepped into (Fig 6,A and C).[25, 26] This directional defect occurs for both initiation of pursuit and steady-state pursuit. The gain (eye velocity/target velocity) during steady-state pursuit is reduced to 0.5. In addition, a unilateral MST lesion causes a retinotopic defect in pursuit for targets stepped into and moved within the visual field contralateral to the lesion (see Fig 6,C and D). In patients, unilateral lesions in occipito-temporal cortex, which may contain the homologue to area

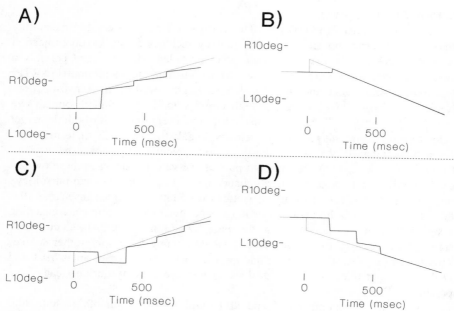

FIG 6.
Schematic of horizontal visual-tracking eye movements to a target moved in a step-ramp trajectory in a monkey 1 day following a right-sided medial superior temporal area lesion. Targets stepped into the intact field elicit accurate saccades but decreased pursuit eye velocity when the target is moved toward the side of the lesion **(A)**, and accurate saccades and pursuit when the target is moved away from the side of the lesion **(B)**. Targets stepped into the defective visual field elicit inaccurate saccades similar to those after a striate cortex lesion **(C and D)**, impaired initiation and steady-state pursuit toward the side of the lesion **(C)**, and impaired initiation but normal steady-state pursuit away from the side of the lesion **(D)**. These findings are consistent with a directional defect for initiation and steady-state pursuit for targets moving toward the side of the lesion, and a retinotopic defect for initiation of pursuit for targets stepped into the contralateral visual field.

MST in the monkey, impair smooth pursuit eye movements similarly to MST lesions in monkeys.[83, 113]

Based on the neural signals processed within area MST, these pursuit deficits are possibly related to a reduction in perceived target velocity. Unfortunately, velocity discrimination has not yet been examined in monkeys with MST lesions. There is one report in human beings, though, in which both perceived target velocity and smooth pursuit eye velocity were measured following a bilateral occipito-temporal lobe lesion, and both were found to be significantly reduced.[137]

Why is there a reduction in smooth pursuit eye velocity in only one direction after a unilateral MST lesion when the proportion of neurons in area MST encoding ipsilateral target motion is only slightly greater than those encoding contralateral target motion? Perhaps the directional deficit occurs owing to the way area

MST neurons project to the cerebellum via DLPN. Although DLPN contains equal numbers of cells encoding ipsilateral and contralateral target motion, only cells encoding ipsilateral target motion may be projecting to the flocculus, a structure where primarily ipsilateral smooth pursuit eye velocity is encoded.[59, 130]

A unilateral lesion of the FEF in monkeys also reduces smooth pursuit eye velocity toward the side of the lesion,[42] and a bilateral lesion results in a severe deficit in both directions.[62] Unlike area MST lesions, FEF lesions do not cause a retinotopic defect in smooth pursuit, i.e., accurate saccades are still made to moving targets (J. C. Lynch, Ph.D., personal communication, 1988). Smooth pursuit deficits have also been reported to occur in patients with frontal lobe lesions.[92, 111]

We have found that hemidecortication in monkeys not only impairs steady-state pursuit toward the side of the lesion but also away from the side of the lesion and vertically.[121] For targets moving toward the side of the lesion or vertically at speeds ranging from 2 to 150 degrees/sec, only saccadic eye movements are used to track the target. For targets moving away from the side of the lesion, smooth pursuit is nearly normal for target speeds of 2 to 20 degrees/sec, but eye velocity does not exceed 20 degrees/sec for targets moving faster than this velocity. Large unilateral cortical lesions in human patients have also been reported to cause bilateral horizontal deficits in smooth pursuit.[8, 52] Based on these studies, it appears that the cortical efferent pursuit pathways within one hemisphere can mediate ipsilateral smooth pursuit at low velocities, but that the efferent pursuit pathways in both hemispheres are required to mediate smooth pursuit at high velocities in both horizontal directions and vertical smooth pursuit at all velocities.

In summary, areas FEF and MST appear to be part of two parallel cortical efferent systems. These two cortical areas may have different roles in the generation of smooth pursuit. We speculate that the FEF may be more involved in the generation of volitional pursuit, which does not necessarily rely on a moving visual stimulus as in predictive smooth pursuit or pursuit of a moving target that transiently disappears.[42, 135] In contrast, MST may be more involved in generating reflexive pursuit, in which a moving visual stimulus is always required to elicit smooth pursuit. This division of labor for the smooth pursuit system is analogous to that suggested for the saccade system.[120, 134]

MST and FEF Chronic Deficits.—The directional pursuit deficit following unilateral lesions in either MST or FEF recovers within several weeks in monkeys.[26, 42] This recovery may occur because the lesions are incomplete or because each cortical area can compensate for the other if damaged. Preliminary data suggest that cortical lesions involving both of these areas impair smooth pursuit much more than a lesion isolated to either area alone.[63] In addition, we found that a second-stage lesion in the FEF reinstated a severe pursuit deficit in a monkey that had previously recovered pursuit following a bilateral occipital lobectomy (unpublished result, 1987).

The directional pursuit deficit found horizontally and vertically following hemidecortication also recovers in 20 to 40 weeks in monkeys.[121] Within this period, normal steady-state pursuit eye velocities can be generated vertically and away from the side of the lesion, but maximum eye velocity only reaches 65% of its preoperative value toward the side of the lesion. These findings in hemidecorticate monkeys are qualitatively similar to the findings in patients studied several years following hemidecortication.[104, 116] This recovery in smooth pursuit eye velocity is probably mediated by cortex in the intact hemisphere, as smooth pursuit in patients with bilateral occipito-temporal cortical lesions is persistently impaired.[137]

Hemidecorticate monkeys also have a persistent spontaneous nystagmus that interferes with smooth pursuit. The slow phases of this nystagmus are directed away from the side of the lesion with a speed of 1 to 2 degrees/sec. Consequently, for targets moving away from the side of the lesion, eye velocity was slightly higher than target velocity, requiring small back-up saccades, and for targets moving toward the lesioned side eye velocity was slightly lower than target velocity, requiring small catch-up saccades. The origin of this spontaneous nystagmus is not clear, though it has been referred to as a "pursuit paretic nystagmus."[104] It is found in patients with pursuit deficits following hemidecortication or unilateral occipito-temporal lobe lesions.[56, 104] Alternatively, it may be due to a defect in the gaze-holding systems mediated by the optokinetic system, as lesions in subcortical structures mediating optokinetic nystagmus (OKN) also result in a similar nystagmus (see "Optokinetic Nystagmus" section).

Spatial Visual Attention

Anatomy and Physiology.—Several cortical areas, including the PP and the prefrontal cortex, have been implicated in mediating spatial visual attention.[74] Visually responsive cells in PP and prefrontal cortex encode the location of visual stimuli in a craniotopic (head-referenced) coordinate system.[3, 29] The neuronal response in these areas is enhanced if the visual stimulus is behaviorally significant to the animal.[16, 30, 131] In PP cortex this enhancement can occur even if there is just a shift of attention to the target without an actual eye movement. Neurons in both PP and prefrontal cortex increase their discharge during attentive fixation of a small target.[4, 96, 108] This "attentive fixation" response has an orbital position component; neural activity increases with eccentricity from midline in one direction and decreases with eccentricity in the other.

Part of the cortical system mediating spatial visual attention is interposed between the cortical afferent and cortical efferent systems mediating smooth pursuit (see Fig 2). Posterior parietal cortex receives a projection from MT and projects to both MST and the FEF.[6, 89, 100, 124] Thus, there is both a direct pathway from the cortical afferent to the cortical efferent pursuit areas and an indirect pathway between these two areas via a cortical spatial attention area. Whether smooth pursuit uses the direct or the indirect pathway or both may depend on the nature of the stimulus. For moving stimuli that occupy much of the visual field, the subject need not selectively attend to the stimulus to the exclusion of other stimuli to generate smooth tracking eye movements.[36] Thus, the attentional system may be bypassed with this stimulus. For small moving targets, by contrast, the subject must attend to a particular target to generate smooth pursuit eye movements.

Lesions.—Patients with hemispatial neglect from unilateral parieto-occipital lobe lesions can generate smooth pursuit and optokinetic slow-phase eye movements directed away from the side of the lesion, but these eye movements do not initially enter into contralateral hemispace.[8, 73, 94] This deficit is thus a spatial defect and is distinct from both the retinotopic and the directional defects in visual tracking described above. We speculate that spatial deficits in smooth pursuit are due to dysfunction in directing visual attention.

More detailed information concerning spatial defects in smooth pursuit and in OKN is known for monkeys. In hemidecorticated monkeys, steady-state pursuit to any size target and slow phases of OKN are generated away from the side of the lesion, but the eyes will not enter into contralateral hemispace during the initial postoperative period. This spatial deficit is in register with the head (craniotopic) and not with the body (somatotopic), i.e., eye movements stop at the midline of the head no matter where the head is positioned with respect to the body. Within one month after hemidecortication, monkeys make smooth pursuit eye movements 20 to 30 degrees into contralateral craniotopic space. This recovery may depend in part on the integrity of cerebral cortex in the intact hemisphere. After recovery of the gaze deviation from a unilateral prefrontal lobe lesion in monkeys or in patients, a subsequent frontal lobe lesion on the intact side results in a prolonged gaze deviation toward the side of the second lesion.[53, 106]

Disconnection Syndromes

Because of the extensive pathways interconnecting the cerebral areas involved in pursuit, smooth pursuit function is susceptible to white matter lesions. Retinotopic, directional, and spatial deficits can occur depending on whether the cortical afferent, cortical efferent, or spatial attention systems have been disconnected, respectively. The white matter pathways interconnecting the cerebral areas in each of these systems will be reviewed along with the smooth pursuit deficits that occur following disruption of these pathways.

Cortical Afferent System

In the monkey, striate cortex projects to area MT, and this area in turn projects to area MST via arcuate or "U" fibers traveling just underneath cerebral cortex (Fig 7).[118] Since smooth pursuit can be generated in any direction for targets located in either the left or right visual hemifields, the efferent pursuit pathway in each hemisphere must get information from both the ipsilateral and contralateral afferent systems. This transfer of information could be mediated via the ipsilateral and interhemispheric projections between MT and MST. The interhemispheric

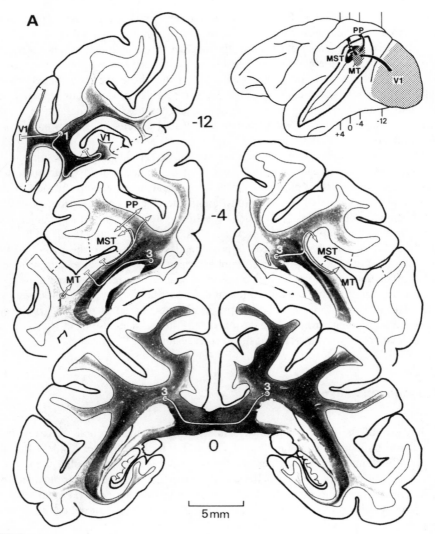

FIG 7.
A and B, summary diagrams schematically illustrating the major pathways interconnecting the areas in occipital cortex, parietal cortex, and the brain stem that are thought to be involved in smooth pursuit eye movements in the monkey. The numeral *1* in the myelin-stained coronal sections indicates arcuate fibers; *2* indicates fibers in the internal sagittal stratum; and *3* indicates fibers in the tapetum/major forceps. The origin of the fiber pathways is indicated by a bar within the cortex, whereas the termination is indicated by an arrowhead. *V1* = striate cortex; *MST* = medial superior temporal; *MT* = middle temporal; *PP* = posterior parietal; *Pul.* = pulvinar; *LTN* = lateral terminal nucleus; *DLPN* = dorsolateral pontine nucleus; *LPN* = lateral pontine nucleus. (Adapted from Tusa RJ, Ungerleider LG: Fiber pathways of cortical areas mediating smooth pursuit eye movements in monkeys. *Ann Neurol* 1988; 23:174–183.)

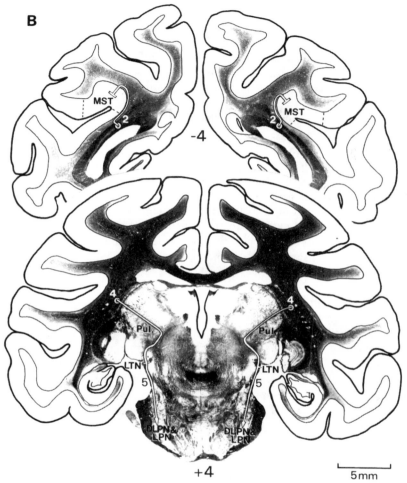

FIGURE 7 (cont.).

projections consist of fibers sequentially passing through the tapetum, major forceps, and the splenium of the corpus callosum. Because area MST is responsible for one direction of pursuit, disconnection of this area from area MT located in both hemispheres should result in a directional deficit in smooth pursuit similar to that produced by a focal lesion in MST. We have found such a deficit in monkeys following a unilateral lesion of striate cortex combined with transection of the splenium of the corpus callosum (unpublished data, 1988). Although area MT also projects to the FEF, the other cortical area throught to be involved in the efferent pursuit pathway, it is not yet known whether the FEF receives a bilateral projection from MT.

Cortical Efferent System

Area MST projects ipsilaterally to DLPN via the internal sagittal stratum, retrolenticular portion of the internal capsule, and cerebral peduncle (see Fig 7).[118] Presumably, a disconnection between MST and DLPN would also impair smooth pursuit, but this has not been specifically examined in the monkey. Brigell et al.[10] have reported a directional deficit in pursuit toward the side of the lesion in a patient with a small posterior thalamic hemorrhage, which they attributed to disruption of the corticofugal fibers passing through either the posterior thalamus or the adjacent retrolenticular portion of the internal capsule. This is the route by which area MST projects to the pontine nuclei. Sharpe and Deck[102] did not find a directional defect in smooth pursuit in a patient with an occipito-parietal hematoma involving the internal sagittal stratum. However, the lesion in their patient may have been located caudal to the critical portion of the pathway. The internal sagittal stratum runs from the most caudal part of the occipital horn to the posterior tip of the internal capsule and carries corticofugal fibers from several different cortical areas. To produce a directional pursuit deficit, a lesion in the internal sagittal stratum would have to disconnect the homologue of area MST from the brain stem.

Spatial Visual Attention System

Precisely which cerebral pathways are involved in mediating visual attention as it involves smooth pursuit is unknown. In monkeys it appears that striate cortex provides essential visual information to cerebral regions involved in visual attention via callosal pathways. Monkeys in which one cerebral hemisphere has been denied access to any information from striate cortex by virtue of a unilateral striate ablation plus corpus callosum splenial section show the same hemispatial deficits for smooth pursuit and OKN as do hemidecorticate monkeys (unpublished finding, 1988).

Basal Ganglia

Patients with basal ganglia disease also have deficits in smooth pursuit eye movements. Pursuit gain to targets moving in periodic, predictable trajectories is significantly reduced in patients with progressive supranuclear palsy and in advanced cases of Huntington's disease.[22, 55, 115] Advanced cases of Parkinson's disease also have decreased pursuit gain to targets moving in a sine-wave trajectory at high frequencies.[103, 105]

It is not known why patients with basal ganglia disease have pursuit deficits. Smooth pursuit eye movements to targets moving in a step-ramp trajectory have not yet been examined in these patients to determine whether they have a retinotopic or a directional pursuit deficit. It is possible that the pursuit deficit they have is not mediated by one of the pathways discussed previously but rather by a parallel pathway through the basal ganglia. In addition to a direct projection from

FEF to NRTP, the FEF also projects to NRTP via a basal ganglia circuit: FEF–caudate nucleus–substantia nigra pars reticulata–pedunculopontine nucleus pars compacta–DLPN.[1, 27] An analogous basal ganglia pathway plays a vital role in saccadic eye movements.[134]

Clinical Implications

Different aspects of the pursuit system can be tested by using targets moving in Rashbass trajectories, step-ramp trajectories confined to one visual hemifield, and periodic, predictable trajectories. Nonpredictable Rashbass trajectories are the best stimuli to examine initiation of pursuit. The eye movements generated during the first 100 msec of pursuit initiation are primarily open loop and so they are uncontaminated by visual feedback and visual prediction. Consequently, this target trajectory also gives the best assessment of pursuit function. Maximum eye acceleration during initiation of pursuit ranges from 100 to 300 degrees/sec^2 depending on the intensity of the target and the velocity and location of the target in the visual field. Maximum eye velocity during a Rashbass trajectory is about 50 degrees/sec. Nonpredictable step-ramp trajectories are the best stimuli to examine smooth pursuit of targets confined to one visual hemifield. During smooth pursuit of targets moving in periodic, predictable trajectories, eye accelerations can reach values as high as 1,250 degrees/sec,^{2} and peak eye velocities to predictable ramp stimuli can reach values as high as 100 degrees/sec. These high eye accelerations and velocities are partially due to the use of prediction, which greatly increases the visual tracking ability.

By determining whether the pursuit defect is retinotopic, directional, or spatial, one can roughly localize the lesion. A retinotopic defect occurs following a lesion within the cerebral afferent system, which includes areas V1, V2, MT, MST, and the arcuate fibers in the white matter that interconnect these areas. A directional defect occurs following a lesion within the cerebral efferent system, which includes two parallel systems: area MST projections to DLPN and area FEF projections to NRTP. Since an area MST lesion causes both a retinotopic and a directional defect, whereas an FEF lesion is only known to cause a directional deficit, one should be able to determine which of these two regions is involved in patients with directional pursuit deficits. A spatial defect occurs following a unilateral lesion within the cerebral attention system, which includes PP and prefrontal cortex.

OPTOKINETIC NYSTAGMUS

Functional Description

Optokinetic nystagmus consists of slow-phase eye movements generated in the direction of a moving visual stimulus and quick-phase eye movements generated in the opposite direction. The optokinetic system works synergistically with the vestibular system to generate compensatory slow phases during self-rotation. The purpose of these eye movements is to stabilize images of the visual environment on the retina during head movements.

The slow phases of optokinetic nystagmus (OKN) in primates consists of two components, an immediate component and a velocity-storage component. In monkeys, the characteristics of these two components are most clearly revealed in response to a full-field optokinetic drum suddenly rotated around the animal at a constant velocity. In response to this stimulus, slow-phase eye movements are immediately generated, reaching a velocity of about 50% of drum velocity (immediate component). This component is thought to be generated by either the smooth pursuit system or some other ocular following system such as a large-field short-latency visual-tracking system recently described in monkeys and human subjects.[19, 79] This is an involuntary response with an extremely short latency (50 msec in monkeys and 75 msec in human subjects). This response is elicited by movement of the entire visual scene, although it is optimally excited by a large moving stimulus (40 degrees across) with the background moving in the opposite direction. It has been suggested that this system is using parallax cues to help individuals moving in space to stabilize eyes on nearby passing objects.

Following the immediate response to an optokinetic drum, slow-phase eye velocity gradually increases to equal drum velocity. This slow rise reflects the velocity-storage component of OKN. The velocity-storage component is thought to be mediated by visual input into a vestibular-optokinetic velocity-storage neural integrator in the brain stem.[20] If during OKN the lights illuminating the drum are then turned off, nystagmus continues but slow-phase eye velocity gradually decays to zero. This is called optokinetic after-nystagmus (OKAN). The slow phases of OKAN are the best measure of the contribution of the velocity-storage system to OKN.

In human beings, the immediate component plays a more important role in the generation of OKN. The slow-phase eye velocity generated by the velocity-storage system, as revealed by OKAN, is variable even in the same subject.[114] The velocity-storage component is perhaps best quantitated by measuring OKAN in successive, brief periods of darkness during the optokinetic response.[98] This procedure reveals a slow rise in slow-phase eye velocity that peaks in the range of 10-20 degrees/sec.[114] Although the velocity-storage system in human subjects saturates at a much lower value than in monkeys, the shape of the retinal-slip nonlinearity, as reflected in the value of OKAN as a function of retinal-slip velocity, is similar. The peak value of OKAN is reached with retinal-slip velocities in the range of 40 to 120 degrees/sec.[28]

Effects of Fixation and Attention on OKN and OKAN

For OKN drum speeds ranging from 10 to 180 degrees/sec, the maximum eye velocity that can be reached is about 60 degrees/sec when the subject does not try actively to pursue the pattern on the OKN drum.[36] Maximum eye velocity increases to about 100 degrees/sec if the subject tries to pursue each pattern on the drum. This increase in slow-phase eye velocity is due to an increase in the immediate component of OKN (unpublished results, 1986). These results are most easily explained if the smooth pursuit system becomes fully engaged when the pattern of the OKN drum is actively fixated.

If the subject fixates a small stationary foveal target at the onset of optokinetic stimulation of the visual surround, the immediate component of OKN is reduced to zero.[28] Some charging of the velocity-storage system still occurs, as reflected in OKAN when the lights are turned out, but to a much smaller degree than when comparable degrees of retinal-slip are presented during active OKN. Thus, fixation of a stationary target prevents information about retinal-slip velocity from being relayed to the velocity-storage mechanism.

Anatomic and Physiologic Description

The cerebral circuit mediating the immediate component of OKN is unknown but most likely overlaps with the smooth pursuit system illustrated in Figure 2. Neurons in areas MT, MST, PP, and DLPN all respond to large targets; some even prefer large stimuli.[40, 48, 84, 112] Certain cells in PP discharge with latencies less than 50 msec to stimuli that elicit the large-field short-latency visual-tracking response.[41] In addition, lesions along the same cortical-subcortical pathway described for the pursuit system result in OKN deficits to a small hand-held drum in human patients.[45]

The cerebral circuit believed to be mediating the velocity-storage component of OKN in monkeys begins with a crossed retinal projection to the nucleus of the optic tract (NOT) and the dorsal terminal nucleus (DTN) of the accessory optic system.[35] (Fig 8) These two subcortical nuclei lie next to each other in the pretectal region of the midbrain near the brachium of the superior colliculus and may functionally represent the same structure. The role of this retinal projection to NOT/DTN in OKN is best appreciated in the Dutch-belted rabbit, a species in which OKN is generated exclusively by subcortical nuclei.[21] In this species of rabbit, neurons in the right NOT/DTN are only driven by retinal-slip velocity information from the left eye, and neurons in the left NOT/DTN are driven only by the right eye. Neurons in NOT/DTN have a baseline level of activity of about 20 spikes per second, and their activity is enhanced for temporal-to-nasal stimuli and inhibited for nasal-to-temporal stimuli. Thus, neurons in the right NOT/DTN are excited by retinal-slip directed to the right, and neurons in the left NOT/DTN are excited by retinal-slip directed to the left. Optimal activation is obtained for retinal-slip velocities of 0.1 to 20 degrees/sec. In this species, the OKN response to a constant-velocity rotating OKN drum shows no immediate tracking response, but rather a slow increase in slow-phase eye velocity that has a strong temporal-nasal asymmetry during monocular viewing. In species with binocular vision and better central vision, such as cats and monkeys, neurons in the right and left NOT/DTN are also excited only by retinal-slip directed to the left and right, respectively. In these species, though, neurons in NOT/DTN respond to retinal-slip velocities up to 100 degrees/sec and respond during stimulation of either eye.[31, 35] This improved response is thought to be mediated by a cerebral cortical projection to NOT/DTN. Behaviorally, this cortical input extends the range of retinal-slip velocities that can elicit the velocity-storage component of OKN, and eliminates the nasal-temporal asymmetry during monocular viewing inherent in the retinal–NOT/DTN pathway. If visual cortex is ablated bilaterally in cats, neurons in DTN only respond to retinal-slip velocities up to about 13 degrees/sec and only respond during stimulation of the contralateral eye.[33]

The cortical circuits modifying the retinal-slip velocity capabilities of NOT/DTN are best known in the cat. Areas within occipito-temporal cortex mediate ipsilateral slow phases of OKN generated from either eye via an ipsilateral projection to NOT/DTN.[34, 66, 117] These cortical areas in turn receive retinal-slip information from both visual hemifields via bilateral projections from areas V1 and V2. We postulate that a similar cerebral projection circuit enhances the retinal-slip velocity of NOT/DTN in the monkey, which partially overlaps with the smooth pursuit cerebral pathway (Fig 8). The cortical afferent system includes a projection from the dLGN to V1 to MT directly and indirectly via V2. This system processes information about target motion in the contralateral visual field. The cortical efferent system includes a projection from the MST to the NOT and the DTN of the accessory optic system. The large arrow below the box enclosing each cortical efferent system indicates the relative extent each hemisphere mediates retinal-slip velocity in the horizontal direction. The cortical efferent system in each hemisphere receives a projection from both the ipsilateral and contralateral cortical afferent systems. For vertical OKN, the cerebral pathway is similar but involves the medial terminal nucleus and the lateral terminal nucleus of the accessory optic system instead of NOT/DTN.[31, 32, 85]

Based on physiologic and lesion studies, the remaining OKN pathway appears to involve a projection from NOT/DTN to the NRTP, which in turn projects to the medial vestibular–propositus hypoglossi (MV/PH) nuclear complex.[91] The MV/PH complex appears to be part of the vestibular-optokinetic velocity-storage system; vestibular and optokinetic signals converge at the level of the vestibular nucleus, and lesions within the MV/PH complex impair the velocity-storage system for both VOR and OKN.[17, 129] Furthermore, electrical stimulation of NOT/DTN in the monkey appears to activate the velocity-storage mechanism to produce the velocity-storage component of OKN. Stimulation of NOT/DTN results in ipsilateral slow phases with velocities that rise slowly to a steady-state level followed by after-nystagmus at the end of stimulation.[97] The maximum slow-phase eye velocity induced by electrical stimulation is the same as that of OKAN found behaviorally.

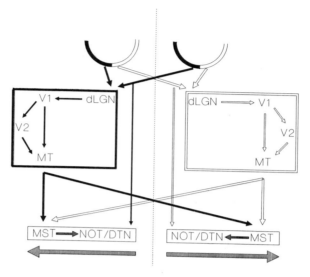

FIG 8.

Schematic diagram illustrating the cerebral systems believed to be involved in the velocity-storage component of optokinetic nystagmus in the monkey. A cortical afferent system includes a projection from the dorsolateral geniculate nucleus *(dLGN)* to striate cortex *(V1)*, which in turn projects to the middle temporal area *(MT)* directly and indirectly via prestriate cortex *(V2)*. This system processes information about target motion in the contralateral visual field. In the schematic, the regions and pathways mediating motion information from the right and left visual hemifields are outlined by thick black lines and open double lines, respectively. The cortical efferent system includes a projection from the medial superior temporal *(MST)* area to the nucleus of the optic tract *(NOT)* and the dorsal terminal nucleus *(DTN)* of the accessory optic system. The cortical efferent system in each hemisphere receives a projection from both the ipsilateral and contralateral cortical afferent systems. Areas NOT and DTN also receive a direct retinal projection from the contralateral eye. Each cerebral hemisphere mediates ipsilateral aptokinetic slow phases, which is indicated by the large arrow below the box enclosing each cortical efferent system.

Lesions

Bilateral Lesions

The most extensive study of OKN following cortical lesions has been made in monkeys following bilateral occipital lobectomies.[135] Despite complete removal of all striate cortex, there is still a residual optokinetic response in monkeys, but it has the characteristics of an afoveate optokinetic system found, for example, in the intact Dutch-belted rabbit. The immediate component of OKN is eliminated. The velocity-storage component gives a poor response to high retinal-slip velocities and shows a temporal-to-nasal bias during monocular viewing. These findings indicate that in intact monkeys, striate cortex makes three major contributions to

OKN. Striate cortex provides afferent input to (1) generate the immediate tracking component of OKN; (2) balance inherent temporal-to-nasal asymmetries in the velocity-storage system; and (3) extend the range of retinal-slip velocities to which the velocity-storage system of OKN can respond. If the lesion extends forward and involves areas MT and MST in occipito-temporal cortex, the qualitative findings are the same, but quantitatively the deficit is more severe.[135] This finding suggests that NOT/DTN probably receives parallel projections from both striate cortex and the MT/MST complex to enhance OKN. A similar effect of lesion has been described in the cat.[107, 117]

Unilateral Lesions

A unilateral V1 ablation in monkeys does not cause a directional defect in full-field OKN (unpublished results, 1988). This is because visual motion in the intact visual hemifield can still be used by area MST in each hemisphere to generate normal optokinetic slow phases in each direction. This motion information may be mediated via the intrahemispheric and interhemispheric projections from the intact MT to MST (see Fig 8).

Hemidecortication in monkeys reduces the gain (slow-phase eye velocity/OKN drum velocity) of the immediate OKN component in both horizontal directions (bidirectional) and reduces the gain of the velocity-storage component toward the side of the lesion (unidirectional; unpublished results, 1988). The degree of the deficit is the same for both binocular and monocular viewing, and there is no temporal-to-nasal preference during monocular viewing. Qualitatively, similar deficits are found following lesions in area MST, but the degree of the deficit is less.[25] Thus, other areas besides area MST are probably involved in generating both components of OKN. Unilateral lesions of frontal cortex in human patients have also been reported to cause a decrease in ipsilateral slow-phase eye velocity.[39]

Unilateral lesions in the NOT/DTN complex or the dorsolateral pontine nucleus in the monkey, the two subcortical projection fields of MST, also cause directional deficits in OKN. A unilateral electrolytic or neurotoxic lesion of NOT/DTN eliminates the velocity-storage component of OKN toward the side of the lesion but leaves intact the immediate tracking component.[38, 97] In addition, this lesion results in a spontaneous horizontal jerk nystagmus found in the dark with a slow-phase eye velocity of about 2 degrees/sec directed away from the lesioned side. Unilateral lesions of the NOT/DTN complex do not cause a monocular asymmetry in OKN or OKAN. A unilateral lesion of DLPN in monkeys apparently does not cause spontaneous nystagmus or affect the velocity-storage system but does cause a bidirectional deficit in the immediate tracking component of OKN.[71]

It is curious why unilateral cerebral lesions do not cause a monocular asymmetry in the velocity-storage component of OKN whereas bilateral lesions do cause an asymmetry. This finding suggests that the NOT/DTN complex on the side of the hemisphere with the unilateral cortical lesion is still getting visual input from both eyes. Either this information comes directly from the retina or possibly indirectly via bilateral cortical projections to NOT/DTN.

Clinical Implications

Since OKN in human beings is primarily mediated by the immediate visual-tracking system, OKN can be used to assess the afferent and efferent cortical smooth pursuit systems. This can be especially useful in inattentive or uncooperative patients. Asymmetries should be looked for in slow-phase eye velocity generated in the two horizontal directions. A unilateral cerebral lesion will reduce slow-phase eye velocity in both directions but more so for slow-phase eye movements directed toward the side of the lesion. Directional deficits will occur following unilateral lesions in occipito-temporal cortex, the dorsolateral pontine nucleus, the flocculus, and the interconnecting pathways.

Although the velocity-storage system contributes little to OKN in human beings, it is useful to know the features of this system, as individuals with certain smooth pursuit disorders have an OKN response that is primarily driven by the velocity-storage system. Certain patients with achromatopsia show a gradual build-up in slow-phase velocity and a temporal-to-nasal directional preference during OKN.[5, 101] This may be due to removal of cone input from the cortical pursuit system. Certain patients with pursuit deficits due to bilateral occipital lobe infarctions and craniocervical junction abnormalities show similar OKN responses.[72, 133] It is important to remember that monocular asymmetry in the velocity-storage component of OKN occurs with dysfunction in the cerebral pursuit pathways in both cerebral hemispheres and not following dysfunction in only one cerebral hemisphere.

A spontaneous horizontal jerk nystagmus can occur in human patients following a unilateral cerebral lesion. The slow phases of this nystagmus are directed away from the side of the lesion. This probably arises from destruction of the homologue of area MST in occipito-temporal cortex (stimulation of this region in monkeys results in ipsilaterally directed slow phases and ablation results in spontaneous nystagmus with contralaterally directed slow phases). Although this nystagmus has been called a "pursuit paretic nystagmus,"[104] it probably arises from an imbalance of spontaneous input into the velocity-storage OKN system. Unilateral ablation of NOT/DTN, which receives projections from area MST and forms the cortical efferent pathway for the velocity-storage component of OKN, also results in a spontaneous nystagmus with slow phases directed away from the side of the lesion. In contrast, ablation of DLPN, the MST-recipient subcortical area mediating smooth pursuit, does not produce nystagmus.

Summary

Optokinetic nystagmus in human beings is generated by a hierarchy of visual-tracking systems that evolved in parallel with binocular vision. The most primitive system is a subcortical system that involves the vestibular-optokinetic velocity-storage system. This is the only system found in the Dutch-belted rabbit. The characteristics of this system are (1) a gradual increase in slow-phase eye velocity in response to a full-field optokinetic drum rotating at a constant velocity, (2) an inability to respond to high retinal-slip velocities, and (3) a nasal-temporal asymmetry during monocular viewing. With the evolution of binocular vision, a parallel visual input involving cerebral cortex was added to this subcortical system. This cortical pathway (1) increases the range of retinal-slip velocities that can drive the subcortical system and (2) balances the nasal-temporal asymmetries during monocular viewing. With the evolution of a fovea, an entirely new immediate visual-tracking system evolved. In response to a full-field optokinetic drum rotating at a constant velocity, this system immediately generates high-speed slow-phase eye movements. This system functions largely involuntarily, i.e., it requires little visual fixation or attention by the subject, although visual fixation of the target can significantly increase slow-phase eye velocity. In human beings, the immediate visual-tracking system overwhelms the more primitive system mediated by the velocity-storage system (the velocity-storage system only accounts for 10 to 20°/sec of eye velocity). The slow phases of OKAN are the best measure of the velocity-storage system since they are uncontaminated by the immediate visual-tracking system.

REFERENCES

1. Alexander GE, DeLong MR, Strick PL: Parallel organization of functionally segregated circuits linking basal ganglia and cortex. *Ann Rev Neurosci* 1986; 9:357–381.
2. Allman J, Miezin F, McGuinness E: Stimulus specific responses from beyond the classical receptive field: Neurophysiological mechanisms for local-global comparisons in visual neurons. *Ann Rev Neurosci* 1985; 8:407–430.
3. Anderson RA, Essick GK, Siegel RM: Encoding of spatial location by posterior parietal neurons. *Science* 1985; 230:456–458.
4. Anderson RA, Mountcastle VB: The influence of the angle of gaze upon the excitability of the light-sensitive neurons of the posterior parietal cortex. *J Neurosci* 1983; 3:532–548.
5. Baloh RW, Yee RD, Honrubia V: Optokinetic asymmetry in patients with maldeveloped foveas. *Brain Res* 1980; 186:211–216.
6. Barbas H, Mesulam MM: Organization of afferent input to subdivisions of area 8 in the rhesus monkey. *J Comp Neurol* 1981; 200:407–431.
7. Becker W, Fuchs AF: Prediction in the oculomotor system: Smooth pursuit during transient disappearance of a visual target. *Exp Brain Res* 1985; 57:562–575.
8. Bogousslavsky J, Regli F: Pursuit gaze defects in acute and chronic unilateral parieto-occipital lesions. *Eur Neurol* 1986; 25:10–18.
9. Boman DK, Hotson JR: Anticipatory slow eye movements follow perceived target motion. *Invest Ophthalmol Vis Sci* 1987; 28(suppl):332.
10. Brigell M, Babikian V, Goodwin JA: Hypometric saccades and low-gain pursuit resulting from a thalamic hemorrhage. *Ann Neurol* 1984; 15:374–378.
11. Brodal P: The corticopontine projection in the rhesus monkey: Origin and principles of organization. *Brain* 1978; 101:251–283.
12. Brodal P: Further observations on the cerebellar projections from the pontine nuclei and the nucleus reticularis tegmenti pontis in the rhesus monkey. *J Comp Neurol* 1982; 204:44–55.

13. Brodmann K: Beitraege zur histologischen Lokalisation der Grosshirnrinde: IIIte Mitteilung: Die Rindenfelder der niederen Affen. *J Psychol Neurol* 1905; 4:177–226.

14. Bruce CJ, Goldberg ME: Primate frontal eye fields: I. Single neurons discharging before saccades. *J Neurophysiol* 1985; 53:603–635.

15. Bunt AH, Minckler DS: New anatomical evidence for bilateral representation of the central retina. *Arch Ophthalmol* 1977; 95:1445–1447.

16. Bushnell MC, Goldberg ME, Robinson DL: Behavioral enhancement of visual responses in monkey cerebral cortex: I. Modulation in posterior parietal cortex related to selective visual attention. *J Neurophysiol* 1981; 46:755–772.

17. Cannon SC, Robinson DA: Loss of the neural integrator of the oculomotor system from brain stem lesions in monkey. *J Neurophysiol* 1987; 57:1383–1409.

18. Carl JR, Gellman RS: Human smooth pursuit: Stimulus-dependent responses. *J Neurophysiol* 1987; 57:1446–1463.

19. Carl JR, Gellman RS, Miles FA: Short latency ocular following responses in humans. *Invest Ophthalmol Vis Sci* 1987; 28(suppl):332.

20. Cohen B, Matsuo V, Raphan T: Quantitative analysis of the velocity characteristics of optokinetic nystagmus and optokinetic after-nystagmus. *J Physiol* 1977; 270:321–344.

21. Collewijn H: Direction-selective units in the rabbit's nucleus of the optic tract. *Brain Res* 1975; 100:489–508.

22. Collewijn H, Went LN, Tamminga EP, et al: Oculomotor defects in patients with Huntington's disease and their offspring. *J Neurol Sci* 1988; 86:307–320.

23. Desimone R, Ungerleider LG: Multiple visual areas in the caudal superior temporal sulcus of the macaque. *J Comp Neurol* 1986; 248:164–189.

24. DeYoe EA, Van Essen DC: Concurrent processing streams in monkey visual cortex. *Trends Neurosci* 1988; 11:219–226.

25. Dursteler MR, Wurtz RH: Pursuit and optokinetic deficits following chemical lesions of cortical areas MT and MST. *J Neurophysiol* 1988; 60:940–965.

26. Dursteler MR, Wurtz RH, Newsome WR: Directional pursuit deficits following lesions of the foveal representation within the superior temporal sulcus. *J Neurophysiol* 1987; 57:1262–1287.

27. Edley SM, Graybiel AM: The afferent and efferent connections of the feline nucleus tegmenti pedunculopontinus, pars compacta. *J Comp Neurol* 1983; 217:187–215.

28. Fletcher WA, Hain TC, Zee DS: Steady-state and dynamic responses of the human optokinetic system. *Invest Ophthalmol Vis Sci* 1987; 28(suppl):332.

29. Gentilucci M, Scandolara C, Pigarev IN, et al: Visual responses in the postarcuate cortex (area 6) of the monkey that are independent of eye position. *Exp Brain Res* 1983; 50:464–468.

30. Goldberg ME, Bushnell MC: Behavioral enhancement of visual responses in monkey cerebral cortex: II. Modulation in frontal eye fields specifically related to saccades. *J Neurophysiol* 1981; 46:773–787.

31. Grasse KL, Cynader MS: Electrophysiology of lateral and dorsal terminal nuclei of the cat accessory optic system. *J Neurophysiol* 1984; 51:292–309.

32. Grasse KL, Cynader MS: Electrophysiology of the medial terminal nucleus of the accessory optic system in the cat. *J Neurophysiol* 1982; 48:490–504.

33. Grasse K, Cynader M, Douglas RM: Alterations in response properties in the lateral and dorsal terminal nuclei of the cat accessory optic system following visual cortex lesions. *Exp Brain Res* 1984; 55:69–80.

34. Herdman SJ, Tusa RJ, Smith CB: Cortical areas involved in horizontal OKN in cats: Metabolic activity. *J Neurosci,* 1989; 9:1150–1162.

35. Hoffmann KP, Distler C: The role of direction selective cells in the nucleus of the optic tract of

cat and monkey during optokinetic nystagmus, in Keller EL, Zee DS (eds): *Adaptive Processes in Visual and Oculomotor Systems*. Elmsford, NY, Pergamon Press Inc, 1986, pp 261–266.

36. Honrubia V, Downey WL, Mitchell DP, et al: Experimental studies on optokinetic nystagmus: II. Normal humans. *Acta Otolaryngol* 1968; 65:441–448.

37. Huber A: Homonymous hemianopia after occipital lobectomy. *Am J Ophthalmol* 1962; 54:623–629.

38. Kato I, Harada K, Hacegawa T, et al: Role of the nucleus of the optic tract in monkeys in relation to optokinetic nystagmus. *Brain Res* 1986; 364:12–22.

39. Kaga K, Suzuki J: Optokinetic pattern asymmetry in patients with cerebral lesions, in Honrubia V, Brazier MAB (eds): *Nystagmus and Vertigo*, New York, Academic Press, 1982, pp 279–286.

40. Kawano K, Sasaki M: Response properties of neurons in posterior parietal cortex of monkey during visual-vestibular stimulation: II. Optokinetic neurons. *J Neurophysiol* 1984; 51:352–360.

41. Kawano K, Watanabe Y, Yamane S: Neuronal activity in the posterior parietal cortex (area PG) of alert monkey during ocular following responses, abstracted. *Soc Neurosci Abstr* 1988; 14:956.

42. Keating EG, Gooley SG, Kenney DV: Impaired tracking and loss of predictive eye movements after removal of the frontal eye fields, abstracted. *Soc Neurosci Abstr* 1985; 11:472.

43. Keller EL: Cerebellar involvement in smooth pursuit eye movement generation: Flocculus and vermis, in Kennard C, Clifford Rose F (eds): *Physiological Aspects of Clinical Neuro-Ophthalmology*. London, Chapman & Hall, 1988, pp 341–355.

44. Keller EL, Crandall WF: Neuronal responses to optokinetic stimuli in pontine nuclei of behaving monkey. *J Neurophysiol* 1983; 49:169–187.

45. Kjallman L, Frisen L: The cerebral ocular pursuit pathways. *J Clin Neuro Ophthalmol* 1986; 6:209–214.

46. Komatsu H, Wurtz RH: Directionally selective effects of electrical stimulation of monkey cerebral cortex on pursuit eye movements. *Invest Ophthalmol Vis Sci* 1987; 28(suppl):316.

47. Komatsu H, Wurtz RH: Relation of cortical areas MT and MST to pursuit eye movements: I. Localization and visual properties of neurons. *J Neurophysiol* 1988; 60:580–603.

48. Komatsu H, Wurtz RH: Relation of cortical areas MT and MST to pursuit eye movements: III. Interaction with full-field visual stimulation. *J Neurophysiol* 1988; 60:621–644.

49. Kowler E, Martins AJ, Pavel M: The effect of expectations on slow oculomotor control: IV. Anticipatory smooth eye movements depend on prior target motions. *Vision Res* 1984; 24:197–210.

50. Langer T, Fuchs AF, Chubb MC, et al: Floccular efferents in the rhesus macaque as revealed by autoradiography and horseradish peroxidase. *J Comp Neurol* 1985; 235:26–37.

51. Langer T, Fuchs AF, Schudder CA, et al: Afferents to the flocculus of the cerebellum in the rhesus macaque as revealed by retrograde transport of horseradish peroxidase. *J Comp Neurol* 1985; 235:1–25.

52. Larmande P, Prier S, Masson M, et al: Pertubations de la poursuite oculaire lesions parieto-occipitales unilaterales. *Rev Neurol* 1980; 136:345–353.

53. Latto R, Cowey A: Fixation changes after frontal eye-field lesions in monkeys. *Brain Res* 1971; 30:25–36.

54. Leichnetz GR, Spencer RF, Smith DJ: Cortical projections to the paramedian tegmental and basilar pons in the monkey. *J Comp Neurol* 1984; 228:388–408.

55. Leigh RJ, Newman SA, Folstein SE, et al: Abnormal ocular motor control in Huntington's disease. *Neurology* 1983; 33:1268–1275.

56. Leigh RJ, Thurston SE: Recovery of ocular motor function in humans with cerebral lesions, in Keller EL, Zee DS (eds): *Adaptive Processes in Visual and Oculomotor Systems*. Elmsford, NY, Pergamon Press Inc, 1986, pp 231–238.

57. Leventhal AG, Ault SJ, Vitek DJ: The nasotemporal division in primate retina: The neural bases of macular sparing and splitting. *Science* 1988; 240:66–67.

58. Lisberger SG, Evinger C, Johanson GW, et al: Relationship between eye acceleration and retinal image velocity during foveal smooth pursuit in man and monkey. *J Neurophysiol* 1981; 46:229–249.

59. Lisberger SG, Fuchs AF: Role of primate flocculus during rapid behavioral modification of vestibuloocular reflex: I. Purkinje cell activity during visually guided horizontal smooth pursuit eye movements and passive head rotation. *J Neurophysiol* 1978; 41:733–763.

60. Lisberger SG, Westbrook LE: Properties of visual inputs that initiate horizontal smooth pursuit eye movements in monkeys. *J Neurosci* 1985; 6:1662–1673.

61. Livingstone MS: Art, illusion and the visual system. *Sci Am* 1988; 258:78–85.

62. Lynch JC: Frontal eye field lesions in monkeys disrupt visual pursuit. *Exp Brain Res* 1987; 68:437–441.

63. Lynch JC, Allison JC, Hines RS, et al: Oculomotor impairment following combined lesions of parieto-occipital cortex and frontal eye fields in rhesus monkeys, abstracted. *Soc Neurosci Abstr* 1986; 12:1086.

64. MacAvoy MG, Bruce CJ, Gottlieb J: Smooth eye movements elicited by microstimulation in the frontal eye fields region of alert macaque monkeys, abstracted. *Soc Neurosci Abstr* 1988; 14:956.

65. McHugh DE, Bahill AT: Learning to track predictable target waveforms without a time delay. *Invest Ophthalmol Vis Sci* 1985; 26:932–937.

66. Marcotte RR, Updyke BV: Cortical visual areas of the cat project differentially onto the nuclei of the accessory optic system. *Brain Res* 1982; 242:205–217.

67. Maunsell JHR, Newsome WT: Visual processing in monkey extrastriate cortex. *Ann Rev Neurosci* 1987; 10:363–401.

68. Maunsell JHR, Van Essen DC: Functional properties of neurons in middle temporal visual area of the macaque monkey. *J Neurophysiol* 1983; 49:1127–1147.

69. May JG, Andersen RA: Different patterns of corticopontine projections from separate cortical fields within the inferior parietal lobule and dorsal prelunate gyrus of the macaque. *Exp Brain Res* 1986; 63:265–278.

70. May JG, Keller EL, Crandall WF: Changes in eye velocity during smooth pursuit tracking induced by microstimulation in the dorsolateral pontine nucleus of the macaque, abstracted. *Soc Neurosci Abstr* 1985; 11:79.

71. May JG, Keller EL, Suzuki DA: Smooth-pursuit eye movement deficits with chemical lesions in the dorsolateral pontine nucleus of the monkey. *J Neurophysiol* 1988; 59:952–977.

72. Mehdorn E: Nasal-temporal asymmetry of the optokinetic nystagmus after bilateral occipital infarction in man, in Lennerstrand G, Zee DS, Keller EL (eds): *Functional Basis of Ocular Motility Disorders,* Elmsford, NY, Pergamon Press Inc, 1982, pp 321–324.

73. Meienberg O, Harrer M, Wehren C: Oculographic diagnosis of hemineglect in patients with homonymous hemianopia. *J Neurol* 1986; 233:97–101.

74. Mesulam MM: A cortical network for directed attention and unilateral neglect. *Ann Neurol* 1981; 10:309–325.

75. Meyer CH, Lasker AG, Robinson DA: The upper limit of human smooth pursuit velocity. *Vision Res* 1985; 25:561–563.

76. Michael JA, Melvill Jones G: Dependence of visual tracking capability upon stimulus predictability. *Vision Res* 1966; 6:707–716.

77. Miezin F, Applegate C, Petersen S, et al: Brain regions in humans activated during smooth pursuit visual tracking, *abstracted. Soc Neurosci Abstr* 1988: 14:795.

78. Miezin FM, Fox PT, Raichle ME, et al: An extrastriate region in human visual cortex sensitive to low contrast moving dots and high temporal frequencies. *Invest Ophthalmol Vis Sci* 1988; 29(suppl):326.

79. Miles FA, Kawano K: Visual stabilization of the eyes. *Trends Neurosci* 1987; 10:153–158.

80. Mohler CW, Goldberg ME, Wurtz RH: Visual receptive fields of frontal eye field neurons. *Brain Res* 1973; 61:385–389.

81. Mohler CW, Wurtz RH: Role of striate cortex and superior colliculus in visual guidance of saccadic eye movements in monkeys. *J Neurophysiol* 1977; 40:74–94.

82. Morris EJ, Lisberger SG: Different responses to small visual errors during initiation and maintenance of smooth-pursuit eye movements in monkeys. *J Neurophysiol* 1987; 58:1351–1369.

83. Morrow MJ, Sharpe JA: Smooth pursuit initiation in humans with cerebral hemispheric lesions, abstracted. *Soc Neurosci Abstr* 1988; 14:612.

84. Mustari MJ, Fuchs AF, Wallman J: Response properties of dorsolateral pontine units during smooth pursuit in the rhesus macaque. *J Neurophysiol* 1988; 60:664–686.

85. Mustari MJ, Fuchs AP, Langer TP, et al: The role of the primate lateral terminal nucleus in visuomotor behavior, in: Hicks TP, Benedek G (eds): *Progress in Brain Research,* vol 75. New York, Elsevier Science Publ, B.V., 1988, pp 121–128

86. Newsome WT, Pare EB: A selective impairment of motion perception following lesions of the middle temporal visual area. *J Neurosci* 1988; 8:2201–2211.

87. Newsome WT, Wurtz RH, Dursteler MR, et al: Deficits in visual motion processing following ibotenic acid lesions of the middle temporal visual area of the macaque monkey. *J Neurosci* 1985; 5:825–840.

88. Newsome WT, Wurtz RH, Komatsu H: Relation of cortical areas MT and MST to pursuit eye movements: II. Differentiation of retinal from extraretinal inputs. *J Neurophysiol* 1988; 60:604–620.

89. Petrides M, Pandya DN: Projections to the frontal cortex from the posterior parietal region in the rhesus monkey. *J Comp Neurol* 1984; 228:105–116.

90. Pola J, Wyatt HJ: Target position and velocity: The stimuli for smooth pursuit eye movements. *Vision Res* 1980; 20:523–534.

91. Precht W: Anatomical and functional organization of optokinetic pathways, in Lennerstrand G, Zee DS, Keller EL (eds): *Functional Basis of Ocular Motility Disorders.* Elmsford, NY, Pergamon Press Inc, 1982, pp 291–302.

92. Pyykko I, Dahlen AI, Schalen L, et al: Eye movement in patients with speech dyspraxia. *Acta Otolaryngol Head Neck Surg* 1984; 98:481–489.

93. Rashbass C: The relationship between saccadic and smooth tracking eye movements. *J Physiol* 1961; 159:326–338.

94. Reeves AG, Perret J, Jenkyn LR, et al: Pursuit gaze and the occipitoparietal region. *Arch Neurol* 1984; 41:83–84.

95. Riddoch G: Dissociation of visual perceptions due to occipital injuries, with especial reference to appreciation of movement. *Brain* 1917; 40:15–57.

96. Sakata H, Shibutani H, Kawano K: Spatial properties of visual fixation neurons in posterior parietal association cortex of the monkey. *J Neurophysiol* 1980; 43:1654–1672.

97. Schiff D, Cohen B, Raphan T: Nystagmus induced by stimulation of the nucleus of the optic tract in the monkey. *Exp Brain Res* 1988; 70:1–14.

98. Segal BN, Liben S: Modulation of human velocity storage sampled during intermittently illuminated optokinetic stimulation. *Exp Brain Res* 1985; 59:515–523.

99. Segraves MA, Goldberg ME, Deng S, et al: The role of striate cortex in the guidance of eye movements in the monkey. *J Neurosci* 1987; 7:3040–3058.

100. Seltzer B, Pandya DN: Converging visual and somatic sensory cortical input to the intraparietal sulcus of the rhesus monkey. *Brain Res* 1980; 192:339–351.

101. Sharpe LT, Collewijn H, Nordby K: Fixation, pursuit and optokinetic nystagmus in a complete achromat. *Clin Vis Sci* 1986; 1:39–49.

102. Sharpe JA, Deck JHN: Destruction of the internal sagittal stratum and normal smooth pursuit. *Ann Neurol* 1978; 4:473–476.

103. Sharpe JA, Fletcher WA, Lang AE, et al: Smooth pursuit during dose-related on-off fluctuations in Parkinson's disease. *Neurology* 1987; 37:1389–1392.

104. Sharpe JA, Lo AW, Rabinovitch HE: Control of the saccadic and smooth pursuit systems after cerebral hemidecortication. *Brain* 1979; 102:387–403.

105. Shibasaki H, Tsuji S, Kuroiwa Y: Oculomotor abnormalities in parkinson's disease. *Arch Neurol* 1979; 36:360–364.

106. Steiner I, Melamed E: Conjugate eye deviation after acute hemispheric stroke: Delayed recovery after previous contralateral frontal lobe damage. *Ann Neurol* 1984; 16:509–510.

107. Strong NP, Malach R, Lee P, et al: Horizontal optokinetic nystagmus in the cat: Recovery from cortical lesions. *Dev Brain Res* 1984; 13:179–192.

108. Suzuki H, Azuma M: Prefrontal neuronal activity during gazing at a light spot in the monkey. *Brain Res* 1977; 126:497–508.

109. Suzuki DA, Keller EL: The role of the posterior vermis of monkey cerebellum in smooth-pursuit eye movement control: II. Target velocity-related Purkinje cell activity. *J Neurophysiol* 1988; 59:19–40.

110. Suzuki DA, Keller EL: Visual signals in the dorsolateral pontine nucleus of the alert monkey: Their relationship to smooth-pursuit eye movements. *Exp Brain Res* 1984; 53:473–478.

111. Takemori S, Ishikawa M, Yamada S: Cerebral control of eye movements. *Otorhinolaryngology* 1981; 43:262–273.

112. Their P, Koehler W, Buettner UW: Neuronal activity in the dorsolateral pontine nucleus of the alert monkey modulated by visual stimuli and eye movements. *Exp Brain Res* 1988; 70:496–512.

113. Thurston SE, Leigh RJ, Crawford T, et al: Two distinct deficits of visual tracking caused by unilateral lesions of cerebral cortex in humans. *Ann Neurol* 1988; 23:266–273.

114. Tijssen MAJ, Straathof CSM, Hain TC, et al: Optokinetic-afternystagmus in humans: Normal values of amplitude, time constant and asymmetry. *Ann Otol Rhinol Laryngol*, in press.

115. Troost BT, Daroff RB: The ocular motor defects in progressive supranuclear palsy. *Ann Neurol* 1977; 2:397–403.

116. Troost BT, Daroff RB, Weber RB, et al: Hemispheric control of eye movements: I. Quantitative analysis of smooth pursuit in a hemispherectomy patient. *Arch Neurol* 1972; 27:449–452.

117. Tusa RJ, Demer JL, Herdman SJ: Cortical areas involved in OKN and VOR in cats: Cortical lesions. *J Neurosci,* 1989; 9:1163–1178.

118. Tusa RJ, Ungerleider LG: Fiber pathways of cortical areas mediating smooth pursuit eye movements in monkeys. *Ann Neurol* 1988; 23:174–183.

119. Tusa RJ, Ungerleider LG: The inferior longitudinal fasciculus: A reexamination in humans and monkeys. *Ann Neurol* 1985; 18:583–591.

120. Tusa RJ, Zee DS, Herdman SJ: Effect of unilateral cerebral cortical lesions in ocular motor behavior in monkeys: Saccades and quick phases. *J Neurophysiol* 1986; 56:1590–1625.

121. Tusa RJ, Zee DS, Herdman SJ: Recovery of oculomotor function in monkeys with large unilateral cortical lesions, in Keller EL, Zee DS (eds): *Adaptive Processes in Visual and Oculomotor Systems.* Elmsford, NY, Pergamon Press Inc, 1986, pp 209–216.

122. Tychsen L, Lisberger SG: Visual motion processing for the initiation of smooth-pursuit eye movements in humans. *J Neurophysiol* 1986; 56:953–968.

123. Tychsen L, Rizzo M, Hurtig RR, et al: Visual motion processing in humans after loss of striate cortex, *abstracted. Soc Neurosci Abstr* 1988; 14:796.

124. Ungerleider LG, Desimone R: Cortical connections of visual area MT in the macaque. *J Comp Neurol* 1986; 248:190–224.

125. Ungerleider LG, Desimone R, Galkin TH, et al: Subcortical projections of area MT in the macaque. *J Comp Neurol* 1984; 223:368–386.

126. Ungerleider LG, Mishkin M: Two cortical visual systems, in Ingle DJ, Goodale MA, Mansfield RJW (eds): *Analysis of Visual Behavior*. Cambridge, Mass, MIT Press, 1982, pp 549–586.

127. Von Bonin G, Bailey P: *The Neocortex of Macaca Mulatta*. Urbana, Ill, University of Illinois Press, 1947, p 163.

128. Von Economo CF: *The Cytoarchitectonics of the Human Cerebral Cortex*. London, Oxford Medical Publications, 1929.

129. Waespe W, Henn V: Neuronal activity in the vestibular nuclei of the alert monkey during vestibular and optokinetic stimulation. *Exp Brain Res* 1977; 27:523–538.

130. Waespe W, Rudinger D, Wolfensberger M: Purkinje cell activity in the flocculus of vestibular neurectomized and normal monkeys during optokinetic nystagmus (OKN) and smooth pursuit eye movements. *Exp Brain Res* 1985; 60:243–262.

131. Wurtz RH, Goldberg ME, Robinson DL: Behavioral modulation of visual responses in the monkey: Stimulus selection for attention and movement, in Sprague JM, Epstein AN (eds): *Progress in Psychobiology and Physiological Psychology*, vol 9. New York, Academic Press, 1980, pp 43–83.

132. Yamada J, Noda H: Afferent and efferent connections of the oculomotor cerebellar vermis in the macaque monkey. *J Comp Neurol* 1987; 265:224–241.

133. Yee RD, Baloh RW, Honrubia V, et al: Slow build-up of optokinetic nystagmus associated with downbeat nystagmus. *Invest Ophthalmol Vis Sci* 1979; 18:622–629.

134. Zee DS: Ocular motor control: The cerebral control of saccadic eye movements, in Lessell S, van Dalen JTW (eds): *Neuro-Ophthalmology*. New York, Elsevier North-Holland, Inc, 1984, pp 141–156.

135. Zee DS, Tusa RJ, Herdman SJ, et al: Effects of occipital lobectomy upon eye movements in primate. *J Neurophysiol* 1987; 58:883–907.

136. Zee DS, Yamazaki A, Butler PH, et al: Effects of ablation of flocculus and paraflocculus on eye movements in primate. *J Neurophysiol* 1981; 46:878–899.

137. Zihl J, Von Cramon D, Mai N: Selective disturbance of movement vision after bilateral brain damage. *Brain* 1983; 106:313–340.

CHAPTER 9

Nystagmus, Saccadic Intrusions/Oscillations, and Oscillopsia

L. F. Dell'Osso, Ph.D.

Professor, Departments of Neurology and Biomedical Engineering, Case Western Reserve University, Director, Ocular Motor Neurophysiology Laboratory, Veterans Administration Medical Center, Cleveland, Ohio

Understanding the pathophysiology of ocular oscillations necessitates differentiation between those involving only the slow system and those that are purely saccadic. Oscillations containing both saccades and slow phases require identification of both the causative phase (i.e., that which takes the eyes away from their intended direction) and the corrective phase. Modern recording methods have made possible these determinations and thereby clarified the underlying ocular motor mechanisms responsible for many oscillations. Table 1 lists 45 types of nystagmus (two of which were not included previously) along with many other terms found in the literature to describe them; similarly, Table 2 lists 16 saccadic oscillations and intrusions with other descriptive terms. The tables evolved from those that appeared in previous book chapters.[1-4]

The definitions and categorizations used herein result from applying criteria derived from accurate ocular motility recordings. They differentiate between nystagmus and saccadic oscillations, and as a result, I have found that some saccadic oscillations were originally described using the word *nystagmus*. Most oscillations were named before the benefits of accurate recordings. Quotation marks are used

Curr Neuro Ophthalmol 2:147–182, 1989
© 1989, Year Book Medical Publishers, Inc.
0893–0147/89/02-147-182-$04.00

TABLE 1.

Forty-five Types of Nystagmus*

Acquired
   "Fixation"
Arthrokinetic
   Induced
   Somatosensory
Associated
   Induced
   Stransky's
Audiokinetic
   Induced
Bartels'
   Induced
Bruns'
Centripetal
Cervical
   Neck torsion
   Vertebrobasilar artery
     insufficiency
Circular/elliptic/oblique
   Alternating windmill
   Circumduction
   Diagonal
   Elliptic
   Gyratory
   Oblique
   Radiary
Congenital
   "Fixation"
   Hereditary
Convergence
Convergence-evoked
Dissociated
   Disjunctive
Downbeat
Drug-induced
   Barbiturate
   Induced
Epileptic
   Ictal
Flash-induced
   Flicker-induced
   Induced
Gaze-evoked
   Deviational
   Gaze-paretic
   "Neurasthenic"
   "Seducible"
   "Setting-in"
Horizontal

(Continued.)

TABLE 1 (cont.).

Forty-five Types of Nystagmus*

Induced
  Provoked
Intermittent vertical
Jerk
Latent/manifest latent
  Monocular "fixation"
  Unimacular
Lateral medullary
Lid
Miner's†
  Occupational
Muscle-paretic
  Myasthenic
Optokinetic
  Induced
  "Kinetic"
  "Optic"
  Optomotor
  Panoramic
  "Railway"
  Sigma
  "Train"
Optokinetic after-nystagmus
  Induced
  Postoptokinetic
  Reverse postoptokinetic
Pendular
Periodic/aperiodic alternating
  Alternans
Physiologic
  End point
  Fatigue
Pursuit after-nystagmus
  Induced
Pursuit-defect†
Rebound
Reflex
  Baer's
See-saw
Somatosensory
  Induced
Spontaneous
Stepping around
  Apparent/real
  Induced
  Somatosensory
Torsional
  Rotary
Uniocular
Upbeat

(Continued.)

TABLE 1 (cont.).

Forty-five Types of Nystagmus*

Vertical
Vestibular
  A(po)geotropic/geotropic
  Alternating current
  Bechterew's
  Caloric/caloric-after
  Compensatory
  Electrical/faradic/galvanic
  Head-shaking
  Induced
  L-
  Labyrinthine
  Perverted
  Pneumatic/compression
  Positional/alcohol
  Positioning
  Postrotational
  Pseudocaloric
  Rotational/perrotary
  Secondary phase

*Synonyms and other terms are indented under either the preferred or the more inclusive designation; some nystagmus types may be acquired or congenital; quoted terms are erroneous or nonspecific.
†May not exist.

for those oscillations that are *not* truly nystagmus or for subjective clinical terms found in the literature that are inadequate, are not clearly defined, or have been misapplied. Since these ambiguous or erroneous terms do not convey accurate information about the basic nature of the movement, they are better left at the bedside. In those cases where historical precedence supports their continued usage (e.g., abduction "nystagmus" and convergence-retraction "nystagmus"), the quotation marks show that these are saccadic oscillations. The best names reflect the mechanism thought to be responsible for the eye movement (e.g., saccadic pulse); such terms maximize the information carried to the reader by describing a movement by its well-defined component parts.

NYSTAGMUS

Nystagmus is defined as a biphasic ocular oscillation containing slow eye movements that are responsible for its genesis and continuation. Fast eye movements (saccades), if they are present, serve a corrective function and do not represent the basic ocular motor dysfunction. The two phases of ocular nystagmus are about equal in amplitude. What follows, in alphabetical order, is a discussion of each

TABLE 2.

Sixteen Saccadic Intrusions and Oscillations*

Bobbing/dipping
  Inverse bobbing
  Reverse bobbing
Convergence-retraction "nystagmus"
  "Nystagmus" retractoris
Double saccadic pulses (single/multiple)
  Saccadic intrusions/oscillations
Dynamic overshoot
  "Quiver"
Dysmetria
Flutter
Flutter dysmetria
Macro–saccadic oscillations
Macro–square-wave jerks (bursts/single)
  Kippdeviationen/"Kippnystagmus"
  "Pendular macro-oscillations"
  Saccadic "nystagmus"
  Saccadic oscillations/intrusions
Myoclonus
  Laryngeal "nystagmus"
  "Lightning eye movements"
  Pharyngeal "nystagmus"
Opsoclonus
  "Dancing eyes"
  "Lightning eye movements"
  Saccadomania

Psychogenic flutter
  Hysterical flutter
  Hysterical "nystagmus"
  "Ocular fibrillation"
  "Ocular shuddering"
  Psychological "nystagmus"
  Voluntary flutter
  Voluntary "nystagmus"
Saccadic lateropulsion
  Ipsipulsion
  Contrapulsion
Saccadic pulses/pulse trains
  Abduction "nystagmus"
  Ataxic "nystagmus"
  Saccadic intrusions/oscillations
  Stepless saccades
Square-wave jerks/oscillations
  Gegenrucke
  Hopping "nystagmus"
  "Lightning eye movements"
  Myoclonus
  Saccadic intrusions/oscillations
  Zickzakbewegungen
Superior oblique myokymia

*Synonyms and other terms are indented under either the preferred or the more inclusive designation; quoted terms are erroneous or nonspecific.

nystagmus type in which significant work has been done in the past 2 years. Discussions of all types of nystagmus may be found in the aforementioned previous publications.[1-4]

Associated Nystagmus

Associated (Stransky's) nystagmus is a high-frequency, induced nystagmus caused by the attempted forceful opening of one eye while the subject continues to keep the eyes closed tightly.[5]

Cervical Nystagmus

Cervical nystagmus is allegedly caused by cervical spondylosis, whiplash, cervical muscle impairment, and cervical cord disease. A recent critical review of the literature has concluded that the entire concept of cervical nystagmus is highly suspect.[6] In our laboratory, we are not convinced that we have ever seen a patient with cervical nystagmus.

Congenital Nystagmus

An excellent article contains illustrations of most of the known characteristics of congenital nystagmus (CN) as well as some new findings.[7] In it are discussions of both the effort to see and state of arousal on the intensity of CN; the presence of CN during various stages of sleep; aperiodic alternating nystagmus; bias reversals during steady fixation; and both accurate and inaccurate foveation during fixation. A dramatic change in waveform was shown for both an adult and an infant when going from fixation to a state of low arousal. During fixation the waveforms were jerk or pseudocycloid with amplitudes up to 4 degrees and frequencies of 2 to 4 Hz, whereas during the low state of arousal the waveform became pendular, the amplitudes rose to 15 degrees to 60 degrees, and the frequency dropped to about 1 Hz. The authors emphasized that although we normally refer to CN as " congenital," it may not be constantly present until many weeks after birth.

In an attempt to determine whether the pendular part of dual jerk waveforms were truly sinusoidal, Reccia et al.[8] used spectral analysis. Unfortunately, the data were obtained using low-bandwidth, bitemporal electro-oculography (EOG). By subtracting the power spectrum of a pure sawtooth waveform from the dual jerk waveform, the authors were able to emphasize the pendular component. Their statistical analysis concluded that a sinusoidal fit would better approximate the data than an exponential fit; the latter was suggested by the model of Optican and Zee.[9]

One problem facing the clinician is the proper diagnosis of nystagmus occurring at birth or early infancy. Distinction must be made among CN, latent/manifest latent nystagmus (LMLN), spasmus nutans, or an acquired nystagmus indicating neurologic pathology. A recent article discussed some of the many pitfalls in distinguishing CN from LMLN and in identifying the nystagmus blockage syndrome in those patients with CN who use an esotropia to damp their CN or convert it to manifest latent nystagmus (MLN).[10] These authors pointed out the problems inherent in many published studies where these distinctions have not been made and where the patient population has included some with each of these conditions. Although both CN and LMLN are congenital types of nystagmus, to avoid confusion, I have deliberately refrained from using the word *congenital* when referring to LMLN. In the aforementioned article, the term *manifest* congenital nystagmus is CN and the term *latent and manifest latent congenital nystagmus* is LMLN. Despite the difference in terminology, this article clearly discusses some of the diagnostic problems. Though a causal relationship between esotropia and LMLN has not been proved, it is my opinion that since all patients with LMLN have strabismus, there is a strong suggestion of a causal (necessary but not sufficient) link.

An attempt has been made to use electromyographic (EMG) recordings to examine the possibility that there are two types of gaze-angle nulls present in CN.[11] One type is attributed to the active blockage of the nystagmus by an increase in the discharge of the synergistic extraocular muscles responsible for the gaze angle adopted. The second type is the classic null position, for which no good explanation has been proved, and is thought to result from an equilibrium position between the forces present in the push-pull ocular motor system. According to this article, the blockage type of null occurs at angles greater than 10 degrees from primary position and the so-called Kestenbaum null occurs closer to primary position. The key to differentiation, according to these authors, is analysis of time histograms of the EMG signal, since ocular motor activity reflected in ENG is the same for both types of nulls. Before discussing this article further, some definitions are in order. For a gaze angle position of low nystagmus to be a true null, the nystagmus must be higher at gaze angles to either side of it. Those patients who turn their heads in one direction so their eyes are in *extreme* lateral deviation do not fulfill this definition. It is well known that many patients with LMLN put the fixating eye in extreme adduction and take advantage of Alexander's law to minimize their nystagmus; this is not a true null angle. Similarly, some patients with CN also adopt an extreme head turn, forcing their eyes laterally and minimizing their nystagmus; this too is not a true null since the eyes cannot be deviated further to test whether the nystagmus increases at those gaze angles. Thus, patient 1 of the six studied in this article could not be said to have a true CN null. This is further evidenced by the observation that he adopted both a right and a left eye turn, during which his nystagmus was minimal; patients with CN with true nulls have only one such position. The other five patients appeared to have true nulls.

The question then remains: Are the differences reflected in EMG histograms indicative of different mechanisms? In the illustrations shown for each type of null, the histograms are peaked in the off-null positions and flatter where the nystagmus is minimal. This is to be expected, even if the nystagmus did not decrease; the increased activity caused by raising the firing level as the eye is deviated into its on direction would tend to broaden the histogram and lower the peak that is a measure of the relative number of intervals with given durations. Thus, even the EMG histograms are qualitatively the same. The authors claim that the difference is because for the Kestenbaum null the flatter curve is "five times faster" than for the other type; the meaning of that statement is obscure. Unfortunately, the two figures that must be compared are on different time scales both for the curve shown in primary position and for that shown at the null position. It is difficult to make comparisons between these two figures, and I was unable to find any measured points to which I could attribute a fivefold difference.

We have measured the CN of patients who have true nulls at most gaze angles as well as some whose nulls were so far in lateral gaze that we could not go further to prove that it was a true null. It is too simplistic to pick a number like 10 degrees and say that true nulls occur at smaller angles and that, beyond 10 degrees, only the so-called blockage null occurs. All nulls will exhibit the change in EMG histograms described above, since increased activity will result in a broader, flatter curve. The widths of the peaks shown in both primary positions and at the null for the two patients illustrated in this article bear the same relationship; the widths of both peaks for patient 5 are greater than those for patient 1. If these authors have uncovered a difference in the types of CN nulls present in the patient population, they have not proved it conclusively in this article. Furthermore, if the mere increase in activity of a muscle can be used to block the nystagmus, then all such patients should be able to do this in both directions. This is not seen with patients with binocular CN; it is with patients with strabismic LMLN. Also, this increase in synergistic activity is not equivalent to the blockage of CN with convergence where the increase in activity is in antagonistic muscles and affects the push-pull system in a different way.

An interesting Japanese pedigree of hereditary CN in five generations was attributed to X-linked irregular dominant transmission.[12] Absence of male-male transmission and generation skipping was noted. The CN waveforms were predominantly pendular, and there was good central vision and an absence of sensory defects in this pedigree. These patients are further examples that waveform cannot be used to classify CN as "sensory-defect" nystagmus. In another article, five male infants who showed findings of abnormal auditory brain-stem response and pendular CN were reported.[13] They also had hypotonia of head and limbs in the early infantile period and later paresis. Unfortunately, the method for recording the eye movements was poor, and it was impossible to identify the CN waveforms from the figures provided. If the time constant given was correct, the recordings more accurately reflect eye velocity than position. Given their other abnormalities, it is possible that these patients had both CN and other neurologic disorders as suggested by the authors. An animal model for CN may have been produced in monkeys by monocularly depriving them of vision at birth, then reversing their sutures 25 days later.[14] A variable nystagmus was observed that could be jerk, pendular, or combinations of both; the slow phases of the jerk nystagmus were of increasing velocity. Also, a latent component was noted on cover testing. At present, there is no known animal model for CN, and if this procedure is repeatable, it may provide one.

In our early studies of CN, we noted that responses to changes in target position were often combinations of hypometric saccades and the slow phases of the CN waveform.[15] This observation led us to hypothesize that CN was caused by an abnormality in the saccadic system; we have long since realized that it is in the slow eye movement system. An excellent article contains the responses to step changes in target position exhibited by subjects with CN.[16] It was found that the hypometric saccades or slow phase responses occurred most frequently when the target was displaced in the direction of the slow phase. Since the retinal stimulus produced by step change in a target position is the same stimulus that normal subjects receive from a step change followed by a ramp motion back toward the fovea, comparison was made with responses of normal subjects to the standard Rashbass stimulus. The authors concluded that the ocular motor responses of patients with CN were *normal saccadic responses* to the sequence of retinal image motion produced by this stimulus and not contributions from the pursuit system in response to position displacements on the retina, as has been suggested by others. The responses of patients with CN with albinism were less likely to contain saccades, and this was attributed to their impaired sensory functioning. Thus, there is now additional evidence supporting the hypothesis that both the saccadic and pursuit systems of subjects with CN *function normally* given the ongoing oscillation; this hypothesis was contained in the earliest model of the saccadic and pursuit systems operating in the presence of an ongoing oscillation.[17] In another article, albinism has been linked with periodic alternating CN.[18]

Two interesting cases of CN that became manifest only during unidirectional pursuit were reported.[19] It is well documented that the attempt to pursue a slowly moving target significantly alters CN. Specifically, the static null is shifted in the direction opposite to the pursuit. Thus, the actual CN amplitude at a given gaze angle is greater during pursuit than when viewing a stationary target since that gaze angle is farther from the null during pursuit than during steady fixation. It is common to record a high-amplitude CN waveform during pursuit of rapidly moving targets across the whole field of gaze, from 20 degrees left to 20 degrees right, despite the fact that the same subject might have a broad null region somewhere in this range when looking at stationary targets. In the two subjects presented in this article, no CN was present during fixation of stationary targets at any gaze angle. However, when pursuing targets moving in one direction, a nystagmus developed that had increasing-velocity exponential slow phases and was diagnosed as being CN. These patients' complaints of oscillopsia (OSOP) only during such pursuit have been with them throughout their lives. It is interesting that the normal suppression of OSOP seen in subjects with CN was not present in these cases where the nystagmus was only manifest during unidirectional pursuit. Given the effects of smooth pursuit on the CN null, the most parsimonious explanation for these observations is that these patients had a very broad null region that encompassed their whole range of gaze angles when viewing static targets. When they attempted to pursue in one direction, that null region was shifted in the opposite direction, causing a nystagmus in the same direction as the pursuit. These would be two extreme examples of the well-known null shift seen in most subjects with CN. Kawai[20] studied the effects of an optokinetic background on CN. He concluded (agreeing with my own observations) that the perceived circular vection is in the proper direction for the background movement and, furthermore, that the optokinetic nystagmus (OKN) dynamics were normal in subjects with CN.

In many subjects with CN, the nystagmus damps and acuity increases with convergence. The variety of clinical conditions under which this occurs suggests that this effect is determined by the convergence angle rather than the state of accommodation. A recent study confirmed this hypothesis and further found that binocular viewing was unnecessary for the damping of CN.[21] Also confirmed were the observations that asymmetric convergence damps CN (this is the basis for the use of composite prisms), and that, once converged, gaze angle plays no important role in CN amplitude (if it did, convergence prisms or bimedial recession operations would not be of much value since real-life situations require looking in all fields of gaze). By carefully controlling each variable, the author clearly demonstrated the importance of convergence.

In the final part of the article, the author attempted to evaluate the effects on visual acuity of prism therapy but neglected to adjust the patients' refractions while in the converged position. She correctly stated that base-out prisms have an identical effect on CN intensity at distance as at near fixation. However, both conditions cause accommodation that is beneficial at near but detrimental at distance. Therefore, the correct ("traditional") method of applying base-out prisms to increase acuity requires the addition of -1.00 diopters to the patient's distance refraction to negate the induced accommodation; this results in the clearest possible vision at distance. By merely adding prisms to the patient's normal distance refraction, the author was effectively "over-plussing" them at distance and requiring them constantly to fight their natural accommodated state induced by convergence; she did *not* duplicate the traditional therapy. This cannot result in optimal acuity and would be uncomfortable in the long term. Reducing CN increases acuity only when the afferent apparatus is functioning correctly. Either afferent defects (like foveal aplasia) or poor refraction will prevent maximal acuity even if the eyes were forcibly held still. Less than optimal refraction reduces acuity in all patients, so it is difficult to understand why an improvement in acuity was expected from patients with CN. The author's use of prisms without minus lenses produced two oppositely directed effects: CN was damped and vision was blurred. The net effect was no increase in acuity with prisms. When acuity is not compromised, the reduction of CN intensity *is* a sufficient condition for an increase in acuity. It is my opinion that both the final conclusion and Figure 10 are invalid and should be ignored by the reader. Unfortunately, this well-done study of the variables involved is marred by the misapplication of its results. Also, the use of Fresnel prisms is *not* the method of choice in these cases. They degrade vision, and, more important, the many vertical lines are very distracting to one whose eyes are constantly oscillating across them; at night any side light causes inordinate glare from the vertical lines. Prisms should be ground from optical-quality plastic or glass.

Von Noorden and Wong[22] recently reported the surgical results in the nystagmus blockage syndrome (NBS). The results of unilateral recession-resection and bimedial recession with or without posterior fixation sutures were comparable and poor. Both over- and under-corrections occurred more frequently, and the number of operations was higher than in a controlled group of essential infantile esotropia without nystagmus. Normal binocular vision was not achieved in a single case. It would appear from these results that NBS is not conducive to simple surgical correction. A spectral analysis of the EOG was used to evaluate CN surgery quantitatively.[23] Unfortunately, the use of AC-coupled, low-pass–filtered, bitemporal EOG severely limits the usefulness of the data gathered. Performing high-powered analysis on such poorly gathered data does not significantly increase the authority of the paper's conclusions. I agree with the authors that spectral analysis can be a useful tool in the quantitative study of CN and its surgery, but it should be applied to accurately measured data.

In response to occasional anecdotal reports of CN damping when contact lenses are inserted, we studied the effects of soft contact lenses on CN amplitude and waveform and on visual acuity.[24] We found that the presence of a contact lens can damp CN, owing to sensory feedback from the inner eyelid, and improve visual acuity. The use of a topical anesthetic abolished the effect; pressure on the eyelid (with no anesthetic) also reduced the CN. This is a new, benign, and potentially useful therapy that expands the population of patients with CN who can be helped to those without gaze-angle or convergence nulls while including those with nulls. Even in those without need for refractive correction, plano contacts should damp their CN and improve their acuity.

In addition to surgery, optical methods, and biofeedback, another treatment for CN has been introduced: acupuncture.[25] Four single needles with a diameter of 0.02 mm and length of 40 mm were inserted about 10 mm through the skin in the distal and proximal points of both sternocleidomastoid muscles. This is not painful (personal observation). The needle tips are stimulated by an electrical current carrying a square wave or by manually beating the needle every 5 minutes, and the duration of the insertion is 20 minutes. The program is repeated two times per month. Acupuncture was effective in eight of 13 cases; there were four young children with poor cooperation and one with cerebral palsy. After treatment, the effects persisted for 4 to 7 days with a reduction in CN amplitude of 50% and frequency of 15%. Acupuncture was also tried in two cases of acquired nystagmus and resulted in a reduced sensation of OSOP.

Jan et al.[26] described a test that is supposed to determine the amblyopic eye in infants with CN and associated sensory loss. The confusing and inaccurate term "sensory nystagmus" should be ignored by the reader; all CN is caused by a motor instability. The authors claim that when fixating with the poorer eye, the nystagmus will be "wider" (higher amplitude?) and slower and, when fixating with the better eye, faster and of smaller amplitude. They cautioned against applying this test in the presence of latent nystagmus (LN) or MLN but neglected CN with a latent component. Without recordings, none of these can be reliably differentiated. Applying this test to unknown types of nystagmus and attempting to evaluate the results without any objective criteria tells us nothing about the relationship (if any) between acuity of the fixating eye and measurable characteristics of CN. My experience has been that no such relationship exists for all patients, although a properly done study may show that many patients conform to the clinical impression of these authors. They have described a way to give parents a "quick answer"; I wonder if we can give them an accurate answer.

Convergence Nystagmus

An uncommon movement disorder (oculomasticatory myorhythmia) was identified in Whipple's disease.[27] It consists of convergence nystagmus and concurrent contractions of the masticatory muscles. The convergence nystagmus had dynamics characteristic of normal vergence movements and there was no palatal myoclonus. The authors concluded that patients with this sign should be treated presumptively for Whipple's disease.

Convergence-Evoked Nystagmus

An interesting case of convergence-evoked pendular nystagmus was reported.[28] Accommodative vergence was identified as the cause of this nystagmus, which only appeared when attempting to fixate a target moving toward the subject and was unaffected by covering one eye. The absence of neurologic or ophthalmologic abnormalities led the authors to classify this as a congenital type of nystagmus. Flutter, including voluntary flutter, was ruled out by the authors.

Dissociated Nystagmus

A common type of dissociated nystagmus (DISN) is that associated with spasmus nutans. Weissman et al.[29] identified the waveform as a pendular DISN whose key characteristic was the variable phase-shift between the oscillations of the two eyes. This study makes it possible to distinguish spasmus nutans from CN without the obligatory wait for the nystagmus to disappear.

An interesting form of DISN has been described in the context of coma.[30] It consisted of a slow divergence from primary position followed by a rapid return to primary position; the entire cycle could last from 4 to 10 seconds and was repeated irregularly every 1 to 15 seconds. The authors termed this "repetitive divergence." Since this was a repetitive oscillation, albeit a very slow one, it can be considered a rare form of DISN.

Downbeat Nystagmus

Gresty et al.[31] investigated otolithic and semicircular canal influences on downbeat nystagmus (DBTN). They concluded that the DBTN in their patient arose from an asymmetry of vertical canal function that became manifest when the otoliths were tilted with respect to gravity. Since, in a second patient, the DBTN was insensitive to tilt, they further concluded that various cases of DBTN lie on a continuum between these extreme examples. Although DBTN is usually associated with Arnold-Chiari malformations, two patients were reported with DBTN and lesions remote from the craniocervical junction.[32] One patient had decompensated aqueductal stenosis and the other had a midbrain infarction. Downbeat nystagmus has also been reported in a patient with vitamin B_{12} deficiency, which presumably resulted in cerebellar or brain-stem lesions,[33] and as a presenting sign in von Hippel-Lindau disease.[34]

A case of DBTN that was diagnosed with magnetic resonance imaging (MRI) and disappeared immediately after surgical treatment was recently described.[35] The responsible lesion was a syringomyelic cyst in the medulla. After the cyst was incised and emptied of fluid, both the nystagmus and the accompanying OSOP disappeared immediately.

Drug-Induced Nystagmus

Diazepam was used to maximally disrupt pursuit performance as part of a study of the effects of training and disruption on smooth pursuit.[36] The authors uncovered inherent asymmetries in vertical smooth eye movements that contribute to drug-induced vertical nystagmus. Downbeat nystagmus was reported with lithium intoxication[37] and secondary to excessive alcohol intake[38]; the latter was reversible after a period of abstinence. More commonly, alcohol produces horizontal gaze-evoked nystagmus, and this has led to a "roadside sobriety" test conducted by law enforcement officers.[39] Using nystagmus as an indicator of alcohol intoxication is an unfortunate choice, since many normal individuals have physiologic end-point nystagmus; small doses of tranquilizers that would not interfere with driving can produce nystagmus; nystagmus may be congenital or consequent to neurologic disease; and without a neuro-ophthalmologist or someone knowledgeable about sophisticated methods of eye movement recordings, it is difficult to determine whether the nystagmus is pathologic. It is unreasonable that such difficult judgments have been placed in the hands of minimally trained law officers.

Epileptic Nystagmus

Lavin[40] reported a case of pupillary oscillations synchronized with epileptic nystagmus. The nystagmus beat with a fast phase that was contralateral to the focus of the abnormality, and the pupils dilated as the eyes moved laterally and constricted when they returned toward the central position. This "clonic" phase lasted about 30 seconds, and the pupils remained symmetric during and after the seizures.

Induced Nystagmus

Electrical stimulation of the nucleus of the optic tract (NOT) resulted in horizontal nystagmus with ipsilateral slow phases followed by after-nystagmus in the same direction.[41] The time course of the slow-phase velocity was similar to that of OKN and optokinetic after-nystagmus (OKAN). Both the rising and falling time constants of the nystagmus and after-nystagmus were sensitive to the frequency and duration of the electrical stimulation. The authors concluded that the NOT stimulation elicited the component of OKN that is responsible for the slow rise in slow-phase velocity and for OKAN. Functionally, NOT was seen as a major source of visual information related to retinal slip. The indirect pathway that excites the velocity storage mechanism in the vestibular system to produce the slow component of OKN and OKAN probably lies in NOT in the monkey as it does for other animals.

Latent/Manifest Latent Nystagmus

Von Noorden et al.[42] recently reported on the successful application of conventional occlusion therapy in patients with LN and strabismic amblyopia. The diagnosis of LN or MLN was made on clinical grounds, and it is therefore possible that some of the patients diagnosed with LN may have had a low-amplitude MLN. It is also possible that some of the patients had CN with a latent component; without accurate eye movement recordings, the waveforms of the nystagmus cannot be determined. I agree with the authors that it is clinically irrelevant to distinguish between LN, MLN, and CN for the purposes of amblyopia treatment, but it is extremely important to make this distinction when considering surgical or other therapy of the nystagmus itself. While it was previously thought that strabismus is almost always present in patients with LMLN, better recording techniques have led us to hypothesize that strabismus is a necessary condition for LMLN and is therefore present in 100% of the cases.[43]

Moidell et al.[44] studied the effect of early enucleation on the position of the egocenter. The egocenter, that is, the origin of judgments of visual direction, is normally located on the median plane of the head midway between the two eyes. The authors found a significant shift of the egocenter toward the remaining eye of the enucleates that was unrelated to the age at enucleation and concluded that egocenter location is plastic and can be modified by the complete monocularity imposed by enucleation. This documentation of egocenter shift is supportive evidence for the hypothesis that it is the inability to reconcile the difference between monocular egocentric direction and binocular egocentric direction that is the primary cause for LMLN.[45] We reported on a case of unidirectional LMLN in a patient with a congenitally blind eye that was replaced by a prosthesis.[46] We found that his unidirectional MLN spontaneously changed direction in the dark and beat toward his blind eye rather than the eye he always used for vision. We concluded that eye dominance was genetically predetermined and not influenced by visual development, this despite the shifting of his egocenter toward his good eye. In another study of children with congenital or early loss of vision in one eye, visual evoked responses (VER) were evaluated.[47] Half of these patients developed a jerky nystagmus whose clinical description strongly suggests MLN. The authors concluded that VER asymmetries correlated with ocular motor disturbances.

Lid Nystagmus

Howard described a case of convergence-evoked lid nystagmus in a patient with a large angiomatous lesion distorting the blood supply to the pontomesencephalic and pontomedullary junctions.[48] In addition, bilateral gaze-evoked and upbeat nystagmus were sometimes present; they were considered to be independent of the lid nystagmus that beat in the upward direction. Owing to the extent of the lesion, precise localization of the site causing dissociation between the lid and ocular nystagmus was not possible.

Optokinetic Nystagmus

Subjects with normal stereopsis will exhibit OKN when viewing moving stereoscopic contours in a dynamic random-dot stereogram. The use of this phenomenon as an objective test of stereopsis requires that stereoblind subjects not develop OKN. Archer et al.[49] recently showed this to be the case. None of their stereoblind subjects had an optomotor response to stereoscopic contours regardless of the alignment angle at which the image pair was presented.

Zee et al.[50] reported the effects of occipital lobectomy on eye movements in rhesus monkeys. They found that OKN was markedly altered but not abolished in all animals. The velocity-storage component of OKN was present, but the immediate-pursuit component was eliminated. The maximum value of OKN that could be achieved was decreased to 10% of the preoperative values. The authors noted that the residual OKN was similar to that of afoveate animals, with a diminished response to high velocities of retinal-image motion and a predominance for temporal-to-nasal motion during monocular viewing. Immediately after occipital lobectomy, the necessity for the occipital cortex in normal primates was evident; it makes the predominant contribution toward the generation of the velocity-storage component of OKN. The long-term changes suggested that monkeys could learn to use extrastriate pathways to generate more volitional types of visual-ocular motor behavior. However, some of the more reflexive mechanisms for stabilizing images on the retina eventually deteriorate, presumably owing to the loss of visual feedback. Finally, the authors noted that as some of the ocular motor functions recovered, others deteriorated. Specifically, spontaneous and gaze-evoked nystagmus developed 3 to 6 months after surgery, and the time constant of the neural integrator dropped to values as low as 2.6 to 4.8 seconds.

In man it is difficult to distinguish true OKN from "pseudo-OKN" that is probably mediated by the pursuit system. Since pursuit is predominantly a foveal reflex, it is interesting to observe OKN in patients with central visual field defects. Crevits and Van Vliet[51] reported on six such patients. They found, in some cases, an inverted OKN. A prerequisite for eliciting this was directing the attention of the subject to the field defect; if attention was directed peripherally, the OKN was normal. In general, the reversed OKN was sporadic and occurred only at stimulus velocities of 120 degrees per second.

Verhagen et al.[52] examined the ocular motor responses of a patient who survived the locked-in syndrome. The patient had a pontine infarction mainly on the right side. There was a lack of cortical OKN and preservation of subcortical OKN in this patient. In contrast to previous studies of OKN in patients with the locked-in syndrome, a full-field stimulus was used rather than the small tape normally employed at the bedside; this may be the reason that OKN has been found to be absent in many of these cases. In addition to OKN, the vestibulo-ocular response (VOR) was measured. Postrotary nystagmus responses revealed vestibular hyperreactivity and short time constants with internuclear ophthalmoplegia (INO) on both sides. Since survival of such patients is rare, the recordings made yielded some insight into the ocular motor subsystems involved.

Yee et al.[53] studied both OKN and the VOR in patients with schizophrenia. They found that mean gains in OKN and pursuit of schizophrenic patients were significantly lower than those of normal subjects. Also, suppression of the VOR by fixation was impaired in this patient population. The authors noted that the groups of patients they studied were taking psychotropic drugs at the time of the study, and these medications could be responsible for the impairment of eye movements found. Though they found some impairment in schizophrenics, they concluded that the magnitude of the impairment was less than suggested in previous studies and that specific eye movement abnormalities might not be a reliable biologic marker for schizophrenia.

Optokinetic After-Nystagmus

Lafortune et al.[54] investigated a dependence of human OKAN, velocity storage, and OKN characteristics on the optokinetic stimulus exposure time. Their results supported the hypothesis of two velocity storage integrators, one responsible for the short time constant decay (pursuit mediated) and the other for the long time constant decay (optokinetic system mediated). They demonstrated a dependence of the long time constant integrator of OKAN on the stimulus exposure time, but the short time constant integrator appeared to be independent of exposure time. They concluded that the charging time course of each component was independent of the other. The decay time constants of each component were found to be invariant. Their data suggested that the integrators were direction sensitive. In a related study, Jell et al.[55] studied the after-effects subsequent to pursuit of a single light-emitting diode (LED) target. Subjects pursued a target moving at 20 degrees per second from 30 degrees left to center gaze and repeated the pursuit after a 3-second period of darkness. The decay of pursuit began about 130 msec after the LED went out, and the authors used this value to obtain all pursuit decay curves. The measured decay time constant was exactly what would have been predicted because of the mechanical and viscoelastic properties of the eyeball in the orbit. The authors concluded that a neural integrator probably does not exist in the system, but if it did, its decay time constant would have to be 0.3 seconds or less.

Himi et al.[56] studied the asymmetry of vertical OKAN in squirrel monkeys. Optokinetic after-nystagmus commonly has two components: OKAN-I is in the same direction as the OKN and OKAN-II is in the opposite direction. These authors found that the slow-phase eye velocity of upward OKAN-I increased with increasing stimulus velocity, whereas that of downward OKAN-I diminished. The time constant of OKAN-I was shortened with an increase in stimulus speed in both directions. With a downward stimulus, a short stimulus duration failed to elicit OKAN-II. With a longer stimulus duration, the appearance of OKAN-II increased in percentage. Their data showed that the asymmetry of OKAN-I and OKAN-II differed.

Optokinetic nystagmus is attenuated by fixation of a stationary target, and illusory induced motion (IM) of that target occurs opposite to the direction of the stimulus motion. It has been proposed that the IM is caused by a perceptually registered efferent signal for pursuit that opposes an unregistered signal for OKN. If this were true, parallel changes in the magnitudes of IM and optokinetic reflexes during and after optokinetic stimulation should occur. Heckmann and Post[57] found that leftward IM magnitude and rightward slow-phase velocity of OKAN increased at similar rates across 90 and 160 seconds of 60 degrees per second motion of background contours and decayed at similar rates after stimulus termination. The close dynamic correlation of OKAN slow-phase velocity with IM of opposite direction parallels previous work studying the effects of stimulus direction, luminance, and velocity. The authors concluded that a voluntary efferent signal, which sums negatively with a signal in the optokinetic system to achieve stable fixation, produces IM of the fixated target. Their hypothesis also applies to the oculogyral illusion, autokinesis, and apparent motion of a fixated target during head movement. This study also contains a general discussion of several other related hypotheses.

Both OKN and OKAN in the vertical direction were studied using three head positions (upright, lateral, and head-hanging).[58] Normal subjects were subjected to full-field OKN stimulation; OKN asymmetry (downbeating greater than upbeating) was noted in the upright position at various stripe velocities. In three subjects this asymmetry was eliminated in the head-hanging position but only slightly reduced in the lateral position; in one subject the asymmetry was reversed in the head-hanging position. Downbeating OKAN was found in half of the subjects in the upright position but was not affected by position change; upbeating OKAN never occurred.

Pendular Nystagmus

Dehaene et al.[59] described a case of acquired pendular nystagmus (PNDN) in a patient with multiple sclerosis. The nystagmus was vertical and uniocular; after eye closure it became binocular. Although the authors stated that PNDN was present only in primary position, during upgaze the PNDN can clearly be seen superimposed on an upbeat jerk nystagmus in their Figure 1, part 3. During exacerbation of the multiple sclerosis, the PNDN disappeared and a bilateral INO and rebound nystagmus were observed. With the disappearance of the INO and rebound nystagmus, the PNDN reappeared. When the PNDN was present, the patient complained of OSOP. Cordonnier et al.[60] described a case of reversible acquired PNDN occurring after brain-stem hemorrhage. Their patient also had bilateral horizontal gaze palsy and skew deviation on downgaze; a pontine lesion was detected. These two cases illustrate the difficulty one encounters in trying to localize the disturbance that might be responsible for acquired PNDN. Pendular oscillations result from instabilities in closed-loop control systems, and therefore, pathology at any of several sites that interrupt or alter a neurologic closed loop can be the cause of the instability.

Periodic/Aperiodic Alternating Nystagmus

Nuti et al.[61] described two cases of aperiodic alternating nystagmus (APAN), one caused by vertebrobasilar insufficiency and the second by a whiplash injury. In addition to APAN, gaze-evoked nystagmus, rebound nystagmus, saccadic dysmetria, square-wave jerks (SWJ), vestibular nystagmus, and OSOP were exhibited at various times by these patients. The first patient was treated with baclofen with satisfactory results. In CN, APAN is common, but the acquired varieties are often much more periodic. The authors pointed out the connection between rebound nystagmus and periodic alternating nystagmus (PAN), with the former due to less severe pathology than the latter. Cohen et al.[62] studied the effects of baclofen on the VOR and velocity storage in rhesus monkeys. They found a reduction in the VOR time constant, reduced off-axis rotary nystagmus slow phases, reduced OKN gain, and reduced peak velocity and falling time constant of OKAN. The effects of baclofen were simulated on a model by reducing the falling time constant of the velocity-storage integrator. Functionally, baclofen reduces the effectiveness of compensatory ocular motor reflexes. Since PAN may result from an inability to stabilize elements of velocity storage, reducing the storage time constant would also shorten the VOR time constant and stabilize the system.

Larmande et al.[63] reported a case of periodic alternating ping-pong gaze (PAPPG). The lesion responsible for the movement was initially unilateral, and the PAPPG was intermittent and associated with Cheyne-Stokes respiration. Since PAPPG is usually observed during coma and in connection with widespread bilateral hemispheric ischemia, this particular manifestation is interesting and necessitates reevaluation of the possible cause of the disorder.

Reflex Nystagmus

Reflex (Baer's) nystagmus is a low-amplitude, high-frequency acquired nystagmus associated with erosion or other superficial lesions of the cornea.[64]

See-Saw Nystagmus

Although see-saw nystagmus (SSN) is usually pendular, a recent case was reported with jerk SSN due to brain-stem infarction.[65] No ocular motility records were presented. Two cases (siblings) of congenital SSN associated with retinitis pigmentosa have also been reported.[66] Although it has previously been reported that in congenital SSN the rising eye extorts and falling eye intorts, these patients exhibited the characteristic rising-eye intorsion and falling-eye extorsion seen in patients with acquired SSN. The authors concluded that it is not possible to diagnose congenital from acquired SSN solely from the torsional component. It was gratifying to read that, despite the presence of retinitis pigmentosa, the authors did not fall into the trap of ascribing this congenital nystagmus to the sensory defect. In another report, SSN was described in a patient who suffered bitemporal hemianopia due to head trauma.[67] Curiously, the SSN ceased temporarily after ingestion of alcohol; it also disappeared during sleep. See-saw nystagmus has been associated with a Chiari malformation.[68] This patient, who complained of OSOP, improved after surgical decompression. The authors pointed out the importance of the association between SSN and Chiari malformations since early diagnosis and decompression might improve neurologic function and prevent further deterioration. Kanter et al.[69] presented a patient with SSN whose lesion was localized by MRI to the paramedian ventral midbrain with involvement of the right interstitial nucleus of Cajal. This was the first MRI study of SSN associated with a presumed brain-stem vascular event.

Torsional Nystagmus

Using the new torsional search coil, Noseworthy et al.[70] reported on a case of torsional nystagmus secondary to a midpontine lesion that was probably a venous angioma. The waveforms had both linear and increasing-velocity slow phases. The nystagmus increased during active pitch rotations of the head and damped with convergence. The authors postulated a disruption of central vestibular connections.

Upbeat Nystagmus

Upbeat nystagmus was described in a family whose members have a dominantly inherited, early onset, nonprogressive syndrome that includes mild cerebellar ataxia associated with cerebellar vermian atrophy seen on MRI.[71] The slow phases were linear and the nystagmus obeyed Alexander's law. Two other patients with upbeat nystagmus were described; they suffered from caudal brain-stem dysfunction.[72] The authors suggested that dorsal paramedian damage in the rostral medulla was probably the critical lesion responsible for the upbeat nystagmus.

Vertical Nystagmus

Ishikawa et al.[73] described a patient with neuro-Behçet syndrome whose vertical nystagmus was upbeat and changed to downbeat with caloric stimulation. Some months later her upbeat nystagmus had decreased and she developed downbeat nystagmus on downgaze. Initially, tilting her head decreased her upbeat nystagmus, but during the latter examination, the tilt caused the downbeat nystagmus to increase. Both findings suggested a vestibular component to the patient's vertical nystagmus. The eye movement recordings revealed slow phases that could be linear, or increasing- or decreasing-velocity waveforms. In another case, a patient exhibited upbeat and downbeat nystagmus as a result of a thalamic arteriovenous malformation and no sign of posterior fossa disease.[74] No eye movement recordings were provided.

Vestibular Nystagmus

Gresty et al.[75] studied eye movement responses to combined linear and angular head movement. The response to linear motion was evaluated by subtracting responses to head-centered angular oscillation about a vertical axis (on-axis) from those evoked by similar oscillation with the head displaced 30 cm eccentrically from the axis (off-axis). This assumes a linear summation of both effects. The eccentric position evoked movements of higher velocity, especially at the higher frequencies and when subjects imagined near targets. The gain of the linear response under this condition was about -1, suggesting that eye velocity compensates for linear head velocity, and is in accord with the thoretical prediction that, when viewing near targets, eye movements compensate for linear head motion. Grossman et al.[76] evaluated frequency and velocity ranges of natural head rotations. They found that the maximum fundamental horizontal frequencies during walking and jogging were 1 and 3 Hz, respectively, whereas the maximum vertical frequencies were 4 and 3 Hz. However, the vertical rotations contained significant harmonic components that could reach 15 to 20 Hz during vigorous jogging. Voluntary horizontal head rotations could produce 5 Hz, while vertical rotations produced up to 4 Hz. Since head velocities during walking and jogging (horizontal and vertical) were less than 160 degrees per second whereas voluntary head shaking could produce velocities greater than 500 degrees per second, it is not surprising that OSOP accompanies vigorous head rotations; they may reflect unnatural demands on the VOR.

Hain et al.[77] studied head-shaking nystagmus (HSN) in patients with unilateral peripheral vestibular lesions. In addition to HSN, whose slow phases are directed toward the side of the lesion, all subjects showed a prolonged, lower-amplitude reversal phase. The authors were able to explain this behavior using a model that included the central velocity-storage mechanism, Ewald's second law, and adaptation of primary vestibular afferent activity. They concluded that, in patients with unilateral peripheral lesions, HSN always has both phases and that the reversal phase does not suggest clinical recovery but rather a short-term adaptive process together with a significant unilateral peripheral lesion. When HSN does not have a reversal phase it may be caused by a central lesion. The authors pointed out that HSN was not specific for vestibular lesions since one of their normal subjects also had HSN. However, Takahashi[78] reported three cases of bidirectional HSN caused by central vestibular disturbance. Thus, both central and peripheral lesions can cause bidirectional HSN.

It has been found that under conditions of microgravity, a nonconvective caloric nystagmus exists. However, under usual clinical conditions (normal gravity), about 85% of the maximal thermal reaction is explained by the convection hypothesis of Bárány.[79] An examination of nystagmus intensity in the supine and prone positions in 22 healthy ears found high interindividual variance and an exceptional case with predominately nonconvectively released nystagmus. A vertical nystagmus or vertical nystagmus component can sometimes be elicited with caloric stimulation of the horizontal canals. Such perverted nystagmus suggests brain-stem pathology. However, a case was presented with confirmed peripheral pathology in which vertical nystagmus was elicited in this way.[80] The author discussed the possibility of dissociated canal dysfunction secondary to a unilateral horizontal semicircular canal. Caloric nystagmus has been demonstrated in a chronic persistent vegetative state with intact brain-stem reflexes. Recently, caloric nystagmus was recorded in a patient with an isoelectric EEG.[81] This is further evidence of the brain-stem nature of the caloric nystagmus reflex.

Lin et al.[82] studied direction-changing positional nystagmus. Although this is commonly considered an indication of central disease, these authors found peripheral vestibular lesions. They also found that apogeotropic nystagmus was no more frequent in central lesions than was geotropic nystagmus. Using a portable recording apparatus, Nishikawa and Nishikawa[83] were able to record the nystagmus in a case of Meniere's disease before, during, and after the vertiginous attack. Before the attack, the nystagmus was toward the affected side, at the onset of the attack, toward the nonaffected side, and both during and after the attack, toward the affected side. No hypothetical mechanisms were proposed to account for this time course. Hain et al.[84] studied postrotary nystagmus in normal subjects and patients with cerebellar lesions. The vestibular response of the normal subjects decayed with a time constant of 19.6 seconds when upright and 7.2 seconds after tilting prone, whereas those with midline cerebellar lesions showed no effect of the tilting. The authors concluded that the midline cerebellum regulates a neural network in the brain stem that perseverates peripheral vestibular input.

Barratt et al.[85] studied responses of patients with neuro-otologic disease to off-axis rotation. Patients with vestibular neurinectomies who had asymmetric responses to on-axis rotation showed greater asymmetry with off-axis rotation at high stimulus frequencies. Some patients with cerebellar lesions showed abnormally enhanced or depressed and asymmetric responses in the off-axis rotation when compared with on-axis rotation. All patients with abnormal off-axis responses had positional nystagmus. In contrast, patients with benign paroxysmal vertigo (BPV) or chronic linear vertigo did not show abnormal off-axis responses. The authors concluded that off-axis testing may be useful in elucidating pathophysiology but is not a decisive clinical test for the presence of otolith dysfunction.

Baloh et al.[86] reported on 240 cases of BPV. A torsional paroxysmal positional nystagmus always occurred after a rapid position change from sitting to head-hanging. Their data suggested a peripheral posterior semicircular canal origin of BPV. The authors noted that unless the patient was tested during the period of acute episodes of vertigo, positional nystagmus was not observed. Lackner and Graybiel[87] found that Coriolis cross-coupled angular acceleration stimulation readily induced motion sickness under terrestrial conditions. This susceptibility was in direct proportion to gravity. These findings explain the low susceptibility of Skylab astronauts to motion sickness during in-flight stimulation. In another study, these authors found that head movements in free fall, especially pitch movements, were provocative until adaptation occurred.[88] They concluded that space motion sickness was a consequence of prolonged exposure to a nonterrestrial force background rather than of exposure to free fall per se. Watt[89] concluded that prolonged exposure to inappropriate VOR will usually lead to motion sickness. He suggested that though VOR gain may be decreased in weightlessness initially, rapid compensatory mechanisms restore it to normal within minutes of reaching weightlessness. This compensation is not enough to protect against the development of motion sickness, however.

SACCADIC INTRUSIONS AND OSCILLATIONS

Nonnystagmic ocular motor intrusions and oscillations represent solely saccadic or saccadically initiated instabilities. I have identified 16 varieties of saccadic intrusions and oscillations that have been characterized in the literature by many other terms, including ten that erroneously contain the term *nystagmus*. This section contains discussions of recent studies of saccadic intrusions and oscillations; they are in alphabetical order. For discussions of other types, see previous reports on the subject.[1-4]

Bobbing/Dipping

Rosa et al.[90] studied five cases of ocular bobbing, with postmortem examination in two. Three of the cases were described as typical, one atypical, and one asymmetric. The commonly damaged nervous structure in four of the five cases was the pons. One of their cases was the first reported case of bobbing in a patient with Creutzfeldt-Jakob disease. The authors hypothesized that both mesencephalic and medullary burst neuron centers played a prevalent part in ocular bobbing. There is some disagreement regarding both the necessity for patients to be comatose to exhibit dipping and whether cerebral structures are involved.[91, 92] Although coma may not be necessary, it is agreed that a reduced level of consciousness is required for dipping to occur. In a report on the clinical spectrum of ocular bobbing and dipping, Mehler[93] reported the first case of reverse dipping. Bobbing begins with a fast downward phase, reversed bobbing with a fast upward phase, and dipping with a slow downward phase; all have been previously described. Reverse dipping begins with a slow upward phase, and its description completes the four possibilities. Rosenberg[94] described two patients who had three of these four types of movements: bobbing, dipping, and reverse bobbing. He suggested that they may all be differing manifestations of the still-unknown pathophysiologic process. The description of a case of atypical bobbing in acute organophosphate poisoning is another instance where a severe intrinsic pontine lesion is not required for atypical bobbing.[95] Dipping has been described in a patient with deafness and pinealoblastoma.[96] Since this was a discrete lesion, the authors discussed possible mechanisms. A clear difference between this and previous cases was that the patient was alert. In this and most other articles on bobbing and dipping, the absence of good ocular motility records weakens speculation and hypotheses on responsible mechanisms.

Convergence-Retraction "Nystagmus"

Oohira et al.[97] studied five patients with convergence-retraction "nystagmus." In four of the five, the waveforms were typical: adducting fast phases and decreasing-velocity slow phases. In the other, the fast phases appeared to be slow saccades possibly because of small or absent innervational pulses. The authors compared the fast phases of convergence-retraction nystagmus with the associated and voluntary adducting movement seen during vertical saccades in normal subjects. They suggested that a disorder in the neural circuitry that regulates the excitability of neurons involved in these eye movements is responsible for convergence nystagmus.

Flutter

Herishanu et al.[98] reported an unusual case of blink-induced flutter in a patient with multiple sclerosis. The flutter was present whenever the patient blinked or attempted to blink while her lids were held open; no spontaneous saccadic intrusions or oscillations were observed during fixation. Furman et al.[99] reported spontaneous remission of ocular flutter and other saccadic intrusions and oscillations in two women. Since their remission preceded the appearance of a primary neoplastic process remote from the nervous system, the authors warned that such remission does not necessarily imply a benign outcome. Bergenius[100] studied the saccadic abnormalities in patients who exhibited ocular flutter. He found opsoclonus, increased frequency of SWJ, high peak velocity of voluntary saccades, and hypermetria. Salonen et al.[101] reported a case of sarcoidosis where flutter was the only neurologic sign. The flutter disappeared in 2 months, and the authors suggested that neurosarcoidosis should be considered as a potential cause.

Hotson investigated the proposal that voluntary flutter is an inherent capability in humans.[101a] He found no difference in saccadic peak velocity between control subjects and those capable of voluntary flutter. With training, control subjects were able to learn to produce runs of voluntary flutter. This learned flutter was composed of recurrent complete saccades rather than saccades interrupted in midflight. He concluded that voluntary flutter is not a genetic trait but a learned event that is usually undeveloped in man.

Macro–Square-Wave Jerks (Bursts/Single)

Fukazawa et al.[102] reported on a patient with marked atrophy of the cerebellum and brain stem. Both macro–square-wave jerks (MSWJ) and macro-saccadic oscillations (MSO) were recorded. By recording both horizontal and vertical eye movements, the authors demonstrated that both these oscillations had a vertical component (i.e., they were diagonal movements). The patient's oscillations almost completely disappeared after administration of several sedative drugs; she denied having OSOP. The discussion of MSWJ, SWJ, and MSO is confused, reflecting the misconception that MSWJ are merely large SWJ; this is an unfortunate and common result of the original naming of MSWJ. Although SWJ are usually of smaller amplitude than MSWJ, we have recorded large SWJ in some patients and small MSWJ in others. Thus, as pointed out in an earlier report,[103] the real difference between MSWJ and SWJ is in the latency between the initial and final saccade. In SWJ it is 200 msec, and in MSWJ it can vary between 50 and 150 msec. The authors also seemed confused about the differences between MSWJ and MSO; these were also pointed out in the earlier study. Table 3 contains the similarities and differences between these three oscillations and square-wave oscillations (SWO), a more recently described phenomenon.[104]

Myoclonus

Myoclonus is a pendular oscillation that conforms to the definition of nystagmus and is so regarded by European writers. It is usually classified separately because of associated rhythmic movements of nonocular muscles in synchrony with the eyes. It was originally referred to as "pharyngeal and laryngeal nystagmus."[105]

TABLE 3.

Characteristics of Square-Wave Instabilities

	SWJ	SWO	MSWJ	MSO
Amplitude, degrees	0.5–5, constant*	0.5–5, constant*	4–30, variable	1–30, increasing then decreasing
Time course	Sporadic/ bursts	Bursts	Bursts/ sporadic	Bursts
Latency, msec	200	200	50–150	200
Foveation	Yes	Yes	Yes	No
Presence in darkness	Yes	Yes	Yes	No

*Amplitudes occasionally may reach 10 degrees.

Ocular myoclonus is a form of segmental myoclonus[106] and is characterized by continuous, rhythmic, to-and-fro pendular oscillation, usually in the vertical plane. Nakada and Kwee[107] pointed out that myoclonus may have oblique and rotary components. They speculated that the generation of myoclonus involved the VOR adaptation mediated by the flocculus and provided a model that might account for it. Myoclonus that is present even during sleep usually persists as a chronic sign until the death of the patient.[108] There have been reports of myoclonus responding to treatment using valproic acid[109] and trihexyphenidyl.[110]

Opsoclonus

Adding to the many substances that have been reported to induce opsoclonus, Dehaene and Van Vleymen[111] presented a case in which phenytoin and diazepam caused opsoclonus. Hunter and Kooistra[112] discussed the neuropathologic findings in a case of opsoclonus. They found structural lesions limited to the cerebellum and inferior olives and severe depletion of Purkinje cells with preservation of granular cells in the neocerebellum and paleocerebellum. Purkinje cells were preserved in the archicerebellum. No abnormalities were found in the paramedian pontine reticular formation of the caudal pons. In a case of opsoclonus associated with adenocarcinoma of the breast, steroid treatment was successful.[113] Ridley et al.[114] looked at omnipause neurons in two cases of opsoclonus associated with oat cell carcinoma of the lung. The light-microscopic appearance of these neurons was normal. The authors concluded that, although the cells appeared normal, it is still possible that their function was disturbed and opsoclonus resulted. Borodic et al. have extensively reviewed the literature of 19 autopsied cases of opsoclonus.[115]

Saccadic Lateropulsion

Benjamin et al.[116] recorded both lateropulsion and upbeat nystagmus as manifestations of central vestibular dysfunction. The patient had a right hemispheric cerebellar infarction. The lateropulsion was contralateral to the side of the lesion. The authors discussed the lesion (shown on a computed tomogram of the brain) as it related to vestibulo-ocular pathways and concluded that the combination of lateropulsion and upbeat nystagmus was caused by an interruption of these pathways.

Saccadic Pulses/Pulse Trains

We hypothesized that the fast phases of so-called abduction nystagmus of INO are really saccadic pulses present in the abducting eye as a result of the weakness in the adducting eye.[117] Zee et al.[118] recently supplied additional evidence in support of that hypothesis. They studied four patients with INO and patched one eye for 1 to 5 days to allow the nervous system time to optimize innervation for the habitually viewing eye. They found that the conjugate adjustment of innervation diminished the abduction overshoot and backward postsaccadic drift made by the habitually viewing eye. The authors conclude that abduction nystagmus is a manifestation of a normal adaptive response in patients with INO.

Square-Wave Jerks/Oscillations

Ohtsuka et al.[119] studied the origin of SWJ under conditions of fixation of targets of variable size. The size of SWJ was found to be directly related to the size of the target; the frequency and duration of SWJ remained constant and were independent of target size. The SWJ within the range of microsaccades disappeared as larger SWJ appeared. The authors concluded that SWJ were enlarged versions of microsaccadic SWJ that appear when viewing very small targets. The authors agreed with Doslak et al.[119a] and concluded that the saccadic intrusion (i.e., the first saccade of a SWJ) is caused by a spurious error signal that takes the eye off the target, creating a real error that is corrected by the return saccade after a normal latency. Even in the dark, the eye position after an SWJ equaled the mean eye position before the SWJ. Thus, SWJ occur normally but are usually of microsaccadic amplitudes. The instability of eye position in the dark in patients with cerebellar degeneration was found to differ from that of normal subjects.[120] In addition to SWJ, unidirectional drifts and corrective saccades were observed. Patients with spinocerebellar degeneration showed unsteadiness in nonvisual eye position control. In normal subjects, both in light and in darkness, saccadic intrusions provoked position error signals, and corrective saccades were elicited producing SWJ. However, in patients with moderate and marked instability, the saccadic intrusions did not elicit corrective saccades, and SWJ were not observed. The authors concluded that a position error signal was not provoked in these patients in the dark. They further hypothesized that proprioceptive afferent information from eye muscles contributes to controlling eye position in the dark through the cerebellum.

Both SWO and SWJ were reported in an infant preceding the appearance of CN 5 months later.[121] No other nervous system abnormalities were found. The authors hypothesized that these saccadic oscillations and intrusions precluded the early appearance of the developing CN. Such oscillations in infancy may be a benign condition.

Superior Oblique Myokymia

Rosenthal and Selhorst[122] studied a patient with adenocarcinoma who exhibited continuous nonrhythmic cycloversions. The amplitudes of these cycloversions were 2 degrees and 5 degrees, and superimposed on them were conjugate jerky clockwise clycloversions up to 30 degrees that lasted 3 to 5 seconds. These occurred with a frequency of one to three per minute. It is possible that this is an uncommon form of superior oblique myokymia. Until more recordings are made (with the torsional eye coil) of superior oblique myokymia, it will not be possible to differentiate cases such as this from those with a more common form of superior oblique myokymia. It is important to know what the waveforms are before attempting to differentiate one eye movement from another. Without such information, it is virtually impossible to determine if an oscillation is different from, or merely an unusual form of, another oscillation. Simple clinical descriptions of oculomotor oscillations are not accurate enough and can be erroneous.

OSCILLOPSIA

Oscillopsia is the subjective, illusory movement of the stationary world.[123] Normal ocular motor control systems can prevent slip of images on the retina from exceeding about 4 degrees per second. When retinal image velocity (RIV), commonly called "retinal slip," exceeds that value, visual acuity begins to decline and OSOP may result. Oscillopsia is a common consequence of acquired nystagmus but not of saccadic intrusions or oscillations. Also, most patients with CN do not experience OSOP despite slow-phase RIV that may exceed 100 degrees per second. This subjective feeling of motion of the environment has been associated with acquired nystagmus caused by an Arnold-Chiari malformation[124] or even carbamazepine therapy.[125] Reduction of the nystagmus has caused an equal diminution of the OSOP.[126] Since any excessive RIV may be related to OSOP, nystagmus need not be present. A change in the VOR gain sufficient to cause high RIV may also result in OSOP. Verhagen et al.[127] reported three cases in a family with congenital vestibular areflexia. There was no nystagmus in these patients, and the OSOP occurred only during head or body movements. Oscillopsia has also been caused by aminoglycoside ototoxicity.[128] The authors referred to this as "subjective oscillopsia," which is redundant since all OSOP is subjective. In these patients, OSOP occurred during movement, and there was no nystagmus or other ocular oscillations.

Although there is a direct relationship between RIV and visual acuity, there is not one with OSOP. The magnitude of OSOP cannot be directly related to RIV; in acquired downbeat nystagmus, the magnitude of OSOP is approximately 0.37 of the nystagmus magnitude. At the far end of the spectrum are those patients with CN in whom there are both high RIV and no OSOP. Brandt and Dieterich[129] proposed that the dissociation between RIV and OSOP can be explained by a combination of two separate mechanisms that involve motion perception. These are a physiologic elevation of thresholds to detect object-motion with moving eyes, and a pathologic elevation of thresholds to detect object-motion with either infranuclear ocular motor palsy or supranuclear ocular oscillations. They found that thresholds for egocentric detection of object motion were higher in patients with downbeat nystagmus than in normal subjects and the thresholds increased with increasing nystagmus amplitude. There was a partial suppression of visual motion perception for both the RIV caused by the nystagmus and for objects moving within the visual scene. During smooth pursuit, the motion detection threshold of the visual background increases proportionally with eye velocity. Thus, there appears to be a visual motion perception suppression during eye movements that may reflect a basic sensorimotor mechanism. It has been suggested that the nervous system contains mechanisms whose tuning characteristics in both space and time can be modified and make it possible to do what a camera cannot: resolve form and motion simultaneously and independently.[130] This independence is used clinically by the oscillatory movement displacement threshold (the smallest amplitude of oscillation that causes the perception of movement) to access ocular neural dysfunction in the presence of media opacities.[131]

In an attempt to further understand the relationship between RIV and OSOP, Leigh et al.[132] studied retinal image stabilization in subjects with CN. All subjects reported OSOP during retinal image stabilization, but the condition of stabilization varied from one individual to another. They concluded that several mechanisms operate to maintain special constancy in CN; some individuals appear to use one more than another. The mechanisms used included extraretinal signals, elevated threshold for motion detection, and "suppression" of visual input except during foveation periods. When only part of the visual field was stabilized, one subject reported OSOP of that stabilized central field while the peripheral surround was perceived as not moving. He could reverse the perceptions, causing OSOP of the surround instead of the central field.

Since RIV is related to OSOP in acquired nystagmus, the effects of retinal image stabilization were studied in nystagmus caused by neurologic disease.[133] The stabilization was progressively increased in eight patients with acquired nystagmus until OSOP was abolished; this was achieved at RIV of 5 degrees per second or less. In five patients, further increases in stabilization caused the OSOP to reappear in the opposite direction. In addition to reducing OSOP, stabilization improved visual acuity in four of five patients tested. Both electronic stabilization and an optical device were used to stabilize images of the real world on the retina.[134, 135] Although the optical device provides stabilization over a small central field, it is useful in helping patients to read or watch television by reducing or eliminating their OSOP.

REFERENCES

1. Dell'Osso LF: Nystagmus and other ocular motor oscillations, in Lessell S, Van Dalen JTW (eds): *Neuro-ophthalmology 1980, vol 1*. Amsterdam, Excerpta Medica, 1980, pp 146–177.

2. Dell'Osso LF: Nystagmus and other ocular motor oscillations, in Lessell S, Van Dalen JTW (eds): *Neuro-ophthalmology 1982, vol 2*. Amsterdam, Excerpta Medica, 1982, pp 148–171.

3. Dell'Osso LF: Nystagmus and other ocular motor oscillations and intrusions, in Lessell S, Van Dalen JTW (eds): *Neuro-ophthalmology 1984, vol 3*. Amsterdam, Excerpta Medica, 1984, pp 157–204.

4. Dell'Osso LF: Nystagmus and other ocular motor oscillations and intrusions, in Lessell S, Van Dalen JTW (eds): *Current Neuro-ophthalmology, vol 1*. Chicago, Year Book Medical Publishers, 1988, pp 139–172.

5. Stransky E: Associierter nystagmus. *Neur Centr* 1901; 20:786.

6. Hamann KF: Kritische Anmerkungen zum sogenannten zervikogenen Schwindel. *Laryngol Rhinol Otol* 1985; 64:156–157.

7. Abadi RV, Dickinson CM: Waveform characteristics in congenital nystagmus. *Doc Ophthalmol* 1986; 64:153–167.

8. Reccia R, Roberti G, Russo P, et al: Spectral analysis of dual jerk waveforms in congenital nystagmus. *Biol Cybern* 1986; 55:211–217.

9. Optican LM, Zee DS: A hypothetical explanation of congenital nystagmus. *Biol Cybern* 1984; 50:119–134.

10. Von Noorden GK, Munoz M, Wong SY: Compensatory mechanisms in congenital nystagmus. *Am J Ophthalmol* 1987; 104:387–397.

11. Bagolini B, Campos EC, Fonda S, et al: Active blockage and rest position nystagmus: Electromyographic demonstration of two types of ocular induced head-turn. *Doc Ophthalmol* 1986; 62:149–159.

12. Hayasaka S: Hereditary congenital nystagmus: A Japanese pedigree. *Ophthalmic Paediatr Genet* 1986; 7:73–76.

13. Kaga K, Yokochi K, Kitazumi E, et al: Absence of later auditory brain stem response components, congenital horizontal nystagmus, and hypotonia in male infants. *Ann Otol Rhinol Laryngol* 1986; 95:203–206.

14. Tusa RJ, Smith CB, Herdman SJ: The development of nystagmus in infant monkeys following visual deprivation, abstracted. *Soc Neurosci Abstr* 1987; 13:172.

15. Dell'Osso LF, Gauthier G, Liberman G, et al: Eye movement recordings as a diagnostic tool in a case of congenital nystagmus. *Am J Optom Physiol* 1972; 49:3–13.

16. Bedell HE, Abplanalp PL, McGuire CA: Oculomotor responses to target displacements by patients with congenital idiopathic nystagmus and nystagmus associated with albinism. *Clin Vis Sci* 1987; 2:21–31.

17. Dell'Osso LF: *A Dual-Mode Model for the Normal Eye Tracking System and the System With Nystagmus,* thesis. Laramie, Wyo, University of Wyoming, Laramie, 1968.

18. Guyer DR, Lessell S: Periodic alternating nystagmus associated with albinism. *J Clin Neuro Ophthalmol* 1986; 6:82–85.

19. Kelly BJ, Rosenberg ML, Zee DS, et al: Unilateral pursuit-induced congenital nystagmus. *Neurology* 1989; 39:414–416.

20. Kawai K: Congenital nystagmus: The interactions between fixation and optokinetic background. *Jpn Rev Clin Ophthalmol* 1985; 79:2036–2039.

21. Dickinson CM: The elucidation and use of the effect of near fixation in congenital nystagmus. *Ophthalmic Physiol Opt* 1986; 6:303–311.

22. Von Noorden GK, Wong SY: Surgical results in nystagmus blockage syndrome. *Ophthalmology* 1986; 93:1028–1031.

23. Roberti G, Russo P, Segré G: Spectral analysis of elector-oculograms in the quantitative evaluation of nystagmus surgery. *Med Biol Eng Comput* 1987; 25:573–576.

24. Dell'Osso LF, Traccis S, Abel LA, et al: Contact lenses and congenital nystagmus. *Clin Vis Sci* 1988; 3:229–232.

25. Ishikawa S, Ozawa H, Fujiyama Y: Treatment of nystagmus by acupuncture, *Highlights in Neuro-ophthalmology: Proceedings of the Sixth Meeting of the International Neuro-ophthalmology Society (INOS).* Amsterdam, Aeolus Press, 1987, pp 227–232.

26. Jan JE, McCormick AQ, Hoyt CS: The unequal nystagmus test. *Dev Med Child Neurol* 1988; 30:441–443.

27. Schwartz MA, Selhorst JB, Ochs AL, et al: Oculomasticatory myorhythmia: A unique movement disorder occurring in Whipple's disease. *Ann Neurol* 1986; 20:677–683.

28. Hara T, Kawazawa S, Abe Y, et al: Conjugate pendular nystagmus evoked by accommodative vergence. *Eur Neurol* 1986; 25:369–372.

29. Weissman BM, Dell'Osso LF, Abel LA, et al: Spasmus nutans: A quantitative prospective study. *Arch Ophthalmol* 1987; 105:525–528.

30. Noda S, Ide K, Umezaki H, et al: Repetitive divergence. *Ann Neurol* 1987; 21:109–110.

31. Gresty MA, Barratt H, Rudge P, et al: Analysis of downbeat nystagmus. *Arch Neurol* 1986; 43:52–55.

32. Slavin ML, Rosenberg ML: Unusual associations of downbeat nystagmus. *Neuro-ophthalmology* 1985; 5:265–270.

33. Mayfrank L, Thoden U: Downbeat nystagmus indicates cerebellar or brain-stem lesions in vitamin B_{12} deficiency. *J Neurol* 1986; 233:145–148.

34. Schmidt D, Neumann HPH, Eggert HR, et al: Neuro-Ophthalmologischer Befund bei Hämangioblastom des Kleinhirns und des Hirnstamms—Downbeat-Nystagmus als Erstsymptom eines Hämangioblastoms bei v. Hippel-Lindau Erkrankung. *Fortschr Ophthalmol* 1988; 85:427–433.

35. Pinel JF, Larmande P, Guegan Y, et al: Down-beat nystagmus: Case report with magnetic resonance imaging and surgical treatment. *Neurosurgery* 1987; 21:736–739.

36. Boman DK, Hotson JR: Smooth pursuit training and disruption: Directional differences and nystagmus. *Neuro Ophthalmology* 1987; 7:185–194.

37. Corbett JJ, Jacobson DM, Thompson HS, et al: Downbeating nystagmus and other ocular motor defects caused by lithium toxicity. *Neurology* 1989; 39:481–487.

38. Rosenberg ML: Reversible downbeat nystagmus secondary to excessive alcohol intake. *J Clin Neuro Opthalmol* 1987; 7:23–25.

39. Good GW, Augsburger AR: Use of horizontal gaze nystagmus as a part of roadside sobriety testing. *Am J Optom Physiol Opt* 1986; 63:467–471.

40. Lavin PJM: Pupillary oscillations synchronous with ictal nystagmus. *Neuro Ophthalmology* 1986; 6:113–116.

41. Schiff D, Cohen B, Raphan T: Nystagmus induced by stimulation of the nucleus of the optic tract in the monkey. *Exp Brain Res* 1988; 70:1–14.

42. Von Noorden GK, Avilla C, Sidikaro Y, et al: Latent nystagmus and strabismic amblyopia. *Am J Ophthalmol* 1987; 103:87–89.

43. Dell'Osso LF, Traccis S, Abel LA: Strabismus: A necessary condition for latent and manifest latent nystagmus. *Neuro Ophthalmology* 1983; 3:247–257.

44. Moidell B, Steinbach MJ, Ono H: Egocenter location in children enucleated at an early age. *Invest Ophthalmol Vis Sci* 1988; 29:1348–1351.

45. Dell'Osso LF, Schmidt D, Daroff RB: Latent, manifest latent and congenital nystagmus. *Arch Ophthalmol* 1979; 97:1877–1885.

46. Dell'Osso LF, Abel LA, Daroff RB: Latent/manifest latent nystagmus reversal using an ocular prosthesis: Implications for vision and ocular dominance. *Invest Ophthalmol Vis Sci* 1987; 28:1873–1876.

47. Ciancia AO: Oculomotor disturbances and VER findings in patients with early monocular loss of vision. *Graefes Arch Clin Exp Ophthalmol* 1988; 226:108–110.

48. Howard RS: A case of convergence evoked eyelid nystagmus. *J Clin Neuro Ophthalmol* 1986; 6:169–171.

49. Archer SM, Miller KK, Helveston EM: Stereoscopic contours and optokinetic nystagmus in normal and stereoblind subjects. *Vision Res* 1987; 27:841–844.

50. Zee DS, Tusa RJ, Herdman SJ, et al: Effects of occipital lobectomy upon eye movements in primate. *J Neurophysiol* 1987; 58:883–907.

51. Crevits L, Van Vliet AGM: Optokinetic nystagmus in patients with defects of the central visual field. *Eur Neurol* 1986; 25:454–457.

52. Verhagen WIM, Huygen PLM, Schulte BPM: Ocular motor responses after locked-in syndrome. *Neuro Ophthalmology* 1987; 7:49–56.

53. Yee RD, Baloh RW, Morder SR, et al: Eye movements in schizophrenia. *Invest Ophthalmol Vis Sci* 1987; 28:366–374.

54. Lafortune S, Ireland DJ, Jell RM, et al: Human optokinetic afternystagmus: Charging characteristics and stimulus exposure time dependence in the two-compartment model. *Acta Otolaryngol* 1986; 101:353–360.

55. Jell RM, Sett S, Ireland DJ: Human optokinetic afternystagmus: Is the fast component of OKAN due to smooth pursuit? *Acta Otolaryngol* 1987; 104:298–306.

56. Himi T, Igarashi M, Kulecz WB, et al: Asymmetry of vertical optokinetic after-nystagmus in squirrel monkeys. *Acta Otolaryngol* 1988; 105:312–317.

57. Heckmann T, Post RB: Induced motion and optokinetic afternystagmus: Parallel response dynamics with prolonged stimulation. *Vision Res* 1988; 28:681–694.

58. LeLiever WC, Correia MJ: Further observations on the effects of head position on vertical OKN and OKAN in normal subjects. *Otolaryngol Head Neck Surg* 1987; 97:275–281.

59. Dehaene I, Van Zandycke M, Appel B: Acquired pendular nystagmus. *Neuro Ophthalmology* 1987; 7:297–300.

60. Cordonnier M, Goldman S, Zegers De Beyl D, et al: Reversible acquired pendular nystagmus after brainstem hemorrhage. *Neuro Ophthalmology* 1984; 4:261–263.

61. Nuti D, Ciacci G, Giannini F, et al: Aperiodic alternating nystagmus: Report of two cases and treatment by baclofen. *Ital J Neurol Sci* 1986; 7:453–459.

62. Cohen B, Helwig D, Raphan T: Baclofen and velocity storage: A model of the effects of the drug on the vestibulo-ocular reflex in the rhesus monkey. *J Physiol* 1987; 393:703–725.

63. Larmande P, Belin C, Limodin J, et al: Grandes oscillations pendulaires lentes des globes oculaires et dyspne'e de Cheyne-Stokes. *Rev Neurol* 1987; 143:768–771.

64. Baer C: D. Reflektorische Nystagmus. *Arch Augenheilk* 1902; 45:5.

65. Dehaene I, Van Zandijcke M: See-saw jerk nystagmus. *Neuro Ophthalmology* 1984; 4:261–263.

66. Bergin DJ, Halpern J: Congenital see-saw nystagmus associated with retinitis pigmentosa. *Ann Ophthalmol* 1986; 18:346–349.

67. Frisén L, Wikkelsø C: Posttraumatic seesaw nystagmus abolished by ethanol ingestion. *Neurology* 1986; 36:841–844.

68. Zimmerman CF, Roach ES, Troost BT: See-saw nystagmus associated with Chiari malformation. *Arch Neurol* 1986; 43:299–300.

69. Kanter DS, Ruff RL, Leigh RJ, et al: See-saw nystagmus and brainstem infarction: MRI findings. *Neuro Ophthalmology* 1987; 7:279–283.

70. Noseworthy JH, Ebers GC, Leigh RJ, et al: Torsional nystagmus: Quantitative features and possible pathogenesis. *Neurology* 1988; 38:992–994.

71. Furman JMR, Baloh RW, Yee RD: Eye movement abnormalities in a family with cerebellar vermian atrophy. *Acta Otolaryngol* 1986; 101:371–377.

72. Keane JR, Itabashi HH: Upbeat nystagmus: Clinicopathologic study of two patients. *Neurology* 1987; 37:491–494.

73. Ishikawa S, Nozaki S, Mukuno K: Upbeat and downbeat nystagmus in a single case. *Neuro Ophthalmology* 1986; 6:95–99.

74. Nowack WJ, Clark GF: Vertical nystagmus and thalamic arteriovenous malformation. *Neuro Ophthalmology* 1986; 6:169–172.

75. Gresty MA, Bronstein AM, Barratt H: Eye movement responses to combined linear and angular head movement. *Exp Brain Res* 1987; 65:377–384.

76. Grossman GE, Abel LA, Thurston SE, et al: Frequency and velocity ranges of natural head rotations, abstracted. *Soc Neurosci Abstr* 1986; 12:251.

77. Hain TC, Fetter M, Zee DS: Head-shaking nystagmus in patients with unilateral peripheral vestibular lesions. *Am J Otolaryngol* 1987; 8:36–47.

78. Takahashi S: Clinical significance of biphasic head-shaking nystagmus. *Auris Nasus Larynx* 1986; 13:S199–S204.

79. Müller-Deile J, Reker U, Zell E: Über die Bedeutung der Konvektions-Hypothese Báránys für den thermischen Nystagmus: Ein quantitativer Vergleich der Intensität des thermischen Nystagmus in Bauch- und Rückenlage. *Laryngol Rhinol Otol* 1986; 65:154–157.

80. Norre ME: Caloric vertical nystagmus: The vertical semicircular canal in caloric testing. *J Otolaryngol* 1987; 16:36–39.

81. Nayyar M, Strobos RJ, Singh BM, et al: Caloric-induced nystagmus with isoelectric electroencephalogram. *Ann Neurol* 1987; 21:98–100.

82. Lin J, Elidan J, Baloh RW, et al: Direction-changing positional nystagmus. *Am J Otolaryngol* 1986; 7:306–310.

83. Nishikawa K, Nishikawa M: Nystagmus during attack in Meniere's disease. *Auris Nasus Larynx* 1986; 13:S147–S151.

84. Hain TC, Zee DS, Maria BL: Tilt suppression of vestibulo-ocular reflex in patients with cerebellar lesions. *Acta Otolaryngol* 1988; 105:13–20.

85. Barratt H, Bronstein AM, Gresty MA: Testing the vestibular-ocular reflexes: Abnormalities of

the otolith contribution in patients with neuro-otological disease. *J Neurol Neurosurg Psychiatry* 1987; 50:1029–1035.

86. Baloh RW, Honrubia V, Jacobson K: Benign positional vertigo: Clinical and oculographic features in 240 cases. *Neurology* 1987; 37:371–378.

87. Lackner JR, Graybiel A: The effective intensity of coriolis, cross-coupling stimulation is gravitoinertial force dependent: Implications for space motion sickness. *Aviat Space Environ Med* 1986; 57:229–235.

88. Lackner JR, Graybiel A: Head movements in non-terrestrial force environments elicit motion sickness: Implications for the etiology of space motion sickness. *Aviat Space Environ Med* 1986; 57:443–448.

89. Watt DGD: The vestibulo-ocular reflex and its possible roles in space motion sickness. *Aviat Space Environ Med* 1987; 58:A170–A174.

90. Rosa A, Masmoudi K, Mizon JP: Typical and atypical ocular bobbing: Pathology through five case reports. *Neuro Ophthalmology* 1987; 7:285–290.

91. Van Weerden TW, Van Woerkom TCAM: Ocular dipping. *Neurology* 1985; 35:135.

92. Stark SR, Masucci EF, Kurtzke JF: Ocular dipping-Reply. *Neurology* 1985; 35:135.

93. Mehler MF: The clinical spectrum of ocular bobbing and ocular dipping. *J Neurol Neurosurg Psychiatry* 1988; 51:725–727.

94. Rosenberg ML: Spontaneous vertical eye movements in coma. *Ann Neurol* 1986; 20:635–637.

95. Hata S, Bernstein E, Davis LE: Atypical ocular bobbing in acute organophosphate poisoning. *Arch Neurol* 1986; 43:185–186.

96. Toshniwal P, Yadava R, Goldbarg H: Presentation of pinealoblastoma with ocular dipping and deafness. *J Clin Neuro Ophthalmol* 1986; 6:128–132.

97. Oohira A, Goto K, Ozawa T: Convergence nystagmus. *Neuro Ophthalmology* 1986; 6:313–320.

98. Herishanu Y, Abarbanel JM, Frisher S: Blink induced ocular flutter. *Neuro Ophthalmology* 1987; 7:175–177.

99. Furman JMR, Eidelman BH, Fromm GH: Spontaneous remission of paraneoplastic ocular flutter and saccadic intrusions. *Neurology* 1988; 38:499–501.

100. Bergenius J: Saccade abnormalities in patients with ocular flutter. *Acta Otolaryngol* 1986; 102:228–233.

101. Salonen R, Nikoskelainen E, Aantaa E, et al: Ocular flutter associated with sarcoidosis. *Neuro Ophthalmology* 1988; 8:77–79.

101a. Hotson JR: Convergence-initiated voluntary flutter: A normal intrinsic capability in man. *Brain Res* 1984; 294:299–304.

102. Fukazawa T, Tashiro K, Hamada T, et al: Multisystem degeneration: Drugs and square wave jerks. *Neurology* 1986; 36:1230–1233.

103. Dell'Osso LF, Abel LA, Daroff RB: "Inverse latent" macro square wave jerks and macro saccadic oscillations. *Ann Neurol* 1977; 2:57–60.

104. Abel LA, Traccis S, Dell'Osso LF, et al: Square wave oscillation: The relationship of saccadic intrusions and oscillations. *Neuro Ophthalmology* 1984; 4:21–25.

105. Spencer HR: Pharyngeal and laryngeal "nystagmus." *Lancet* 1886; 2:702.

106. Jankovic J, Pardo R: Segmental myoclonus: Clinical and pharmacologic study. *Arch Neurol* 1986; 43:1025–1031.

107. Nakada T, Kwee IL: Oculopalatal myoclonus. *Brain* 1986; 109:431–441.

108. Keane JR: Acute vertical ocular myoclonus. *Neurology* 1986; 36:86–89.

109. Lefkowitz D, Harpold G: Treatment of ocular myoclonus with valproic acid. *Ann Neurol* 1985; 17:103–104.

110. Jabbari B, Rosenberg M, Scherokman B, et al: Effectiveness of trihexyphenidyl against pendular

nystagmus and palatal myoclonus: Evidence of cholinergic dysfunction. *Movement Disord* 1987; 2:93–98.

111. Dehaene I, Van Vleymen B: Opsoclonus induced by phenytoin and diazepam. *Ann Neurol* 1987; 21:216.

112. Hunter S, Kooistra C: Neuropathologic findings in idiopathic opsoclonus and myoclonus: Their similarity to those in paraneoplastic cerebellar cortical degeneration. *J Clin Neuro Ophthalmol* 1986; 6:236–241.

113. Herishanu Y, Apte R, Kuperman O: Immunological abnormalities in opsoclonus cerebellopathy. *Neuro Ophthalmology* 1985; 5:271–276.

114. Ridley A, Kennard C, Scholtz CL, et al: Omnipause neurons in two cases of opsoclonus associated with oat cell carcinoma of the lung. *Brain* 1987; 110:1699–1709.

115. Borodic GE, Miller DC, Bienfang DC: Opsoclonus: Three autopsied cases and review of the literature, in Smith JL (ed): *Intraocular Lens Complications and Their Management*. Thorofare, New Jersey, Charles B. Slack, in press.

116. Benjamin EE, Zimmerman CF, Troost BT: Lateropulsion and upbeat nystagmus are manifestations of central vestibular dysfunction. *Arch Neurol* 1986; 43:962–964.

117. Dell'Osso LF, Daroff RB: Clinical disorders of ocular movement, in Zuber BL (ed): *Models of Oculomotor Behavior and Control*. Boca Raton, Fla, CRC Press Inc, 1981, pp 233–256.

118. Zee DS, Hain TC, Carl JR: Abduction nystagmus in internuclear ophthalmoplegia. *Ann Neurol* 1987; 21:383–388.

119. Ohtsuka K, Mukuno K, Ukai K, et al: The origin of square wave jerks: Conditions of fixation and microsaccades. *Jpn J Ophthalmol* 1986; 30:209–215.

119a. Doslak MJ, Dell'Osso LF, Daroff RB: Multiple double saccadic pulses occurring with other saccadic intrusions and oscillations. *Neuro-ophthalmology* 1983; 3:109–116.

120. Ohtsuka K, Mukuno K, Sakai H, et al: Instability of eye position in the dark in cerebellar degeneration. *Ophthalmologica* 1988; 196:35–39.

121. Hertle RW, Tabuchi A, Dell'Osso LF, et al: Saccadic oscillations and intrusions preceding the postnatal appearance of congenital nystagmus. *Neuro Ophthalmology* 1988; 8:37–42.

122. Rosenthal GJ, Selhorst JB: Continuous non-rhythmic cycloversion: A possible paraneoplastic disorder. *Neuro Ophthalmology* 1987; 7:291–295.

123. Brickner R: Oscillopsia: New symptom commonly occurring in multiple sclerosis. *Arch Neurol Psychiatry* 1936; 36:586.

124. Bell WO, Charney EB, Bruce DA, et al: Symptomatic Arnold-Chiari malformation: Review of experience with 22 cases. *J Neurosurg* 1987; 66:812–816.

125. Chrousos GA, Cowdry R, Schuelein M, et al: Two cases of downbeat nystagmus and oscillopsia associated with carbamazepine. *Am J Ophthalmol* 1987; 103:221–224.

126. Pedersen RA, Troost BT, Abel LA, et al: Intermittent downbeat nystagmus and oscillopsia reversed by suboccipital craniectomy. *Neurology* 1980; 30:1239–1242.

127. Verhagen WIM, Huygen PLM, Horstink MWIM: Familial congenital vestibular areflexia. *J Neurol Neurosurg Psychiatry* 1987; 50:933–935.

128. Marra TR, Reynolds Jr NC, Stoddard JJ: Subjective oscillopsia ("jiggling" vision) presumably due to aminoglycoside ototoxicity: A report of two cases. *Neuro Ophthalmology* 1988; 8:35–38.

129. Brandt T, Dieterich M: Oscillopsia and motion perception, in Kennard C, Rose FC (eds): *Physiological Aspects of Clinical Neuro-ophthalmology*. London, Chapman and Hall, 1988, pp 321–339.

130. Burr D, Ross J: Visual processing of motion. *Trends Neurosci* 1986; 9:304–307.

131. Whitaker D, Buckingham T: Oscillatory movement displacement thresholds: Resistance to optical image degradation. *Ophthalmic Physiol Opt* 1987; 7:121–125.

132. Leigh RJ, Dell'Osso LF, Yaniglos SS, et al: Oscillopsia, retinal image stabilization and congenital nystagmus. *Invest Ophthalmol Vis Sci* 1988; 29:279–282.

133. Leigh RJ, Rushton DN, Thurston SE, et al: Effects of retinal image stabilization in acquired nystagmus due to neurological disease. *Neurology* 1988; 38:122–127.

134. Rushton DN, Rushton RH: An optical method for approximate stabilization of vision of the real world. *J Physiol* 1984; 357:3P.

135. Rushton D, Cox N: A new optical treatment for oscillopsia. *J Neurol Neurosurg Psychiatry* 1987; 50:411–455.

CHAPTER 10

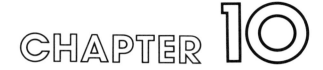

Supranuclear and Nuclear Disorders of Eye Movement

Ekkehard Mehdorn, M.D.

Professor of Ophthalmology, Medical University of Lübeck, Lübeck, Federal Republic of Germany

TOPOLOGY AND PATHOLOGY

Paramedian Pontine Reticular Formation

Monkeys with bilateral lesions of the paramedian pontine reticular formation (PPRF) are unable to generate any type of rapid eye movement, but vestibulo-ocular reflex and smooth pursuit are preserved in these preparations.[1] The clinical picture of bilateral PPRF lesions closely resembles the experimental situation. Hanson et al. described two patients who suffered a selective deficit of voluntary horizontal and vertical saccades and quick phases of nystagmus after hypoxic-ischemic insults during open heart surgery.[2] Smooth pursuit, the vestibulo-ocular reflex, and vergence eye movements were all preserved. Pathologic studies in one patient confirmed an ischemic lesion of the median and PPRF. In another case of bilateral horizontal saccadic palsy with preservation of smooth pursuit, the lesion was caused by a rather large adenocarcinoma metastatic to the pons, and regressed temporarily after corticosteroid treatment.[3]

After unilateral PPRF lesions monkeys demonstrate a selective saccadic deficit, but preservation of smooth pursuit as with bilateral PPRF lesions has not as yet been observed. Therefore, the observation of preserved smooth pursuit in a patient

Curr Neuro Ophthalmol 2:183–198, 1989
© 1989, Year Book Medical Publishers, Inc.
0893–0147/89/02-183-198-$04.00

with a unilateral PPRF lesion after pontine hemorrhage is especially interesting, since it definitely proves that the PPRF is not involved in the generation of smooth pursuit.[4] The patient of Kommerell et al.[4] and the two patients of Hanson et al.[2] were able to hold eccentric gaze ipsilateral to the PPRF lesion once the eyes had been brought into the eccentric position by a smooth pursuit movement. Thus the PPRF is not necessary for holding ipsilateral eccentric gaze. In other words, the PPRF does not participate in the neural integration of the velocity command.

As discussed in the last review,[5] rostral PPRF lesions are not accompanied by a loss of vertical saccadic eye movements,[6] whereas lesions that extend into the caudal PPRF do affect vertical saccades. The involvement of the caudal PPRF in vertical saccade generation explains why vertical saccades are sometimes affected in abducens nucleus lesions.[7, 8] In a patient with a bilateral horizontal and vertical gaze palsy, the attempt to look at either side or to look up and down elicited convergent eye movements that were not accompanied by miosis.[8] The authors could not explain the convergence. Bogousslavsky and Meienberg reviewed the various eye movement disorders resulting from brain-stem and cerebellar stroke, and discussed their localizing values.[9] Several papers have demonstrated that brain-stem and cerebellar lesions can now be localized rather accurately with nuclear magnetic resonance imaging (MRI).[10–15]

Internuclear Ophthalmoplegia and One-and-a-Half Syndrome

Internuclear ophthalmoplegia (INO) is characterized by slow adduction and dissociated nystagmus of the abducting eye. It is well established that the adduction weakness is the immediate consequence of a lesion affecting the medial longitudinal fasciculus (MLF), but the origin of the dissociated abduction nystagmus remains controversial. However, the hypothesis of Baloh et al. has received further support.[16] These authors had suggested that the abduction nystagmus reflects an adaptation of the saccadic system to overcome the adduction weakness. To test this hypothesis, Zee et al. patched the paretic eyes in four patients with unilateral or bilateral INO.[17] In three of their patients the dissociated abduction nystagmus disappeared after 1 to 5 days. These results indicate a role for adaptation in the abduction nystagmus of INO. Therefore, in the presence of dissociated nystagmus, it is not necessary to assume other brain-stem lesions. A lesion of excitatory MLF fibers seems sufficient explanation.

The same conclusion was drawn in another paper, which demonstrated that the ocular motor anomalies observed in INO are principally the same as those seen with peripheral paresis.[18] The authors of both papers[17, 18] are aware of the possibility that in patients and monkeys[19] with INO, more than the MLF may be affected, and other mechanisms may play a role in the dissociated nystagmus. Nevertheless, one should recall that the adduction weakness represents the only constant finding in monkeys[17] and in patients[5] with MLF lesions. The presence or absence of dissociated nystagmus does not represent a reliable criterion to differentiate between INO and infranuclear medial rectus palsy. Further experiments are necessary to explain why some patients have dissociated nystagmus and others do not.

Trauma is an uncommon cause of INO,[20] as are systemic lupus erythematosus,[21] and migraine and supratentorial arteriovenous malformation.[22] Speculation about the mechanism of paralytic pontine exotropia in association with INO or in association with the one-and-a-half syndrome has continued, but no substantially new aspects have been presented.[23, 24] A peculiar type of pseudo-INO with downshoot of the adducting eye in two patients with myasthenia gravis has been added to the potpourri of pseudo-INO.[25] Reports of pseudo-INO remind us that one should be very cautious before assuming a supranuclear origin for a patient's motility disorder.

Disturbances of Vertical Gaze

In a large study of patients with thalamic infarcts, Bogousslavsky et al. attempted to delineate four major syndromes corresponding to the four main arterial territories of the thalamus.[26] The paramedian choroidal artery infarction was the second most common syndrome in their series and the only one accompanied by vertical gaze palsies.

There is now general agreement that the rostral interstitial nucleus of the medial longitudinal fasciculus (riMLF) represents the pulse generator for vertical saccades.[27] Previous clinical pathologic studies suggested that bilateral lesions of the lateral riMLF produce an isolated downgaze palsy, whereas bilateral lesions of the medial riMLF result in upgaze and downgaze palsies.[5, 27] In agreement with these observations was the report of a selective downgaze palsy with bilateral thalamic infarction of Kobari et al.[28] So far, isolated upgaze palsies have been observed only with lesions of the posterior commissure. With the report of Ranalli et al. we must accept that lesions of the posterior commissure are not the only source of upgaze palsies.[29] Ranalli et al. described a patient with a unilateral midbrain infarct that enclosed the right riMLF but spared the posterior commissure. In contrast to previous clinical pathologic descriptions of midbrain infarcts, their report contained a careful analysis of all types of vertical and horizontal eye movements, which were recorded by a search-coil technique. Their patient exhibited a complete upgaze palsy and slowing of vertical saccades in a range of 15 degrees below the midposition. During pursuit and vestibulo-ocular reflex (VOR), the eyes could be elevated a few degrees above the midline. Vertical pursuit and VOR gain were reduced. Horizontal saccades were slowed, although less than vertical saccades. Horizontal pursuit gain was reduced, and only horizontal VOR gain was within the normal range. These observations demonstrate that the riMLF is a critical structure not only for downward saccades, but for vertical saccades in both directions. The patient's saccadic palsy was probably caused by the complete destruction of burst neurons within the right riMLF and of fibers originating from the left riMLF and passing through or near the right riMLF.

Unlike previous reports, the publication of Ranalli et al.[29] presented quantitative data for the impairment of vertical pursuit and VOR, which is often associated with vertical saccadic palsies.[30] Future search-coil studies are necessary to better define the contribution of the rostral midbrain to vertical pursuit and VOR.

Bilateral chemical lesions of the nucleus prepositus hypoglossi and the adjacent vestibular nuclei impair vertical gaze-holding, but the impairment is less pronounced than for horizontal gaze.[31] It appears that the nucleus prepositus hypoglossi and the adjacent vestibular nuclei are part of the vertical neural integrator. Another part of the vertical integration could take place in the rostral midbrain itself. It also seems possible that the neural integrator for upward movements is different from that for downward movement, both anatomically and, perhaps, pharmacologically.[32] The latter speculation is supported by the observation that during an attack of oculogyric crisis, the eyes could not be brought below the horizontal meridian except during a blink.[33] The three patients described in this report had normal conjugate movements in the upper field of gaze. The authors therefore assumed an "offset" in the vertical neural integrator. The oculogyric attacks and the disorders of thought accompanying the attacks could be terminated by administration of an anticholinergic drug, suggesting that pathways subserving upward and downward gaze utilize different neurotransmitters.

Spontaneous nonhypertensive hemorrhages arising in the mesencephalic tectum were described as an unusual cause of vertical gaze disorder.[34] Unilateral oculomotor palsy is the most frequent eye movement disorder after tentorial herniation, but a combination of third nerve nucleus lesion, INO, and vertical gaze paresis may result from midbrain compression.[35] Upgaze palsy with tonic downward deviation (the "setting sun sign") and esotropia was observed after intraventricular hemorrhages in premature infants.[36] The recovery of the upgaze palsy usually was good.

Skew deviation was observed by Ranalli et al.[29] in a patient with midbrain infarction, and a recent review of alternating skew deviation suggested that this eye movement disorder was a localizing sign of the midbrain pretectum.[37] This conclusion was challenged by a more recent report of 33 patients in whom lesions of the cerebellar pathways or the cervicomedullary junction were more often diagnosed.[38]

Oculomotor Nucleus Syndrome

In agreement with our present knowledge of oculomotor subnuclei[39] is the observation of a patient with a unilateral nuclear oculomotor palsy with bilateral superior rectus palsy but normal levator and pupillary function.[40] An isolated unilateral inferior rectus muscle palsy could be correlated by nuclear MRI and histopathologically with a solitary metastasis to the oculomotor nucleus.[41] To our knowledge, this is the first pathologically confirmed report of an isolated nuclear inferior rectus palsy.

Unilateral oculomotor nucleus lesions may be caused by relatively small midbrain infarctions, and additional neurological symptoms may be absent. However, a unilateral fascicular third nerve palsy accompanied by somnolent mutism was recently described by Zermeno et al.[42] Usually, mental disturbances result from bilateral, more widespread infarcts of the midbrain, with bilateral third nerve palsy.[43]

Four cases with a unilateral nuclear oculomotor palsy and an additional abduction palsy of the contralateral eye were described by Masdeu and Rosenberg.[44] The abduction deficit was of supranuclear origin and could be overcome by the vestibulo-ocular reflex. The most probable explanation of this syndrome is an interruption of corticopontine fibers at the oculomotor nucleus level.

HEMISPHERIC CONTROL OF SACCADES

The latencies of visually guided saccades were studied in 60 patients without hemianopia who had *unilateral* lesions variously located in both cerebral hemispheres.[45] In agreement with earlier observations[5] was the finding that lesions confined to the frontal eye fields (FEF) did not cause asymmetric latencies. The latencies of contralateral saccades were significantly increased only in patients with deep and posterior lesions near the corpus callosum and/or the anterior part of the internal capsule that had damaged a certain portion of the efferent pathways descending from the FEF. As opposed to lesions of the FEF, lesions of the posterior part of the parietal cortex or the underlying white matter were accompanied by a significant increase of latencies for contralateral *and* ipsilateral saccades. The authors therefore assumed that the parietal lobe exerted an excitatory and the frontal lobe a predominantly inhibitory bilateral action on the triggering of visually guided saccades. In a patient with a unilateral parietal malignant glioma, voluntary contralateral saccades that were initiated on command without presentation of a visual target had normal velocities, but visually guided contralateral saccades elicited by a peripheral luminous spot had decreased velocities and amplitudes.[46] This case supports previous observations[5] that the parietal-occipital region may be critical for the generation of contralateral visually guided saccades. In the same patient, full-field optokinetic pursuit was more affected than foveal pursuit; the authors speculated on whether this was due to an interhemispheric disconnection. Future studies of saccades in patients with cerebral lesions could be a very interesting supplement to ongoing research in behaving monkeys[47] if they included more detailed analyses of various saccadic tasks.

Are saccadic eye movements in the absence of the geniculocalcarine projection really generated by subcortical centers in man? This question continues to stimulate experiments of hemianopic subjects.[48] I still have some difficulty understanding the research of "blindsight." Principally, what is the definition of "blind"? In the experiments cited the subject was said to have a complete homonymous hemianopia.[48] Perimetry was performed with small (0.8 × 0.8 degrees) and dark targets (12 cd/m²) on a bright (109 cd/m²) background, but the saccades into the perimetrically defined blind hemifield were elicited by larger (1-degree diameter) and much brighter (139 cd/m²) targets. The subject could not "see" these targets, but he was "aware" of these targets. I wonder about the perimetric result if the same targets had been used for perimetry. Nevertheless, research on residual vision of hemianopic patients and on adaptive mechanisms of these patients[49] is fascinating—and it is of practical importance to know whether residual vision within the hemianopic field is of sufficient quality to help circumvent obstacles or to make driving a motor vehicle possible (in Europe, hemianopic persons are not allowed to drive a car).

Forced head and eye turning is often observed in seizures originating from a focus in the frontal or temporal lobe. Simultaneous electroencephalograph and video tape recordings showed that the initial version prior to secondary generalization was a reliable lateralizing sign, but that the late version was not.[50] It could be shown in some patients that the late version originated from the hemisphere involved by secondary generalization. Late version must therefore be cautiously interpreted if it is witnessed during isolated observation of the final minutes of a generalized convulsion.

The eye-head coordination and the interaction of the vestibulo-ocular reflex with the saccadic movement during orienting movements within and beyond the oculomotor range was investigated in two papers.[51, 52] Experiments suggested that in humans the gaze-control system can mobilize all of its available components to facilitate the motion of the visual axis toward the goal. Thus, visually triggered ocular saccades, vestibulo-ocular slow and quick phases, may be used synergistically to attain a desired target. The experiments confirmed that the vestibulo-ocular reflex was inhibited during saccadic eye movements. However, this inhibition was not absolute, but increased with gaze saccade amplitude in most subjects.

Patients with acquired[53] and congenital[54–56] oculomotor apraxia demonstrated that saccade generation and VOR inhibition during gaze shifts were closely related. A patient in whom probably both frontal eye fields and both inferior parietal lobules had been destroyed by infarcts showed the gaze strategy typical of congenital ocular motor apraxia.[53] With the head fixed he was unable to generate visually or command saccades, but with the head free he immediately moved his head so that the vestibulo-ocular reflex drove the eyes into the opposite direction. Finally a slow saccade brought the eyes back onto the target. Obviously the frontoparietal infarcts did not abolish the complete gaze movement, but only the saccade and the inhibition of the VOR. Therefore, the elaboration and initiation of the combined eye head movement must take place outside the lesioned areas. In contrast to the patient with acquired oculomotor apraxia,[53] patients with the congenital form typically show the apraxia in the horizontal[54-56] or vertical planes[5] only; but I have recently seen a combined horizontal and vertical congenital apraxia. The neuropathological origin of congenital ocular motor apraxia remains unclear, although the corpus callosum has again been implicated.[54]

HEMISPHERIC CONTROL OF PURSUIT

Using step-ramp stimuli to control the location of targets in the visual fields of patients with posterior cortical lesions, Thurston et al. could define two distinct deficits of visual tracking.[57] The first, most frequently encountered, deficit was unidirectional toward the side of the cerebral lesion and was present for visual stimuli in both visual hemifields. This deficit is the basis for the smooth pursuit asymmetry one usually observes on bedside testing, and probably represents a deficit on the efferent or motor side of the pursuit system feedback loop. This deficit parallels the tracking deficit that has been found in monkeys with lesions of the medial superior temporal area.[58] The second deficit was a bidirectional inability to estimate the speed of a moving target in the visual hemifield contralateral to the side of the lesion. This inability affected not only smooth pursuit initiation but also the accuracy of catch-up saccades onto moving targets, in the same way that lesions of the middle temporal area do in the monkey.[57] An involvement of Brodmann's areas 19, 39, and 40 was common in patients with pursuit deficits, but some patients with similar lesions had no deficits. Perhaps the FEF that were recently shown to be involved in the generation of smooth pursuit eye movements in monkeys[58] can take over much of the task if the parieto-occipital region is damaged.

In the monkey we are discovering the fiber pathways by which the cortical areas mediating smooth pursuit eye movements are interconnected, and by which pathways the brain stem receives its pursuit commands.[59] Human cases often present with complex pathologies, and if the authors are not aware of modern neurophysiologic findings, interpretations become vague. In a case of locked-in syndrome due to pontine infarction, lack of cortical optokinetic nystagmus and preservation of subcortical optokinetic nystagmus were assumed, although the slow buildup characteristic of subcortical optokinetic nystagmus was not observed and the nasal-temporal asymmetry was not tested for with monocular optokinetic stimulation.[60] Otherwise, how can one speculate about the trajectory of the pursuit pathways, if one considers the PPRF as the final target of the corticopontine pursuit pathways?[61]

An analysis of smooth pursuit eye movements in patients with acute or chronic lesions is facilitated if we know how the pursuit system performs in normal subjects. Studies of the pursuit system in normal human subjects with modern techniques that allow a precise recording of horizontal and vertical eye movements are very useful.[62, 63]

DISEASES OF THE NERVOUS SYSTEM CAUSING DISORDERS OF EYE MOVEMENT

Fisher's Syndrome

The controversy about the lesion site in Fisher's syndrome continues.[64, 65] We will not discuss the arguments in favor of brain stem[64] or peripheral[65] involvement. Unlike previous clinicopathologic studies, that of Dehaene et al includes a neuropathologic examination of the whole central nervous system (CNS), oculomotor nerves from brain stem to eye muscles, facial nerve, spinal ganglia and roots, median nerve, ulnar nerve, and peroneal nerve.[66] In this extensively examined case of Guillain-Barré syndrome the CNS was normal. A purely peripheral nerve involvement without any indication of CNS dysfunction was also documented in three other cases by a comprehensive serial neurophysiologic examination.[67]

A case of Fisher's syndrome 1 month after an influenza vaccination in a 72-year-old man,[68] and another associated with *Campylobacter jejuni* infection[69] contributed no new arguments to the current controversy about the lesion site.

Spasm of the Near Reflex

Spasm of the near reflex, defined as intermittent episodes of convergence, miosis, and accommodation, represents a peculiar type of supranuclear eye movement disorder. It is often confused with abducens paresis and may even mimic myasthenia.[70] The spasm often affects the near triad completely, but isolated spasms of accommodation, convergence, and miosis can be seen as discrete entities.[71] Generally, spasm of the near reflex is considered as having a functional basis, extensive neuroradiologic examinations are not conducted, and therapy is symptomatic.[71] Therefore, cases in which the spasms were associated with definite neurologic disease are worth reporting. In a series of seven patients, two had posterior fossa abnormalities (cerebellar tumor, Arnold-Chiari malformation), two had pituitary tumor, one had a vestibulopathy, and two had a history of head trauma.[72] None of these seven patients had signs of overt personality disorders, and none complained of significant disability. Most of my patients with spasm of the near reflex report antecedent head trauma, and recently I observed the syndrome in a patient with a tumor of the posterior fossa. Although the association with neurologic abnormalities was striking in this personal case and in those cited,[72] a pathogenetic link could not be found. The lack of a common neurophysiologic mechanism should not be taken as an argument against an organic basis for these cases of spasm. On the other hand, the history of head trauma or the presence of an intracranial tumor do not rule out the psychogenic nature of the motility disorder. A causal relationship between head trauma and spasm of the near reflex is especially difficult to accept when the spasm begins several months after an accident.[72, 73]

Neurodegenerative Diseases

In *Parkinson's disease* the loss of nigrostriatal dopamine is now widely recognized as being directly related to the motor symptoms. The loss of nigrostriatal dopamine was hypothesized to be secondary to hypothalamic dysfunction in one study.[74] Smooth pursuit eye movements were severely affected in patients with Parkinson's disease, but the smooth pursuit deficits did not parallel short-term, drug-related on-and-off periods of skeletal motor performance.[75] These results indicated that neural circuits that subserve pursuit were pharmacologically segregated from dopaminergic mechanisms that mediate short- and medium-duration dose-related fluctuations in Parkinson's disease. Parkinson's disease was shown not only to affect the pursuit system, but also to impair the motor programming of coordinated eye-head movements and their interaction with the vestibulo-ocular reflex during gaze shifts.[76]

The clinical features and the neuropharmacology of *progressive supranuclear palsy* (PSP) were reviewed by Duvoisin et al.[77] The natural histories (but not the evolution of ocular motor disturbances) of 52 consecutive patients with PSP were reported in another paper.[78] About half of these patients had an additional horizontal gaze palsy at the time of examination, whereas other motility problems, such as blepharospasm, ptosis, internuclear ophthalmoplegia, nystagmus, lid retraction, and apraxia of eyelid opening or eyelid closure, were rare. A severe disturbance of saccades and pursuit in the vertical and horizontal plane, and absent caloric responses despite preservation of the vestibulo-ocular reflexes, were documented electro-oculographically in three patients with PSP.[79]

The dysfunction of saccadic and smooth pursuit eye movements in *Alzheimer's disease* was analyzed by Fletcher and Sharpe using a magnetic search-coil technique.[80, 81] Saccadic latencies were significantly prolonged, and peak velocities were reduced, only when the timing of the target motion was unpredictable. Saccades to predictable amplitude targets were abnormally hypometric. Several patients showed impersistences of gaze with frequent saccades away from the fixation point, and others could not make saccades away from a target flash, a behavior similar to that of patients with frontal lobe lesions[5] and Huntington's disease.[83, 84] Smooth eye movement gain was uniformly reduced in 13 patients with Alzheimer's disease at all target velocities for several frequencies of sinusoidal target motion, necessitating frequent and large catch-up saccades.[81] Smooth pursuit gain decreased significantly in response to small increments in target acceleration, indicating involvement of an acceleration-saturating nonlinear element that limits smooth pursuit. The use of accelerating targets (e.g., sinusoidal instead of triangular pursuit) obviously represents a more physiologic and sensitive way of testing the pursuit system.[82, 86] The performance of Alzheimer's patients was considerably different from elderly subjects without this disease.[83] Large saccades intruded on the ongoing smooth pursuit movement and appeared to anticipate the target trajectory. Smooth eye movements sometimes resumed immediately after a large intrusion as if the eyes pursued the peripheral retinal target.

Difficulties with initiation of saccades and maintenance of steady fixation were observed in patients with *Huntington's disease*.[84] Saccadic latencies were longer for command saccades than for reflexive, visually guided saccades. As was found in patients with Alzheimer's disease, the authors found an excessive distractibility with difficulties in suppressing saccades toward a suddenly appearing visual target. Another feature restricted to patients who acquired Huntington's disease before the age of 30 years was shown to be a slowing of saccades.[85] The slowing of saccades may not be due to brain stem pathology, but may reflect inhibition of the superior colliculus or other structures involved in the generation of saccades.

Degenerative Diseases Affecting the Brain Stem and Cerebellum

The cerebellar vermis appears to be essential for both horizontal and vertical smooth pursuit and for visual-vestibular interaction, but not for the generation of saccades.[86] To better define the role of the cerebellum in oculomotor control in man, Baloh et al. performed a quantitative study of ten patients with sporadic late cortical cerebellar atrophy, which is known to affect mainly the vermis and flocculonodular lobe, but not or less so the deep cerebellar nuclei.[87] A uniform picture emerged: the main deficit in all patients was impairment of foveal pursuit and a closely related impairment of fixation suppression of the vestibulo-ocular reflex. Full-field optokinetic nystagmus showed a gradual buildup of about 15 degrees/second (final slow-phase velocity minus initial slow-phase velocity) with an early slow-phase velocity saturation (20 to 40 degrees/second). This unusual optokinetic response indicated that the direct visual pursuit pathway that normally bypasses the velocity storage element in humans travels through the cerebellum. Saccades were normal, except in three patients with dysmetria. Increased gain of the vestibulo-ocular reflex (1.5 to 1.7 times), gaze-evoked nystagmus and rebound nystagmus were other prominent features in most of these patients.

A still higher (twofold) increase in vestibulo-ocular reflex gain in a patient with cerebellar degeneration was documented by Thurston et al.[88] The authors speculated that the climbing fiber input from the inferior olivary nuclei, by which the flocculi receive the retinal image slip information they need to adapt the vestibulo-ocular reflex, was affected in this patient, and that the patient might benefit from blocking the acetylcholinesterase within the dorsal cap of the inferior olive. Indeed, physostigmine significantly reduced the gain of the vestibulo-ocular reflex. This study opens an interesting perspective to a pharmacologic modulation of hyperactive or underactive vestibulo-ocular reflex.

The combination of saccadic hypermetria in one horizontal direction, hypometria in the opposite direction, and a horizontal saccadic bias during vertical saccades in patients with lateral medullary infarction was first described by Hagström et al.[89] Kommerell and Hoyt analyzed this peculiar eye movement disorder in depth and coined the term "lateropulsion of saccadic eye movements."[90] As opposed to lateropulsion, which is ipsilateral to the medullary infarction, *contrapulsion* of saccades accompanying a unilateral ischemic lesion of the rostral cerebellum was described by Ranalli and Sharpe.[91] Instead of vertical saccades the subject made oblique saccades away from the lesion. Interestingly, the horizontal and vertical vectors of these saccades were temporally linked, as in normal oblique saccades. The finding suggested that the transformation from the spatial coding within the colliculus into the temporal coding of brain stem burst neurons was disturbed by the cerebellar lesion as if the spatial map had been shifted contralaterally. An analogous vertical bias of horizontal saccades in several members of a family with vestibulocerebellar ataxia was described by Farris et al.[92] It appears that "pulsion" of saccades is worth studying in more detail for further information about the spatial-temporal transformation that occurs during the coding of saccades.

Several eye movement disorders, which improved with thyrotropin-releasing hormones, were found in patients with various spinocerebellar degenerations.[93] Adult-onset progressive supranuclear ophthalmoplegia, cerebellar ataxia, and neurogenic proximal muscle weakness were detected in an unusual syndrome caused by hexosaminidase A deficiency in a brother and sister.[94]

REFERENCES

1. Henn V, Lang W, Hepp K, et al: Experimental gaze palsies in monkeys and their relation to human pathology. *Brain* 1984; 107:619–636.

2. Hanson MR, Hamid MA, Tomsak RL, et al: Selective saccadic palsy caused by pontine lesions: Clinical, physiological, and pathological correlations. *Ann Neurol* 1986; 20:209–217.

3. Nishida T, Tychsen L, Corbett JJ: Resolution of saccadic palsy after treatment of brain-stem metastasis. *Arch Neurol* 1986; 43:1196–1197.

4. Kommerell G, Henn V, Bach M, et al: Unilateral lesion of the paramedian pontine reticular formation. Loss of rapid eye movements with preservation of vestibulo-ocular reflex and pursuit. *Neuro-Ophthalmol* 1987; 7:93–98.

5. Mehdorn E: Supranuclear and nuclear disorders of eye movement. *Curr Neuro-Ophthalmol* 1988; 1:173–184.

6. Morgan DW, Honan W: Lateral gaze palsy due to giant aneurysm of the posterior fossa. *J Neurol Neurosurg Psychiatry* 1988; 52:883–884.

7. Dominguez RO, Bronstein AM: Complete gaze palsy in pontine haemorrhage. *J Neurol Neurosurg Psychiatry* 1988; 52:150–151.

8. Brusa G, Meneghini S, Piccardo A, et al: Regressive pattern of horizontal gaze palsy. Case report. *Neuro-Ophthalmol* 1987; 7:301–306.

9. Bogousslavsky J, Meienberg O: Eye movement disorders in brain-stem and cerebellar stroke. *Arch Neurol* 1987; 44:141–148.

10. Bogousslavsky J, Fox AJ, Carey LS, et al: Correlates of brain-stem oculomotor disorders in multiple sclerosis. Magnetic resonance imaging. *Arch Neurol* 1986; 43:460–463.

11. Dubin L, Quencer RM: Brain-stem infarct. *J Clin Neuro Ophthalmol* 1987; 7:112–113.

12. Hommel M, Gato JM, Pollack P, et al: Magnetic resonance imaging and the "one-and-a-half" syndrome: A case report. *J Clin Neuro Ophthalmol* 1987; 7:161–164.

13. Hommel M, Besson G, Tarel V, et al: L'imagerie par résonance magnétique dans les paralysies de l'oculomotricité horizontale par infarctus. *Rev Neurol* 1988; 144:18–24.

14. Lewis MA, Goldstein S, Baker RS: Magnetic resonance imaging of the posterior fossa in ocular motility disorders—four case studies. *J Clin Neuro Ophthalmol* 1987; 7:235–240.

15. Martyn CN, Kean D: The one-and-a-half syndrome. Clinical correlation with a pontine lesion demonstrated by nuclear magnetic resonance imaging in a case of multiple sclerosis. *Br J Ophthalmol* 1988; 72:515–517.

16. Baloh RW, Yee RD, Honrubia V: Internuclear ophthalmoplegia. I. Saccades and dissociated nystagmus. *Arch Neurol* 1978; 35:484–489.

17. Zee DS, Hain TC, Carl JR: Abduction nystagmus in internuclear ophthalmoplegia. *Ann Neurol* 1987; 21:383–388.

18. Mehdorn E: Dissociated nystagmus in internuclear ophthalmoplegia—Consequence of prenuclear medial rectus palsy. *Fortschr Ophthalmol* 1987; 84:212–214.

19. Burde RM: Internuclear ophthalmoplegia (letter). *Ann Neurol* 1987; 22:668–669.

20. Keane JR: Traumatic internuclear ophthalmoplegia. *J Clin Neuro Ophthalmol* 1987; 7:165–166.

21. Cogen MS, Kline LB, Duvall ER: Bilateral internuclear ophthalmoplegia in systemic lupus erythematosus. *J Clin Neuro Ophthalmol* 1987; 7:69–73.

22. Coppeto JR, Greco P: Unilateral internuclear ophthalmoplegia, migraine, and supratentorial arteriovenous malformation. *Am J Ophthalmol* 1987; 104:191–192.

23. Delreux V, Ghilain S, Laterre C: Internuclear ophthalmoplegia and non-paralytic pontine exotropia. *Acta Neurol Belg* 1987; 87:191–196.

24. Blondel M, Defoort S, Bouchez B, et al: Fisher's one-and-a-half syndrome. Involvement of the 6th cranial nerve nucleus and association with paralytic pontine exotropia. *Acta Neurol Belg* 1986; 86:217–223.

25. Jay WM, Nazarian SM, Underwood DW: Pseudo-internuclear ophthalmoplegia with downshoot in myasthenia gravis. *J Clin Neuro Ophthalmol* 1987; 7:74–76.

26. Bogousslavsky J, Regli F, Uske A: Thalamic infarcts: Clinical syndromes, etiology, and prognosis. *Neurology* 1988; 38:837–848.

27. Büttner-Ennever JA, Büttner U, Cohen B, Baumgartner G: Vertical gaze paralysis and the rostral interstitial nucleus of the medial longitudinal fasciculus. *Brain* 1982; 105:125–149.

28. Kobari M, Ishihara N, Yunoki K: Bilateral thalamic infarction associated with selective downward gaze paralysis. *Eur Neurol* 1987; 26:246–251.

29. Ranalli PJ, Sharpe JA, Fletcher WA: Palsy of upward and downward saccadic, pursuit, and vestibular movements with a unilateral midbrain lesion: Pathophysiological correlations. *Neurology* 1988; 38:114–122.

30. Wall M, Slamovits TL, Weisberg LA, et al: Vertical gaze ophthalmoplegia from infarction in the area of the posterior thalamo-subthalamic paramedian artery. *Stroke* 1986; 17:546–555.

31. Cannon SC, Robinson DA: Neural integrator failure from brain stem lesions in monkey. *Invest Ophthalmol Vis Sci [Suppl]* 1985; 26:3–47.

32. Leigh RJ: Brainstem control of vertical gaze, in Kennard C and Rose FC (eds): *Physiological Aspects of Clinical Neuro-Ophthalmology*. London, Chapman and Hall, 1988, pp 237–248.

33. Leigh RJ, Foley JM, Remler BF, et al: Oculogyric crisis: A syndrome of thought disorder and ocular deviation. *Ann Neurol* 1987; 22:13–17.

34. Sand JJ, Biller J, Corbett JJ, et al: Partial dorsal mesencephalic hemorrhages: Report of three cases. *Neurology* 1986; 36:529–533.

35. Keane JR: Bilateral ocular motor signs after tentorial herniation in 25 patients. *Arch Neurol* 1986; 43:806–807.

36. Tamura EE, Hoyt CS: Oculomotor consequences of intraventricular hemorrhages in premature infants. *Arch Ophthalmol* 1987; 105:533–535.

37. Keane JR: Alternating skew deviation: 47 patients. *Neurology* 1985; 35:725–728.

38. Moster ML, Schatz NJ, Savino PJ, et al: Alternating skew on lateral gaze (bilateral abducting hypertropia). *Ann Neurol* 1988; 23:190–192.

39. Büttner-Ennever JA: Anatomy of the ocular motor nuclei, Kennard C, Rose FC (eds): *Physiological Aspects of Clinical Neuro-Ophthalmology*. London, Chapman and Hall, 1988, pp 200–208.

40. Dehaene I, Marchau M, VanHooren G: Nuclear oculomotor nerve paralysis. *Neuro-Ophthalmol* 1987; 7:219–222.

41. Pusateri TJ, Sedwick LA, Margo CE: Isolated inferior rectus muscle palsy from a solitary metastasis to the oculomotor nucleus. *Arch Ophthalmol* 1987; 105:675–677.

42. Zermeno F, Del Brutto OH, Wielink GV, et al: Unilateral third nerve palsy and somnolent mutism. *J Clin Neuro Ophthalmol* 1987; 7:93–95.

43. Kömpf D, Erbguth F, Kreiten K, et al: Bilateral third nerve palsy in basilar vertebral artery disease. Report of three cases with survival and review of the literature. *Neuro-Ophthalmol* 1987; 7:355–362.

44. Masdeu JC, Rosenberg M: Midbrain-diencephalic horizontal gaze paresis. *J Clin Neuro Ophthalmol* 1987; 7:227–234.

45. Pierrot-Deseilligny C, Rivaud S, Penet C, et al: Latencies of visually guided saccades in unilateral hemispheric cerebral lesions. *Ann Neurol* 1987; 21:138–148.

46. Bogousslavsky J: Impairment of visually evoked eye movements with a unilateral parieto-occipital lesion. *J Neurol* 1987; 234:160–162.

47. Segraves MA, Goldberg ME: Functional properties of corticotectal neurons in the monkey's frontal eye field. *J Neurophysiol* 1987; 58:1387–1419.

48. Barbur JL, Forsyth PM, Findlay JM: Human saccadic eye movements in the absence of the geniculocalcarine projection. *Brain* 1988; 111:63–82.

49. Meienberg O, Wehren C: Oculographic diagnosis of hemineglect in patients with homonymous hemianopia. *J Neurol* 1986; 233:97–101.

50. Wyllie E, Lüders H, Morris HH, et al: Ipsilateral forced head and eye turning at the end of the generalized tonic-clonic phase of versive seizures. *Neurology* 1986; 36:1212–1217.

51. Guitton D, Volle M: Gaze control in humans: Eye-head coordination during orienting movements to targets within and beyond the oculomotor range. *J Neurophysiol* 1987; 58:427–459.

52. Pelisson D, Prablanc C, Urquizar C: Vestibulo-ocular reflex inhibition and gaze saccade control characteristics during eye-head orientation in humans. *J Neurophysiol* 1988; 59:997–1013.

53. Pierrot-Desilligny C, Gautier JC, Loron P: Acquired ocular motor apraxia due to bilateral fronto-parietal infarcts. *Ann Neurol* 1988; 23:199–202.

54. Borchert MS, Sadun AA, Sommers JD, et al: Congenital ocular motor apraxia in twins. *J Clin Neuro Ophthalmol* 1987; 7:104–107.

55. Rosenberg ML, Wilson E: Congenital ocular motor apraxia without head thrusts. *J Clin Neuro Ophthalmol* 1987; 7:26–28.

56. Spiritus M, Waterschoot MP, Bottu J, et al: Eye anomalies and ocular motor disorders in the oro-facial-digital syndrome type II. *Neuro-Ophthalmology* 1987; 7:223–226.

57. Thurston SE, Leigh RJ, Crawford T, et al: Two distinct deficits of visual tracking caused by unilateral lesions of cerebral cortex in humans. *Ann Neurol* 198; 23:266–273.

58. Lynch JC: Frontal eye field lesions in monkeys disrupt visual pursuit. *Exp Brain Res* 1987; 68:437–441.

59. Tusa RJ, Ungerleider LG: Fiber pathways of cortical areas mediating smooth pursuit eye movements in monkeys. *Ann Neurol* 1988; 23:174–183.

60. Verhagen WIM, Huygen PLM, Schulte BPM: Ocular motor responses after locked-in syndrome: Sparing of subcortical optokinetic nystagmus? *Neuro-Ophthalmol* 1987; 7:49–56.

61. Bolling J, Lavin PJM: Combined gaze palsy of horizontal saccades and pursuit contralateral to a midbrain haemorrhage. *J Neurol Neurosurg Psychiatry* 1987; 50:789–791.

62. Berg AV van den, Collewijn H: Directional asymmetries of human optokinetic nystagmus. *Exp Brain Res* 1988; 70:597–604.

63. Boman DK, Hotson JR: Smooth pursuit training and disruption, directional differences and nystagmus. *Neuro-Ophthalmol* 1987; 7:185–194.

64. Al-Din ASN: Controversy about Fisher's syndrome (letter). *Arch Neurol* 1987; 43:543.

65. Ropper AH: Reply to Al-Din. *Arch Neurol* 1987; 43:543–544.

66. Dehaene I, Martin JJ, Genes K, et al: Guillain-Barré syndrome with ophthalmoplegia: Clinicopathologic study of the central and peripheral nervous systems, including the oculomotor nerves. *Neurology* 1986; 36:851–854.

67. Jamal GA, Ballantyne JP: The localization of the lesion in patients with acute ophthalmoplegia, ataxia and areflexia (Miller Fisher syndrome). A serial multimodal neurophysiological study. *Brain* 1988; 111:95–114.

68. Pinchoff BS, Slavin ML, Rosenstein D, et al: Divergence paralysis as the initial sign in the Miller Fisher syndrome. *Am J Ophthalmol* 1986; 101:741–742.

69. Kohler A, Torrente A de, Inderwildi B: Fisher's syndrome associated with campylobacter jejuni infection. *Eur Neurol* 1988; 28:150–151.

70. Rosenberg ML: Spasm of the near reflex mimicking myasthenia gravis. *J Clin Neuro Ophthalmol* 1986; 6:106–108.

71. Smith JL: Accommodative spasm versus spasm of the near reflex. *J Clin Neuro Ophthalmol* 1987; 7:132–134.

72. Dagi LR, Chrousos GA, Cogan DC: Spasm of the near reflex associated with organic disease. *Am J Ophthalmol* 1987; 103:582–585.

73. Bohlmann BJ, France TD: Persistent accommodative spasm nine years after head trauma. *J Clin Neuro Ophthalmol* 1987; 7:129–131.

74. Sandyk R, Iacono RP, Bamford CR: The hypothalamus in Parkinson's disease. *Ital J Neurol Sci* 1987; 8:227–234.

75. Sharpe JA, Fletcher WA, Lang AE, et al: Smooth pursuit during dose-related on-off fluctuations in Parkinson's disease. *Neurology* 1987; 37:1389–1392.

76. White OB, Saint-Cyr JA, Tomlinson RD, et al: Ocular motor deficits in Parkinson's disease. III. Coordination of eye and head movements. *Brain* 1988; 111:115–129.

77. Duvoisin RC, Golbe LI, Lepore FE: Progressive supranuclear palsy. *Can J Neurol Sci* 1987; 14(3):547–554.

78. Maher ER, Lees AJ: The clinical features and natural history of the Steele-Richardson-Olszewski syndrome (progressive supranuclear palsy). *Neurology* 1986; 36:1005–1008.

79. Breuer TJ, Wuisman PG, Korten JJ: Electrooculographic findings in progressive supranuclear palsy. *Clin Neurol Neurosurg* 1987; 89:87–95.

80. Fletcher WA, Sharpe JA: Saccadic eye movement dysfunction in Alzheimer's disease. *Ann Neurol* 1986; 20:464–471.

81. Fletcher WA, Sharpe JA: Smooth pursuit dysfunction in Alzheimer's disease. *Ann Neurol* 1988; 38:272–277.

82. Langenegger T, Meienberg O: Slow conjugate eye movements. Normative data for routine diagnosis of ophthalmo-neurological disorders. *Neuro-Ophthalmol* 1988; 8:53–76.

83. Zackon DH, Sharpe JA: Smooth pursuit in senescence. *Acta Otolaryngol (Stockh)* 1987; 104:290–297.

84. Lasker AG, Zee DS, Hain TC, et al: Saccades in Huntington's disease: Initiation defects and distractibility. *Neurology* 1987; 37:364–370.

85. Lasker AG, Zee DS, Hain TC, et al: Saccades in Huntington's disease: Slowing and dysmetria. *Neurology* 1988; 38:427–431.

86. Furman JM, Baloh RW, Yee RD: Eye movement abnormalities in a family with cerebellar vermian atrophy. *Acta Otolaryngol (Stockh)* 1986; 101:371–377.

87. Baloh RW, Yee RD, Honrubia V: Late cortical cerebellar atrophy. Clinical and oculographic features. *Brain* 1986; 109:159–180.

88. Thurston SE, Leigh RJ, Abel LA, et al: Hyperactive vestibuloocular reflex in cerebellar degeneration: Pathogenesis and treatment. *Neurology* 1987; 37:53–57.

89. Hagström L, Hörnsten G, Silfverskiöld BP: Oculostatic and visual phenomena occurring in association with Wallenberg's syndrome. *Acta Neurol Scand* 1969; 45:568–582.

90. Kommerell G, Hoyt WF: Lateropulsion of saccadic eye movements: Electro-oculographic studies in a patient with Wallenberg's syndrome. *Arch Neurol* 1973; 28:313–318.

91. Ranalli PJ, Sharpe JA: Contrapulsion of saccades and ipsilateral ataxia: A unilateral disorder of the rostral cerebellum. *Ann Neurol* 1986; 20:311–316.

92. Farris BK, Smith JL, Ayyar DR: Neuro-ophthalmologic findings in vestibulocerebellar ataxia. *Arch Neurol* 1986; 43:1050–1053.

93. Yamamoto H, Saito S, Sobue I: Bedside and electro-oculographic analysis of abnormal ocular movements in spinocerebellar degenerations: Effects of thyrotropin-releasing hormone. *Neurology* 1988; 38:110–114.

94. Harding AE, Young EP, Schon F: Adult onset supranuclear ophthalmoplegia, cerebellar ataxia, and neurogenic proximal muscle weakness were in a brother and sister: Another hexosaminidase A deficiency syndrome. *J Neurol Neurosurg Psychiatry* 1987; 50:687–690.

CHAPTER 11

Nonmyasthenic Ophthalmoplegia

John W. Gittinger, Jr., M.D.

Professor of Surgery and Neurology, University of Massachusetts Medical School, Worcester, Massachusetts

ACQUIRED MULTIPLE CRANIAL NEUROPATHY

Multiple ocular motor cranial neuropathies, with or without pain and with or without optic and trigeminal nerve involvement, continue to be both diagnostic and nosologic problems. Campbell and Okazaki report a case in which an elderly man developed pain and ophthalmoplegia on the right.[1] A necrotizing vasculitis led to carotid rupture and death, and at autopsy nongranulomatous inflammation was found in the orbit and in the walls of the cavernous sinus. These authors review previous pathologically verified cases of the Tolosa-Hunt syndrome (THS) and note that most, including the initial report of Tolosa, describe granulation tissue and not granulomas (i.e., with epithelioid cells).

Lapresle and Lasjaunias review the arterial anatomy of the cranial nerve vascular supply and point out that all three ocular motor nerves are supplied by the inferolateral trunk, an intracavernous branch of the internal carotid artery.[2] Bruyn and Buruma believe that many cases of recurrent benign multiple cranial neuropathies (which they call the Charles Symonds syndrome), as well as instances of THS, represent arteritis in the inferolateral trunk and its branches.[3] After looking at the Massachusetts General Hospital's experience with multiple idiopathic cranial neuropathy, Juncos and Beal conclude that those that cannot tentatively be assigned to specific diagnostic categories (including Guillain-Barré syndrome, THS, and mycoplasma encephalitis) may represent indolent multifocal pachymeningitis incited by viruses.[4]

In a previous review, I expressed a preference for designations such as recurrent multiple cranial neuropathies over eponyms such as Tolosa-Hunt.[5] Barontini and co-workers conclude that THS is just one variant of the recurrent cranial neuropathy syndrome.[6] Recurrent facial and ocular motor palsies in one family developed after the age of 40 years, often in individuals who also had diabetes, suggesting microvascular disease as an etiology.[7] Recurrent painful ophthalmoplegia may respond dramatically to steroids, and this has been considered one of the major criteria for the diagnosis of THS. Kwan and co-workers[8] believe that abnormalities of the soft tissue in the orbital apex and cavernous sinus visualized by computed tomography (CT) that resolve with systemic corticosteroids should make THS a diagnosis of inclusion rather than exclusion, but they include cases of presumed cavernous sinus epidermoid and of probable sarcoidosis in their own series of five patients. Both radiation therapy[9] and tonsillectomy[10] are offered as potential treatment modalities in chronic THS. (Incidentally, with the last reference, the slightly misspelled "Tolusa-Hunt syndrome" probably is now permanently embedded in the otolaryngology literature, having now been described in two different journals.)

The period under review has seen the publication of case reports of various cavernous sinus and orbital apex syndromes: some with relatively well-known causes such as mucormycosis,[11] zoster,[12] and metastatic breast carcinoma,[13] and some with rare etiologies such as actinomycosis,[14] rheumatoid nodules,[15] and a nail.[16] Two types of primary cartilagenous tumors of the region are described, one benign (chondromyofibroma)[17] and one malignant (chondrosarcoma).[18] Viswanathan and co-workers point out that such tumors may be associated with carotid occlusion or agenesis.[17] Posteriorly draining carotid-cavernous fistulas may not have typical ophthalmic findings of venous engorgement and exophthalmos, but do cause painful ophthalmoplegia.[19] A large, but not giant, intracavernous aneurysm thrombosed, producing complete unilateral ophthalmoplegia and contralateral hemiparesis—but sparing vision.[20]

The mechanism for complete external ophthalmoplegia in a patient with pseudotumor cerebri is not obvious, nor is the justification for bilateral optic nerve sheath fenestration when there is improvement on conservative therapy.[21] A complex ophthalmoplegia is attributed to fibrous dysplasia of the skull involving the orbits.[22] A diabetic with a sensory-motor polyneuropathy developed complete external ophthalmoplegia with ptosis, with recovery in 4 months, and recurrence a year later.[23] Cammarata and co-workers exclude the Fisher syndrome because the cerebrospinal fluid is normal, but I find their explanation—ischemia—unsatisfying.[23]

ACQUIRED LESIONS OF THE OCULAR MOTOR NERVES

Third Nerve Palsies

Two studies using horseradish peroxidase in laboratory animals who had chronic surgical oculomotor nerve lesions have finally elucidated the mechanism of aberrant regeneration of the third nerve. Sibony and co-workers[24] used the cat, and Fernandez and co-workers[25] the rat, to trace a regenerated axon from an extraocular muscle to the third nerve nucleus, providing strong evidence that what has clinically been called aberrant regeneration is in fact aberrant regeneration (in the sense of reconnection of the proximal ends of cut axons with distal portions innervating another muscle) and not ephaptic transmission or central synaptic reorganization. The subject is not completely closed, however, since Fernandez and co-workers explain bilateral labeling after unilateral lesions and injections of horseradish peroxidase as collateral sprouting from the homologous contralateral muscle, whereas Sibony and associates use such bilateral labeling after injection of the superior rectus muscle as their primary evidence for aberrant reinnervation, and argue that mammals normally lack reinnervational specificity. I favor the latter explanation because it is simpler.

Two probably related disorders of eye movement that may still leave a place for ephaptic transmission or central reorganization are oculomotor neuromyotonia (which may also affect the abducens and trochlear nerves) and oculomotor nerve palsy with cyclic spasms. The intermittent, nonperiodic spasm of various extraocular muscles called neuromyotonia seems most likely to develop after radiation therapy to tumors in the region of the cavernous sinus, and may respond to carbamazepine.[26, 27] Cyclic spasms are attributed to chronic peripheral nerve injury.[28]

Brain stem lesions producing third nerve palsies are being identified more often, in part because of better imaging techniques. A brain stem infarct produced unilateral third nerve palsy and somnolent mutism.[29] Bilateral third nerve palsy is a persistent feature of some basilar territory upper brain stem infarcts,[30] which may be a consequence of trauma.[31] Ipsilateral third nerve palsy and contralateral hemiparesis were the presentation of a brain stem abscess in a 16-year-old boy.[32] A tumor was initially suspected, but surgical drainage yielded *Streptococcus milleri*. Metastatic squamous cell carcinoma of the esophagus produced an isolated inferior rectus palsy.[33] The clinicopathologic correlation in this case is unequivocal. Dehaene and co-workers describe a case consistent with pure nuclear involvement, but the photographs provided are not completely convincing.[34]

The clue to a partial third nerve palsy as the presentation of an internal carotid-posterior communicating aneurysm in an 18-year-old girl was the history that her mother's aneurysm had presented as a complete third nerve palsy 6 months earlier.[35] A less obvious clue was anisocoria and diplopia after meperidine injection for pain in a Canadian emergency room; the probably irrelevant discussion of the effect of opiates on the pupil in this letter is mercifully brief.[36] Partial third nerve palsies as the presenting signs of basilar aneurysms have been less emphasized than those that accompany internal carotid-posterior communicating aneurysms, but represent 6 of a series of 12 cases from the Mayo Clinic[37] and are the subject of a case report from Italy.[38] Bartleson and co-workers conclude that vertebral injections should be considered when angiography is undertaken.[37] A transient third nerve palsy followed rather than preceded clipping of an internal carotid aneurysm; vasospasm is postulated.[39]

The conclusion that early surgery on the causative posterior communicating aneurysm confers a good prognosis for the ophthalmoplegia is probably correct, but is hardly supported by the data in a small series.[40] Even when the ophthalmoplegia persists, relatively few acquired third nerve palsies come to corrective strabismus surgery. Three quarters of 20 patients who had surgery for blepharoptosis had congenital palsies; 6 of the 20 developed corneal exposure.[41]

Neuroimaging of traumatic third nerve palsies does not always demonstrate an anatomic lesion,[42] but CT may reveal evidence of avulsion[43] or an enlarged posterior communicating artery as the result of carotid agenesis.[44] Three radiologists and a neuro-ophthalmologist offer a diagnostic approach to third nerve palsies.[45] Their categories do not include cases of partial third nerve palsy without pupillary involvement, which are the most difficult. Trobe addresses this question again in a short review.[46] In the same journal number, Keene offers some trenchant comments on the partial third nerve palsy question.[47]

Keane also found both unilateral and bilateral third nerve palsies common as sequelae of tentorial herniation.[48] In an article from China, dilated pupils are cited as characteristic of diabetic ophthalmoplegia, although the perspicacious reader will note that the pupils were normal in all five cases described.[49]

Asymptomatic areas of cerebral hypodensity were found on the CT of a 23-year-old woman with a headache and left third nerve palsy, attributed to ophthalmoplegic migraine, but with no mention of cardiac ultrasound to exclude atrial myxoma.[50] A more typical case is reported in a child,[51] and ophthalmoplegic migraine appears to be the correct diagnosis in a patient previously reported as having oculomotor palsy from measles immunization.[52]

What remains are reports of unusual cases: two instances where third nerve palsy was the presentation of multiple sclerosis,[53, 54] an infant found to have a papillary meningioma,[55] a young man with a cavernous hemangioma of the oculomotor nerve,[56] and a superior division palsy after extraction of a mandibular third molar.[57] The spectrum of neuro-ophthalmic findings in pial-dural arteriovenous malformation is expanded by the report of a 62-year-old man with papilledema and a partial third nerve palsy, both responsive to selective embolization.[58] The link of third nerve palsy with recurrent herpes labialis remains to be clearly established,[59] but third nerve palsy may be one manifestation of a mononeuritis multiplex produced by macroglobulinemia.[60] A prolactin determination prior to treatment or biopsy is warranted in any sellar or parasellar mass presenting as a third nerve palsy.[61] And no modern review is complete without a case of acquired immune deficiency syndrome (AIDS).[62]

Fourth Nerve Palsies

Superior oblique palsies are one area where strabismologists and neuro-ophthalmologists share a common ground. Both are interested in diagnosis, and Metz reviews some of the potential pitfalls in recognizing superior oblique palsy.[63] The strabismologists are particularly interested in recognizing bilateral superior oblique palsy, since when the palsy is asymmetrical, the side with the lesser involvement may be "masked."[64, 65] This is important because it affects the choice of surgical technique. Neuro-ophthalmologists, on the other hand, are interested in etiology. Keane describes three cases with abnormal CT: a traumatic contusion, a bullet fragment, and a cysticercal cyst.[66] Other unusual causes defined during the period of this review are trochlear neurinoma,[67] cavernous sinus meningioma,[68] and lumbar puncture (in association with the more common sixth nerve palsy).[69]

Sixth Nerve Palsies

The publication of three articles on the combination of a sixth nerve palsy and Horner's syndrome may indicate that this is not so much rare, as rarely looked for.[70–72] The offending lesion is in or compressing the cavernous sinus. One of these cases represents the most indolent septic cavernous sinus thrombosis on record,[71] which prompts me to question the diagnosis.

A contralateral sixth nerve palsy is associated with cluster headache.[73] A patient with a 40-year history of headache and recurrent sixth nerve palsy responded to steroids,[74] again raising the question as to what is ophthalmoplegic migraine and what is THS.[75]

Savino's brief review is characteristically clear, but I would point out that most medial rectus entrapments produce more limitation of adduction than of abduction (see following).[76] Sixth nerve palsies after treatment for cervical fractures are probably produced by stretching of the brain stem, a mechanism similar to that producing palsies post-lumbar puncture and with increased intracranial pressure.[77]

Slavin and Abramson review the anatomy of the pterygopalatine fossa in their discussion of a squamous cell carcinoma causing trigeminal, abducens, and then oculomotor involvement.[78] Because the pterygopalatine fossa also contains the parasympathetic ganglion of the lacrimal gland—the sphenopalatine ganglion—decreased tearing would be expected, but was not observed. Two other tumors that produce sixth nerve palsies are clivus chordoma and prolactinoma.[79, 80] The latter developed ophthalmoplegia as the tumor shrank in response to bromocriptine.

Bilateral sixth nerve palsies developing a year apart were the presentation for bilateral giant intracavernous aneurysms.[81] One was successfully approached surgically through the cavernous sinus; the other was left alone. Kobayashi and co-workers wisely refuse to speculate as to the mechanism of a sixth nerve palsy seen in a patient with an ipsilateral cavernous sinus subarachnoid diverticulum.[82]

A sixth nerve palsy was one component of a bilateral, multiple cranial neuropathy in a patient with amyloidosis associated with plasma cell dyscrasia.[83] Bilateral sixth nerve palsy and cerebellar ataxia resolved after chemotherapy with cytosine arabinoside and mitoxantrone for promyelocytic leukemia was stopped.[84] Since the patient could not abduct either eye past the midline, the discussion of divergence paralysis in this paper is superfluous. Limitation of abduction developed in an 8-year-old boy with lactic acidosis and cytochrome c oxidase deficiency, who also had the more characteristic optic atrophy.[85]

ACQUIRED NEUROMUSCULAR OPHTHALMOPLEGIA

Despite a clinico-pathological conference in the *New England Journal of Medicine*,[86] a review in *Brain*,[87] and continued biochemical and morphologic studies,[88, 89] there is little to add to my last review regarding the understanding of chronic progressive external ophthalmoplegia (CPEO).[90] A study of 89 family histories leads to the unsurprising conclusion that mitochondrial DNA is not involved in the inheritance of CPEO.[91] The endocrinologic[92-94] and cardiac[95] manifestations continue to be of interest to physicians outside neurology and ophthalmology. The only effective treatment remains cautious ptosis surgery in selected cases.[96]

Amyloidosis of the medial rectus muscle was found in a case of loss of adduction and exotropia.[97] Another case of linear scleroderma (called morphoea) with ophthalmoplegia—in this instance, an acquired Brown's tendon sheath syndrome—has been reported.[98] Acquired Brown's syndromes also develop after trauma, both with[99] and without[100] orbital fractures. Entrapment of the medial rectus producing an acquired retraction syndrome may be more common in young black males because of anatomic factors.[101] The ophthalmoplegia observed with blow-out fractures may have both a mechanical and neurologic component.[102]

CONGENITAL NEUROMUSCULAR OPHTHALMOPLEGIA

The congenital form of Brown's syndrome runs in families and may manifest in both monozygotic and dizygotic twins.[103-105] Panhypopituitarism was found in a child with bilateral Duane's retraction syndrome and non-hypoplastic disks.[106] Three more cases of synergistic divergence occasion a discussion of innervational abnormalities in Duane's syndrome.[107] This subject has been addressed at length in a previous review.[5] Kommerell and Bach apply similar reasoning to explain "twitch abduction" in what appears to be a *forme fruste* of Duane's syndrome.[108]

In a familial case, the jaw moved to the appropriate side on attempts at lateral gaze.[109] I wonder if this is not just an effort artifact in this 7-year-old boy rather than anomalous innervation.

Houtman and co-workers have collected a large pedigree from Holland with the general fibrosis syndrome.[110] Another family, from Lebanon, is said to manifest a progressive form of this autosomal dominant disorder, but the evidence offered is weak.[111] These individuals are also said to have disk colobomas, but no illustration is offered, which may be understandable, considering the limits on medical care in this troubled country. General fibrosis was also encountered in an infant with the Prader-Willi syndrome, leading to the suggestion that the gene for general fibrosis lies on the long arm of chromosome 15, where that of the Prader-Willi syndrome usually is found.[112] Bilateral absence of the superior rectus probably represents a partial form of general fibrosis.[113]

Feeding difficulties and chronic aspiration bring children with Möbius syndrome to the attention of otolaryngologists, who may divert the trachea to the skin to prevent recurrent pneumonia.[114] In some patients with congenital paralysis of conjugate gaze, there is little or no facial weakness, but there may be pendular nystagmus and associated scoliosis or kyphoscoliosis.[115]

REFERENCES

1. Campbell RJ, Okazaki H: Painful ophthalmoplegia (Tolosa-Hunt variant): Autopsy findings in a patient with necrotizing intracavernous vasculitis and inflammatory disease of the orbit. *Mayo Clin Proc* 1987; 62:520–526.

2. Lapresle J, Lasjaunias P: Cranial nerve ischaemic arterial syndromes: A review. *Brain* 1986; 109; 207–215.

3. Bruyn GW, Buruma OJS: Multiple cranial neuropathy: The recurrent and non-recurrent non-familial forms. *Handb Clin Neurol* 1987; 7:569–573.

4. Juncos JL, Beal MF: Idiopathic cranial polyneuropathy: A fifteen-year experience. *Brain* 1987; 110:197–211.

5. Gittinger JW Jr: Non-myasthenic ophthalmoplegias, in Lessell S, van Dalen JTW (eds): *Neuro-Ophthalmology*, vol 2. Amsterdam, Excerpta Medica, 1982, pp 207–225.

6. Barontini F, Maurri S, Marrapodi E: Tolosa-Hunt syndrome versus recurrent cranial neuropathy. *J Neurol* 1987; 234:112–115.

7. Aldrich MS, Beck RW, Albers JW: Familial recurrent Bell's palsy with ocular motor palsies. *Neurology* 1987; 37:1369–1371.

8. Kwan ESK, Wolpert SM, Hedges TR III, et al: Tolosa-Hunt syndrome revisited: Not necessarily a diagnosis of exclusion. *AJNR* 1987; 8:1067–1072.

9. Nasr YG, Boghen D, Vézina J: Tolosa-Hunt syndrome with a prolonged course: Successful treatment with radiotherapy. *Neuro-Ophthalmol* 1987; 7:57–60.

10. Fraible MAS, Myer EC: Tolusa-Hunt syndrome: Resolution of a 12-year course after tonsillectomy. *Laryngoscope* 1987; 97:334–335.

11. Bray WH, Giangiacomo J, Ide CH: Orbital apex syndrome. *Surv Ophthalmol* 1987; 32:136–140.

12. Gupta D, Vishwakarma SK: Superior orbital fissure syndrome in trigemino-facial zoster. *J Laryngol Otol* 1987; 101:975–977.

13. Nelson PB, Robinson AG, Martinez AJ: Metastatic tumor of the pituitary gland. *Neurosurgery* 1987; 6:941–944.

14. Leigh RJ, Good EF, Rudy RP: Ophthalmoplegia due to actinomycosis. *J Clin Neuro-Ophthalmol* 1986; 6:157–159.

15. Konishi T, Saida T, Nishitani H: Orbital apex syndrome caused by rheumatoid nodules. *J Neurol Neurosurg Psychiatry* 1986; 49:460–462.

16. Vander JF, Nelson CC: Penetrating orbital injury with cavernous sinus involvement. *Ophthalmic Surg* 1988; 19:328–330.

17. Viswanathan R, Jegathraman AR, Ganapathy K, et al: Parasellar chondromyxofibroma with ipsilateral total internal carotid artery occlusion. *Surg Neurol* 1987; 28:141–144.

18. Ashworth B, Gordan A: Ophthalmoplegia due to chondrosarcoma in the cavernous sinus. *Neuro-Ophthalmol* 1986; 6:1435–151.

19. Kosmorsky GS, Hanson MR, Tomsak RL: Carotid-cavernous fistulae presenting as painful ophthalmoplegia without external ocular signs. *J Clin Neuro-Ophthalmol* 1988; 8:131–135.

20. Gautier JC, Awada A, Majdalani A: Ophthalmoplegia with contralateral hemiplegia. Occlusion of the internal carotid artery due to thrombosis of an intracavernous aneurysm. *Stroke* 1986; 17:1321–1322.

21. Landan I, Policheria H, McLaurin J: Complete external ophthalmoplegia in a case of pseudotumor cerebri. *Headache* 1987; 27:573–574.

22. Barontini F, Mauri S, Sità D: Peripheral ophthalmoplegia as the only sign of late-onset fibrous dysplasia of the skull. *J Clin Neuro-Ophthalmol* 1986; 6:109–112.

23. Cammarata S, Schenone A, Pasquali GF, et al: Complete bilateral relapsing ophthalmoplegia in a diabetic patient with a sensory-motor distal polyneuropathy. *Eur Neurol* 1986; 25:278–280.

24. Sibony PA, Eviger C, Lessell S: Retrograde horseradish peroxidase transport after oculomotor nerve injury. *Invest Ophthalmol Vis Sci* 1986; 27:975–980.

25. Fernandez E, Pallini R, Gangitano C, et al: Oculomotor nerve regeneration in rats: Functional, histological, and neuroanatomical studies. *J Neurosurg* 1987; 67:428–437.

26. Shults WT, Hoyt WF, Behrens M, et al: Ocular neuromyotonia: A clinical description of six patients. *Arch Ophthalmol* 1986; 104:1028–1034.

27. Lessell S, Lessell IM, Rizzo JF III: Ocular neuromyotonia after radiation therapy. *Am J Ophthalmol* 1986; 102:766–770.

28. Kommerell G, Mehdorn E, Ketelsen UP, et al: Oculomotor palsy with cyclic spasms: Electromyographic and electron microscopic evidence of chronic peripheral neuronal involvement. *Neuro-Ophthalmol* 1988; 8:9–21.

29. Zermeño F, Del Brutto OH, Van Wielink G, et al: Unilateral third nerve palsy and somnolent mutism. *J Clin Neuro-Ophthalmol* 1987; 7:93–95.

30. Kömpf D, Erbguth F, Kreiten K, et al: Bilateral third nerve palsy in basilar vertebral artery disease: Report of three cases with survival and review of the literature. *Neuro-Ophthalmol* 1987; 7:355–362.

31. Tognetti F, Godano U, Galassi E: Bilateral traumatic third nerve palsy. *Surg Neurol* 1988; 29:120–124.

32. Kashiwagi S, Abiko S, Aoki H: Brainstem abscess. *Surg Neurol* 1987; 28:63–66.

33. Pasateri TJ, Sedwick LA, Margo CE: Isolated inferior rectus muscle palsy from a solitary metastasis to the oculomotor nucleus. *Arch Ophthalmol* 1987; 105:675–677.

34. Dehaene I, Marchau M, Vanhooren G: Nuclear oculomotor nerve paralysis. *Neuro-Ophthalmol* 1987; 7:219–22.

35. Brodsky MC, Frenkel REP, Spoor TC: Familial intracranial aneurysm presenting as a subtle stable third nerve palsy. *Arch Ophthalmol* 1988; 106:173.

36. Jones BH, Mendelson M: Oculomotor nerve compression. *Ann Emerg Med* 1986; 15:1255–1256.

37. Bartleson JD, Trautmann JC, Sundt TM Jr: Minimal oculomotor nerve paresis secondary to unruptured intracranial aneurysms. *Arch Neurol* 1986; 43:1015–1020.

38. Boccardo M, Ruelle A, Banchero MA: Isolated oculomotor palsy caused by aneurysm of the basilar artery bifurcation. *J Neurol* 1986; 233:61–62.

39. Kudo T: Postoperative oculomotor palsy due to vasospasm in a patient with a ruptured internal carotid artery aneurysm. *Neurosurgery* 1986; 19:274–277.

40. Feely M, Kapoor S: Third nerve palsy due to posterior communicating artery aneurysm: The importance of early surgery. *J Neurol Neurosurg Psychiatry* 1987; 50:1051–1052.

41. Malone TJ, Nerad JA: The surgical treatment of blepharoptosis in oculomotor nerve palsy. *Am J Ophthalmol* 1988; 105:57–64.

42. Kruger M, Noel P, Ectors P: Bilateral primary traumatic oculomotor nerve palsy. *J Trauma* 1986; 26:1151–1153.

43. Asari S, Yamamoto Y, Satoh T: Direct CT demonstration suggesting oculomotor nerve avulsion following minor head trauma: Case report. *Comput Radiol* 1987; 11:131–134.

44. Wakai S, Watnanabe N, Inoh S, et al: Agenesis of internal carotid artery presenting with oculomotor nerve palsy after minor head injury. *Neurosurgery* 1987; 20:794–796.

45. Kwan ESK, Laucella M, Hedges TR III, et al: A cliniconeuroradiologic approach to third cranial nerve palsies. *AJNR* 1987; 8:459–468.

46. Trobe JD: Isolated third nerve palsies. *Semin Neurol* 1986; 6:135–141.

47. Keane JR: Vertical diplopia. *Semin Neurol* 1986; 6:147–154.

48. Keane JR: Bilateral ocular motor signs after tentorial herniation in 25 patients. *Arch Neurol* 1986; 43:806–807.

49. Shu-ping W, Lian-fang G, Bo M, et al: Diabetic oculomotor palsy: Report of 5 cases. *Chinese Med J* 1985; 98:524–527.

50. Moretti G, Scoditti U, Rustichelli P, et al: A case of ophthalmoplegic migraine with ipsilateral CT-documented hypodense lesions. *Headache* 1985; 25:372–375.

51. Amit R, Benezra D: Oculomotor ophthalmoplegic migraine in an infant. *Headache* 1987; 27:390–391.

52. Uitti RJ, Rajput AH: Multiple sclerosis presenting as isolated oculomotor nerve palsy. *Can J Neurol Sci* 1986; 13:270–272.

53. Hassin H: Ophthalmoplegic migraine wrongly attributed to measles immunization. *Am J Ophthalmol* 1988; 104:192–193.

54. Desai HB, MacFadyen DJ: Multiple sclerosis presenting as third nerve palsy. *Can J Neurol Sci* 1987; 14:178–179.

55. Piatt JH Jr, Campbell GA, Oakes WJ: Papillary meningioma involving the oculomotor nerve in an infant. *J Neurosurg* 1986; 64:808–812.

56. Yamada T, Nishio S, Matsunaga M, et al: Cavernous haemangioma in the oculomotor nerve: A case report. *J Neurol Sci* 1986; 233:63–64.

57. Burke RH, Adams JL: Immediate cranial nerve paralysis during removal of a mandibular third molar. *Oral Surg Oral Med Oral Pathol* 1987; 63:172–174.

58. Nazarian SM, Janati A, Angtuaco EJ, et al: Oculomotor palsy and papilledema with pial-dural arteriovenous malformation. *J Clin Neuro Ophthalmol* 1987; 7:98–103.

59. Sekizawa T, Nakamura S, Kogure K, et al: Idiopathic third cranial nerve palsy associated with herpes simplex virus infection. *Br Med J* 1987; 295:813.

60. Lamarca J, Casquero P, Pou A: Mononeuritis multiplex in Waldenström's macroglobulinemia. *Ann Neurol* 1987; 22:268–272.

61. Wykes WN: Prolactinoma presenting with intermittent third nerve palsy. *Br J Ophthalmol* 1986; 70:706–707.

62. Antworth MV, Beck RW: Third nerve palsy as a presenting sign of acquired immune deficiency syndrome. *J Clin Neuro-Ophthalmol* 1987; 7:125–128.

63. Metz HS: Think superior oblique palsy. *J Pediatr Ophthalmol Strabismus* 1986; 23:166–169.

64. Kraft SP, Scott WE: Masked bilateral superior oblique palsy: Clinical features and diagnosis. *J Pediatr Ophthalmol Strabismus* 1986; 23:264–272.

65. Price NC, Vickers S, Lee JP, et al: The diagnosis and surgical management of acquired bilateral superior oblique palsy. *Eye* 1987; 1:78–85.

66. Keane JR: Trochlear nerve pareses with brainstem lesions. *J Clin Neuro Ophthalmol* 1986; 6:242–256.

67. Yamamoto M, Jimbo M, Ide M, et al: Trochlear neurinoma. *Surg Neurol* 1987; 28:287–290.

68. Slavin ML: Isolated trochlear nerve palsy secondary to cavernous sinus meningioma. *Am J Ophthalmol* 1987; 104:433–434.

69. King RA, Calhoun JH: Fourth cranial nerve palsy following spinal anesthesia: A case report. *J Clin Neuro Ophthalmol* 1987; 7:20–22.

70. Gutman I, Levartovski S, Goldhammer Y, et al: Sixth nerve palsy and unilateral Horner's syndrome. *Ophthalmology* 1986; 93:913–916.

71. Hartmann B, Kremer I, Gutman I, et al: Cavernous sinus infection manifested by Horner's syndrome and ipsilateral sixth nerve palsy. *J Clin Neuro Ophthalmol* 1987; 7:223–226.

72. Striph GG, Burde RM: Abducens nerve palsy and Horner's syndrome revisited. *J Clin Neuro Ophthalmol* 1988; 8:13–17.

73. Peatfield RC: Recurrent VI nerve palsy in cluster headache. *Headache* 1985; 25:325–327.

74. Smith CD, Reeves AG: Amelioration of ophthalmoplegic migraine by prednisone: A case report. *Headache* 1986; 26:94–94.

75. Kandt RS: Can we reliably differentiate Tolosa-Hunt syndrome from ophthalmoplegic migraine? *Headache* 1986; 27:436–437.

76. Savino PJ: Diplopia and sixth nerve palsies. *Sem Neurol* 1986; 6:142–146.

77. Nabors MW, McCrary ME, Fischer BA, et al: Delayed abducens nerve palsies associated with cervical spine fractures. *Neurology* 1987; 37:1565.

78. Slavin ML, Abramson AL: Squamous cell carcinoma of the pterygopalatine fossa (retroantral space). *J Clin Neuro Ophthalmol* 1986; 6:254–257.

79. Handa J, Suzuki F, Nioka H, et al: Clivus chordoma in childhood. *Surg Neurol* 1987; 28:58–62.

80. Dunne JW, Stewart-Synne EG, Pullan PT: Abducent palsy after rapid shrinkage of a prolactinoma. *J Neurol Neurosurg Psychiatry* 1987; 50:496–498.

81. Sano H, Jain VK, Kato Y, et al: Bilateral giant intracavernous aneurysms: Technique of unilateral operation. *Surg Neurol* 1988; 29:35–38.

82. Kobayashi T, Negoro M, Awaya S: Cavernous sinus subarachnoid diverticulum and sixth nerve palsy. *Neuroradiology* 1987; 29:306–307.

83. Little KH, Lee EL, Frenkel EP: Cranial nerve deficits due to amyloidosis associated with plasma cell dyscrasia. *South Med J* 1986; 79:677–681.

84. Ventura GJ, Keating MJ, Castellano AM, et al: Reversible bilateral lateral rectus palsy associated with high-dose cytosine arabinoside and mitontrone therapy. *Cancer* 1986; 58:1633–1635.

85. Hayasaka S, Yamaguchi K, Mizuno K, et al: Ocular findings in childhood lactic acidosis. *Arch Ophthalmol* 1986; 104:1656–1658.

86. Case Records of the Massachusetts General Hospital (Case 34–1987). *N Engl J Med* 1987; 317:493–501.

87. Petty RKH, Hardin AE, Morgan-Hughes JA: The clinical features of mitochondrial myopathy. *Brain* 1986; 109:915–938.

88. Bresolin N, Moggio M, Bet L, et al: Progressive cytochrome c oxidase deficiency in a case of

Kearns-Sayre syndrome: Morphological, immunological, and biochemical studies in muscle biopsies and autopsy tissues. *Ann Neurol* 1987; 21:564–572.

89. Byrne E, Marzuki S, Sattayasai N, et al: Mitochondrial studies in Kearns-Sayre syndrome: Normal respiratory chain function with absence of a mitochondial translation product. *Neurology* 1987; 37:1530–1534.

90. Gittinger JW Jr: Nonmyasthenic ophthalmoplegia, in Lessell S, van Dalen JTW (eds): *Current Neuro-Ophthalmology,* vol 1. Chicago, Year Book Medical Publishers, Inc, 1988, pp 185–197.

91. Bastiaensen LAK: On the hereditary of mitochondrial cytopathies. *Neuro-Ophthalmol* 1987; 7:151–157.

92. Dewhurst AG, Hall D, Schwartz MS, et al: Kearns-Sayre syndrome, hypoparathyroidism, and basal ganglia calcification. *J Neurol Neurosurg Psychiatry* 1986; 1323–1324.

93. Wortsman J, Posillico JT, Brown EM, et al: Letter to the editor. *N Engl J Med* 1988; 318:857.

94. Nubiola A, Vendrell J, Gomis R, et al: Letter to the editor. *N Engl J Med* 1988; 318:857–858.

95. Gallastegui J, Hariman RJ, Handler B, et al: Cardiac involvement in the Kearns-Sayre syndrome. *Am J Cardiol* 1987; 60:385–388.

96. Lane CM, Collin JRO: Treatment of ptosis in chronic progressive external ophthalmoplegia. *Br J Ophthalmol* 1987; 71:290–294.

97. Holmstrom GE, Nyman KG: Primary orbital amyloidosis localized to an extraocular muscle. *Br J Ophthalmol* 1987; 71:32–33.

98. Olver J, Laidler P: Acquired Brown's syndrome in a patient with combined lichen sclerosus et atrophicus and morphoea. *Br J Ophthalmol* 1988; 72:552–557.

99. Baldwin L, Baker RS: Acquired Brown's syndrome in a patient with an orbital roof fracture. *J Clin Neuro Ophthalmol* 1988; 8:127–130.

100. Baker RS, Conklin JD Jr: Acquired Brown's syndrome from blunt orbital trauma. *J Pediatr Ophthalmol Strabismus* 1987; 24:17–21.

101. Gittinger JW Jr, Hughes JP, Suran EP: Medial orbital wall blow-out fracture producing an acquired retraction syndrome. *J Clin Neuro Ophthalmol* 1986; 6:153–156.

102. Wojno TH: The incidence of extraocular muscle and cranial nerve palsy in orbital floor blow-out fractures. *Ophthalmology* 1987; 94:682–687.

103. Magli A, Fusco R, Chiosi E, et al: Inheritance of Brown's syndrome. *Ophthalmologica* 1986; 192:82–87.

104. Moore AT, Walker J, Taylor D: Familial Brown's syndrome. *J Pediatr Ophthalmol Strabismus* 1988; 25:202–204.

105. Wortham EV, Crawford JS: Brown's syndrome in twins. *Am J Ophthalmol* 1988; 105:562–563.

106. Cruysberg JRM, Mitanda AT, Duinkerke-Eerola KU, et al: Bilateral Duane's retraction syndrome associated with congenital panhypopituitarism. *Neuro-Ophthalmol* 1986; 6:165–168.

107. Wagner RS, Caputo AR, Frohman LP: Congenital unilateral adduction deficit with simultaneous abduction: A variant of Duane's retraction syndrome. *Ophthalmology* 1987; 94:1049–1053.

108. Kommerell G, Bach M: A new type of Duane's syndrome: Twitch abduction of attempted upgaze and V-incomitance due to misinnervation of the lateral rectus by superior rectus neurons. *Neuro-Ophthalmol* 1986; 6:159–164.

109. Emre M, Henn V: Familial Duane syndrome with synkinetic jaw movements. *Neuro-Ophthalmol* 1987; 7:211–218.

110. Houtman WA, van Weerden TW, Robinson PH, et al: Hereditary congenital external ophthalmoplegia. *Ophthalmologica* 1986; 193:207–218.

111. Khawam E, Azar D, Shami M, et al: Progressive congenital familae ophthalmoplegia with optic nerve coloboma: Report of a family. *Binoc Vis* 1987; 2:223–231.

112. Kalpakian B, Bateman JB, Sparkes RS, et al: Congenital ocular fibrosis syndrome associated with the Prader-Willi syndrome. *J Pediatr Ophthalmol Strabismus* 1986; 23:170–173.

113. Mather TR, Saunders RA: Congenital absence of the superior rectus muscle: A case report. *J Pediatr Ophthalmol Strabismus* 1987; 24:291–295.

114. Cohen SR, Thompson JW: Variants of Möbius' syndrome and central neurologic impairment: Lindeman procedure in children. *Ann Otol Rhinol Laryngol* 1987; 96:93–100.

115. Kruis JA, Houtman WA, van Weerden TW: Congenital absence of conjugate horizontal eye movements. *Doc Ophthalmol* 1987; 67:13–18.

PART THREE

THE PUPIL

CHAPTER 12

The Pupil

H. Stanley Thompson, M.D.

Professor, Ophthalmology, Department of Ophthalmology, University of Iowa, Iowa City, Iowa

ANISOCORIA

It has been suggested more than once that, in dim light, about 20% of us have clinically visible anisocoria (0.4 mm or more) at any given moment, and this has again been confirmed.[1] But how constant is this anisocoria? Does the pupillary inequality come and go? What percentage of normal subjects might be expected to slip into an anisocoria of 0.4 mm or more if the whole group were watched carefully for several days? These questions have now been addressed by photographing 128 normal subjects, morning and afternoon, for 5 consecutive days,[1] and it seems that the subjects with anisocoria at any given moment (20%) are part of a larger group (40%) seen at least once over the 5 days to have an anisocoria of 0.4 mm or more. Only 3% of the subjects had a constant anisocoria of this size. It can be seen in Fig 1 that these percentages change dramatically with the definition of anisocoria, so that at "0.3 mm or more" most of us drift occasionally into anisocoria, and at "0.2 mm or more" it is hard to find anyone who does *not* have unequal pupils at one time or another. This suggests that the size of our pupils is not set with any more precision than is demanded by visual function—another example of "economy of construction. . . in the pupil apparatus."[2]

Curr Neuro Ophthalmol 2:213–220, 1989
© 1989, Year Book Medical Publishers, Inc.
0893–0147/89/02-213-220-$04.00

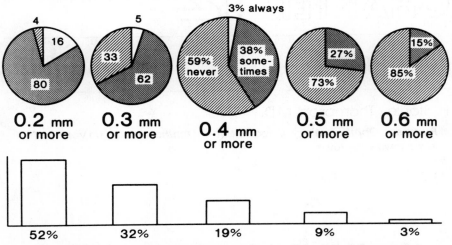

FIG 1.

Prevalence of simple anisocoria based on the data of Lam et al.,[1] showing the percentages of normal subjects with anisocoria at any given moment *(bar graph)* and at least once in a 5-day period for various degrees of anisocoria from 0.2 to 0.6 mm *(pie charts)*.

RELATIVE AFFERENT PUPILLARY DEFECTS

Cox[3] has suggested that a bright direct ophthalmoscope can be used to check a small child for a relative afferent pupillary defect (RAPD). He steps back to about a meter away and just lets the child accommodate on the light as it switches from one eye to the other. I have tried this and it works very well. The pupils seem very small at that distance, but they can still be seen because of the red reflex. A neutral density filter can be held in the light path to one eye without inducing switches in accommodation.

It was suggested[4] that quantitation of the RAPD with neutral density filters can be affected by the intensity of the light stimulus used, a brighter stimulus producing a greater asymmetry. This brought out one response[5] suggesting that, within the range of brightness commonly used, the stimulus intensity did not affect the measurement of the RAPD to a clinically significant degree, and a further reaction[6] that there were situations in which a relatively dim stimulus showed a greater asymmetry of pupillomotor input than a bright stimulus. If, when doing the alternating light test, the pupils seem to be so immobile that the thought crosses your mind that they just might be painted on the iris, then consider the possibility that your light may be too bright. Just turning down the stimulus intensity sometimes improves pupillary mobility, and this may bring a clean end point within your grasp.

The generally positive correlation between the size of the RAPD and the asymmetry of the visual field loss was confirmed in two studies. Using Octopus automated static perimetry,[7] it was seen that patients with an RAPD had much more asymmetry of the visual fields than patients without an RAPD. When measured with filters, the RAPD correlated well with the difference in field loss, but not so well with the difference in the cup-disk ratio between the two eyes. Another group[8] used the Humphrey automated perimeter, added up the sensitivity at each location in each eye, and also found that the difference in total sensitivity between the two eyes (that is, the relative field loss) was proportional to the measured RAPD. Estimating the difference in mean sensitivity, in decibels, has since been made much easier by Humphrey's Statpac software.

The RAPD was measured in 38 patients with retinal detachment.[9] There was a clear, but not very precise, correlation between the pupillary input asymmetry and the extent of the detachment. Each "macula-on" quadrant detached produced approximately 0.35 log units of RAPD, and when the macula came off, the RAPD jumped up by 0.7 log units. The preoperative RAPD averaged 1.4 log units (± 0.7 log), and after successful surgery the mean RAPD was 0.4 log (± 0.3 log).

Another case has been reported[10] of a patient with no visual field loss who had an RAPD contralateral to an area of pretectal damage The assumption in these cases is that the patient has a homonymous pupillary field loss and that, as in a tract lesion, there is a greater defect in the contralateral eye.

Stimulated by a challenge from Landau,[11] Thompson and Corbett[12] reviewed the advantages of the alternating light test, gave a detailed account of how to measure the RAPD with filters, and summarized the clinical value of the test.

PUPIL CONSTRICTION TO DARKNESS

Cox[3] also suggests using a direct ophthalmoscope to look for a paradoxical constriction to darkness. He keeps the ophthalmoscope light just off the visual axis and at less-than-full brightness while he watches the red reflex of the pupils; then an assistant holds the child's attention in the distance while the room lights are turned on and off. Pediatric ophthalmologists have the child look at a cartoon movie in the distance while the room lights are suddenly dimmed.[13] There is no doubt that this odd pupillary constriction can be seen clinically without special equipment; Frank, et al.[13] have described 29 patients who show the phenomenon. They are a strangely mixed group and do not all have retinal disease. Twenty-five of the 29 patients had some abnormality of the optic nerve or retina or had nystagmus, but, interestingly, the other four patients had nothing but amblyopia or a motility problem. I have no doubt that some unifying theory that will explain why the phenomenon can be seen in all these different conditions is just around the corner.

HORNER'S SYNDROME

This year, as in every other year, the vulnerability of the oculosympathetic pathway has been repeatedly rediscovered. For example, after epidural lumbar block, the local anesthetic can find its way up to at least T-1[14, 15]; it can even get across to the other side.[16] Chest tubes that reach to the pulmonary apex likely to damage the sympathetic path, so as a matter of policy they should not go any higher than the third posterior rib.[17] In a series of 1,585 medial sternotomies for heart surgery,[18] 1.39% had some surgical damage to the lower brachial plexus, and about half of these (0.76% of the total) developed a Horner's syndrome on the same side. Placing a line in the jugular vein[19] brings the needle close to the oculosympathetic pathway. A neurofibroma[20] can develop in the cervical sympathetic chain, or a benign goiter,[21] a malignant neoplasm,[22] a giant cell inflammation,[23] or a hematoma after chiropractic manipulation[24] can all press on the carotid sheath to produce a Horner's syndrome. A 13-year-old girl inadvertently swallowed a sewing needle with her food and the needle penetrated the pharyngeal wall. Two months later she sought medical attention for a ptosis, and the needle was seen on roentgenography alongside her left carotid artery. Three months after surgical removal of the needle, the Horner's syndrome had almost disappeared.[25]

A 55-year-old woman with a congenital Horner's syndrome[26] found that she was able to lift her ptotic left lid for 20 to 30 seconds by coughing. A vigorous Valsalva maneuver would not do it. If she had a really severe bout of coughing, the anisocoria would also disappear. She was, however, not able to influence her iris heterochromia. It is interesting to speculate on how this might have happened: (1) the coughing might have irritated the remaining fibers in the left oculosympathetic pathway, lifting the lid and dilating the pupil, (2) the coughing might have produced a transient Horner's syndrome on the other side, balancing up the two eyes, or (3) the coughing might have produced a sufficient rise in blood catecholamine levels to affect the supersensitive, sympathetically denervated Müller muscle in the left lid and eventually the dilator muscle in the iris.

Parkinson[27] has been emphasizing that a postganglionic Horner's syndrome, when combined with a lateral rectus palsy, suggests trouble in the cavernous sinus. A clear case of cavernous sinus infection[28] can now be added to the six other cases that have appeared in the literature in the last decade in response to Parkinson's challenge.[29] After dissecting a cavernous sinus for myself, I am inclined to go along with Parkinson's assessment[27] that the oculosympathetic fibers leave the carotid artery at the level of the gasserian ganglion and rise to flirt briefly with the abducens nerve before clinging to the ophthalmic nerve and going off into the orbit. But do the sympathetic branches to the eyelids follow the nerves or do they follow the vessels to the periphery?

Ten children with Horner's syndrome were studied in Toronto.[30] Two of them had neuroblastoma, and the authors recommended that screening tests for this treatable tumor be done in any child whose Horner's syndrome was not obviously the result of thoracic surgery.

A patient, injured or not, who gets a new postganglionic Horner's syndrome associated with unusual pains in face, head, or neck may have a carotid artery dissection. Kline et al.[31] have done a careful review of this entity for the ophthalmologist. The hazard to the patient is clot formation in the narrowed lumen of the carotid artery. Some of these dissections have probably been reported in the past as Raeder's syndrome.[32] The term *Raeder's syndrome,* if it is to be used at all, should probably be limited to those cases with an undoubted middle-fossa lesion and clear trigeminal nerve dysfunction. It would, of course, be possible for a carotid dissection to extend up to the siphon and, once there, it might conceivably damage the ophthalmic nerve, producing both a postganglionic Horner's and fifth-nerve dysfunction. This I would call a true Raeder's syndrome due to a dissection, but I suspect that most dissections damage the carotid plexus (or the "carotid sympathetic nerve" as Parkinson likes to call it) along the extracranial internal carotid artery. Any fresh postganglionic Horner's in this location would produce vasomotor changes in the forehead that stop at the midline. This might easily be misinterpreted as involvement of the fifth nerve. Thermography of the face can be helpful in localizing the lesion in Horner's syndrome.[33]

In 1983, Coppeto[34] described two patients who appeared to have a lesion at the pontomesencephalic junction who presented with a superior oblique palsy and a contralateral Horner's syndrome; two more such cases have been reported.[35] It seems there is a point low in the dorsal midbrain where the descending oculosympathetic fibers are close to the fasicles of the contralateral fourth nerve.

Carotid arteriosclerosis may contribute to a postganglionic Horner's syndrome.[36] Further confirmation is offered[37] that "enophthalmos" should be struck from the list of the features of Horner's syndrome. Van der Wiel and Van Gijn[38] studied cocaine mydriasis in patients with Horner's syndrome and noted that the affected pupil did not dilate any more in central Horner's than in preganglionic Horner's, confirming the impression that cocaine mydriasis is not a good localizing test in Horner's syndrome.

THIRD-NERVE PALSY

An interesting case was reported by Lustbader and Miller.[39] A 65-year-old hypertensive woman had a pupil-sparing oculomotor palsy with all the appropriate extraocular muscles completely paralyzed. Two months after the onset of symptoms, there was no sign of recovery, and an angiogram was done that showed a potentially treatable interpeduncular basilar aneurysm. Since this case proved to be an exception to so many well-established rules, the authors wondered whether they should be doing a CT scan on every third-nerve palsy that comes in, pupil-sparing or not, and just set aside that old clinical rule: "Pupil spared, wait and watch; pupil involved, angiogram." Trobe's reaction[40] to this case was to say that a good clinical rule should not be abandoned just because you occasionally stub your toe on an exception. He suggested that the rule should be qualified by limiting its applicability to isolated oculomotor-nerve palsies in patients over 50 who have complete extraocular muscle involvement and complete pupil sparing.

A careful study from the New England Medical Center in Boston[41] analyzed a series of third-nerve palsies and came to similar conclusions: when the extraocular muscle palsy is complete and the pupil sparing is also complete, or almost complete, you may safely assume that the third-nerve palsy is due to microvascular disease.

REFERENCES

1. Lam BL, Thompson HS, Corbett JJ: The prevalence of simple anisocoria. *Am J Ophthalmol* 1987; 104:69–73.

2. Stark L, Campbell FW, Atwood J: Pupil unrest: An example of noise in a biological servomechanism. *Nature* 1958; 182:857.

3. Cox TA: Pupillary testing using the direct ophthalmoscope. *Am J Ophthalmol* 1988; 105:427–428.

4. Browning DJ, Tiedeman JS: The test light affects quantitation of the afferent pupillary defect. *Ophthalmology* 1987; 94:53–55.

5. Thompson HS, Jiang MQ: Letter to the editor. *Ophthalmology* 1987; 94:1360–1362.

6. Borchert M, Sadun AA: Bright light stimuli may mask relative afferent pupillary defects. *Am J Ophthalmol* 1988; 106:98–99.

7. Brown RH, Zillis JD, Lynch MG, et al: The afferent pupillary defect in asymmetric glaucoma. *Arch Ophthalmol* 1988; 105:1540–1543.

8. Johnson LN, Hill RA, Bartholomew MJ: Correlation of afferent pupillary defect with visual field loss on automated perimetry. *Ophthalmology* 1988; 95:1649–1655.

9. Folk JC, Thompson HS, Farmer SG, et al: Relative afferent pupillary defect in eyes with retinal detachment. *Ophthalmic Surg* 1987; 18:757–759.

10. Johnson RE, Bell RA: Relative afferent pupillary defect in a lesion of the pretectal afferent pupillary pathway. *Can J Ophthalmol* 1987; 22:282–284.

11. Landau WM: Clinical neuromythology: I. The Marcus Gunn phenomenon: Loose canon of neuro-ophthalmology. *Neurology* 1988; 38:1141–1142.

12. Thompson HS, Corbett JJ: Letter to the editor. *Neurology* 1989; 39:154–156.

13. Frank JW, Kushner BJ, France TD: Paradoxical pupillary phenomena: A review of patients with pupillary constriction to darkness. *Arch Ophthalmol* 1988; 106:1564–1566.

14. Wills MH, Korbon GA, Arasi R: Horner's syndrome resulting from a lumbar sympathetic block. *Anesthesiology* 1988; 68:613–614.

15. McDonald NJ, Stritch M, MacEvilly M: Extradural bupivacaine: A neurological complication. *Irish J Med Sci* 1987; 156:288–289.

16. Schnapp M, Mays KS: Contralateral spread of local anaesthetic solutions. *Can Anaesth Soc J* 1986; 33:828–829.

17. Bertino RE, Wesbey GE, Johnson RJ: Horner syndrome occurring as a complication of chest tube placement. *Radiology* 1987; 164:745.

18. Benecke R, Klingelhöfer J, Rieke H, et al: Manifestationsform und Verlauf von Plexusläsionen nach medianer Sternotomie. *Nervenarzt* 1988; 59:388–392.

19. Prenzel E, Prenzel R, Ketscher KD: Horner-Syndrom nach perkutaner Punktion der Vena jugularis interna: Ein kasuistischer Beitrag. *Anesthesiol Reanimat* 1986; 11:365–367.

20. Ruckley RW, Blair RL: Neurofibroma of the cervical sympathetic chain presenting with Horner's syndrome. *J Laryngol Otol* 1986; 100:1433–1436.

21. Lowrey SR, Shinton RA, Jamieson G, et al: Benign multinodular goitre and reversible Horner's syndrome. *Br J Ophthalmol* 1988; 296:529–530.

22. Savoury LW, Heeneman H: Horner's syndrome: Teaching rounds at Victoria Hospital, University of Western Ontario. *J Otolaryngol* 1988; 17:145–149.

23. Bromfield EB, Slakter JS: Horner's syndrome in temporal arteritis, letter to editor. *Arch Neurol* 1988; 45:604.

24. Grayson MF: Horner's syndrome after manipulation of the neck. *Br J Ophthalmol* 1987; 295:1381–1382.

25. Bazak I, Miller A, Uri N: Oculosympathetic paresis caused by foreign body perforation of pharyngeal wall. *Postgrad Med J* 1987; 63:681–683.

26. Hatt M: Horner-Syndrom, durch Husten reversibel. *Klin Monatsbl Augenheilkd* 1988; 192:143–144.

27. Parkinson D: Further observations on the sympathetic pathways to the pupil. *Anat Rec* 1988; 220:108–109.

28. Hartmann B, Kremer I, Gutman I, et al: Cavernous sinus infection manifested by Horner's syndrome and ipsilateral sixth nerve palsy. *J Clin Neuro Ophthalmol* 1987; 7:223–226.

29. Thompson HS: The pupil and accommodation, in Lessell S, Van Dalen JTW (eds): *Neuro-ophthalmology,* vol 1. Amsterdam, Excerpta Medica, 1980, p 236.

30. Woodruff G, Buncic JR, Morin JD: Horner's syndrome in children. *J Pediatr Ophthalmol Strabismus* 1988; 25:40–44.

31. Kline LB, Vitek JJ, Raymon BC: Painful Horner's syndrome due to spontaneous carotid artery dissection. *Ophthalmology* 1987; 94:226–230.

32. Brandel JP, Chapon F, Viader F, et al: Syndrome de Raeder dû à une dissection carotidienne. *Presse Med* 1987; 16:541.

33. Harada T: Congenital Horner's syndrome in otolaryngologic practice. *Auris Nasus Larynx* 1986; 13:91–95.

34. Coppetto JR: Superior oblique paresis and contralateral Horner's syndrome. *Ann Ophthalmol* 1983; 15:681–683.

35. Guy J, Day AL, Mickle JP, et al: Contralateral trochlear nerve paresis and ipsilateral Horner's syndrome. *Am J Ophthalmol* 1988; 107:73–76.

36. Monteiro MLR, Coppeto JR: Horner's syndrome associated with carotid artery atherosclerosis. *Am J Ophthalmol* 1988; 105:93–94.

37. Van der Wiel HL, Van Gijn J: No enophthalmos in Horner's syndrome. *J Neurol Neurosurg Psychiatry* 1987; 50:498–499.

38. Van der Wiel HL, Van Gijn J: Diagnosis of Horner's syndrome: Use and limitations of the cocaine test. *J Neurol Sci* 1986; 73:311–316.

39. Lustbader JM, Miller NR: Painless, pupil-sparing but otherwise complete oculomotor paresis caused by basilar artery aneurysm. *Arch Ophthalmol* 1988; 106:583–584.

40. Trobe J: Third nerve palsy and the pupil: Footnotes to the rule. *Arch Ophthalmol* 1988; 106:601–602.

41. Kwan ESK, Laucella M, Hedges TR III, et al: A cliniconeuroradiologic approach to third cranial nerve palsies. *Am J Neuroradiol* 1987; 8:459–468.

THE RETINA

PART FOUR

THE RETINA

CHAPTER 13

The Retina

Joseph Rizzo, M.D.

Massachusetts Eye and Ear Infirmary, Department of Ophthalmology, Harvard Medical School, Boston, Massachusetts

Basic scientific research continues to have an impact on clinical neuro-ophthalmology. I have included a basic science section in this chapter that presents information that is, or may be, clinically relevant. For practical reasons, certain generalizations were necessary. References are provided that will permit the interested reader to pursue topics in greater detail. Clinically, an emphasis was placed on retinal vascular disease (amaurosis fugax in particular) because of the ongoing controversy regarding the appropriateness of surgical intervention for carotid artery disease.

GANGLION CELLS

Recent advances in retinal anatomy are revealing spectacular intricacies.[1, 2] For the neuro-ophthalmologist, this knowledge permits a greater sophistication in the understanding of afferent visual disease. I will detail several basic science findings that I believe may have a clinical impact.

The characterization of ganglion cell subtypes has been especially important. Researchers have been able to recognize and define "populations" of ganglion cells by employing methods such as immunohistochemistry, in vivo neurotransmitter labeling, and single-cell injection.[1, 3] Traditional cell staining methods (i.e., Nissl, Golgi) produce either nonspecific or erratic labeling. However, the

Curr Neuro Ophthalmol 2:223–240, 1989

newer methods selectively stain families of cells, frequently portraying the family traits in exquisite detail. These cell families may share a common neurotransmitter, express a common antigen, or have a common feature that is not understood.[4]

Depending on the species, there may be as many as 20 or more subpopulations of ganglion cells.[5] In the primate the number may be half that.[6, 7] From a clinical perspective, the most relevant studies may be of the primate ganglion cells that project to the geniculocortical pathway, the parvocellular (P) and magnocellular (M) cells. The P cells are color-opponent, have small receptive fields and low contrast sensitivity, and include the midget cells that are presumed to be important for central visual acuity. The M cells are spectrally broad-band and have larger receptive fields and high contrast sensitivity. There are claims that M cells are rare in the central retina.[8, 9]

The cellular dichotomy just described is clinically relevant. For instance, the frequent coexistence of central acuity loss and dyschromatopsia in acquired optic neuropathy is assumed to reflect a disruption of the ganglion cells in central retina. Also, contrast sensitivity testing is used to physiologically "isolate" the M-cell pathway. Indeed, there is a body of literature that attests to this approach, as well as to other more sophisticated paradigms. The most convincing reports are for patients with glaucoma,[10, 11] but data for patients with optic neuritis,[12, 13] pseudotumor cerebri,[14-16] compressive lesions of the anterior visual pathway,[17] and Alzheimer's disease[18, 19] reflect a similar theme. The rationale for the use of contrast sensitivity in this way has good basic science support, but it should be recognized that this psychophysical "isolation" is not absolute—the responses probably reflect a preponderance of one pathway over the other. Two critical reviews of contrast sensitivity testing methods are available.[20, 21]

Information obtained from research on monkeys is thought to be particularly valuable because of the remarkable similarity of the monkey to the human.[22, 23] Although it is tempting to extrapolate from the basic science literature to human disease states, one must be cautious, as many studies demonstrate significant cross-species differences.[24]

For example, the most well-characterized ganglion cells in the cat are the X and Y cells. The X cells are linear for spatial summation, exhibit sustained responses, and are thought to be specialized for the transmission of spatial information. The second type of ganglion cell, the Y cell, is nonlinear for spatial summation, exhibits transient response characteristics, and is thought to be specialized for the transmission of motion information.[25] The other ganglion cell types have not been as well studied, and many have more elaborate response characteristics.

It has been assumed that the X cell of the cat is analogous to the P cell of the monkey, and likewise the Y cell to the M cell of the monkey.[26] However, both cat ganglion cell types are highly sensitive to contrast, whereas the monkey's P cell is relatively insensitive to contrast.[24-27] Further, a majority of the M cells are known to have linear response characteristics, a feature previously held to be X-like.[28, 29] These important distinctions exemplify the risk in extending data from one species to another.

RETINAL ANATOMY AND NEUROTRANSMITTERS

The recognition of the diversity of amacrine cells has caused a restructuring of traditional teaching on retinal anatomy, and the influential role of these cells is becoming increasingly apparent. Although diseases resulting from amacrine cell pathology have not been recognized, there is good reason to speculate on their existence. I will outline some features of amacrine cells that may be clinically relevant.

The time-honored concept of a three-neuron pathway from the retina to visual cortex (and its analogy to other primary sensory systems) has been disproved, at least for the rod pathway. One of the most numerous amacrine cells is the A_2 cell. This cell is a link within the rod pathway and is positioned between the rod bipolar and ganglion cells.[30] These cells probably have a significant impact on retinal functioning since over 95% of human photoreceptors are rods. Further, the A_2 cell has an electrical synapse on cone bipolar cells and also forms synapses with the sparsely populated dopaminergic amacrine cells and indoleamine-accumulating amacrine cells.[31] Dopamine is thought to be a "neuromodulator" in the retina[32] and, in consort with the A_2, is apparently capable of gaiting rod signal transmission. An interesting example of a specific defect in rod transmission is included in the section on paraneoplastic syndromes.

Perhaps the most extensively studied amacrine cell in the vertebrate retina is the cholinergic amacrine cell.[33] This cell, together with the γ-aminobutyric acid (GABA) amacrine cell,[34] is essential for the functioning of some of the motion-detecting ganglion cells of the rabbit retina.[35] The motion-detecting pathway has also been studied at higher levels, including the visual association cortices.[36, 37] Psychophysical experiments in primates are able to distinguish this pathway from other "parallel" visual pathways (i.e., form, color).[38, 39] Humans with parieto-occipital lesions demonstrate specific abnormalities of motion detection.[40] Retinal diseases that selectively disrupt motion detection have not been recognized. Although it is speculative to suppose the presence of such diseases, experiments in rabbits have demonstrated that motion detection can be selectively abolished at the retinal level.[41, 42]

A RETINAL EXPLANATION FOR MACULAR SPARING?

A retinal explanation for "macular sparing" was reported over 10 years ago.[43] A recent study demonstrates similar findings, but some of the conclusions may be unjustified.[44] In this latter study, injection of a tracer into the lateral geniculate nucleus of the monkey labeled cells in both retinae, but in the ipsilateral eye the labeling was present on both sides of the macula. On this basis, the authors suggest that macula sparing may be seen unilaterally, which is not consistent with clinical experience.

Although the results seem to suggest that both sides of the macula project ipsilaterally, the staining pattern can be interpreted otherwise. Ganglion cells within the primate macula are displaced laterally relative to the photoreceptors that drive them. Resultingly, cells located on the nasal side of the fovea may actually be connected to photoreceptors on the temporal side.[45] This arrangement could explain the staining pattern that was obtained. For these reasons, this study should probably not be accepted as a mechanism for macular sparing.

RETINAL TRANSPLANTATION AND OPTIC NERVE REGENERATION

Newsstand headlines recently sensationalized a report of a successful transplantation of a monkey head to a human (*World Weekly News*, Oct. 18, 1988). Indeed, neural transplanation, once assumed to be fictional, is a subject of intense basic science and clinical investigation.[46, 47] Although neural transplantation seems to be avant garde, we are in fact approaching the centennial of the first "successful" brain transplant.[48]

Retinal cells will survive and differentiate after transplantation[49–51] and even display physiological responses.[52] Although these reports are intriguing, the disorganized state of the transplants is problematic. The tissue is typically injected into the subretinal space and becomes disfigured in the process. Preservation of anatomic integrity would seem to be a prerequisite for a normally functioning retina.

Despite being in its infancy, the field of neural transplantation is producing astonishing results, almost surreal. A French team was able to modify the behavior of a chick by transplanting part of the brain of a quail; the chick then crowed in a fashion typical of the quail![53]

The field of neural regeneration is beginning to show signs of new life. The dogma that central nervous system axons cannot regenerate has been disproved, at least for the rat visual system. Villegas-Perez and colleagues[54] demonstrated regeneration of up to 20% of retinal ganglion cell axons by grafting sciatic nerve to the transected end of the optic nerve. One aspect is sobering: many of the regenerated axons wither with time.

Success in both regeneration and transplantation strategies would be necessary to restore vision to patients with disease of the afferent visual pathway. Unfortunately, this is not likely to be realized in the near future.

Regeneration of another primary afferent sensory neuron, the acoustic hair cells of adult birds, has also been reported.[55, 56]

RETINAL VASCULAR DISEASE

Amaurosis Fugax

Amaurosis fugax (AF) represents the most common manifestation of carotid artery disease that is referred to neuro-ophthalmologists. Patients with AF are of significant concern because of the implications for stroke, blindness, and death. The approach to the management of this problem is in a state of change.

The enthusiastic, at times impetuous, support for carotid endarterectomy has faded. Several recent publications have questioned the wisdom of this procedure at a time when its widespread use has resulted in it being the third most frequently performed operation in the United States.[57-60] Judging the appropriateness of carotid surgery is not straightforward, and the existing literature is not decisive in this regard.[61-63] One study suggested that carotid endarterectomy was performed for equivocal or "inappropriate" reasons in 64% of cases.[60]

To date, there are no prospective, randomized, controlled studies of the natural history of the atherosclerotic form of AF. Most studies of carotid vascular disease are concerned with cerebral events, and there is a suggestion that AF is associated with different risks than a first attack of ischemia involving the brain.[64-66] A prospective study by Hurwitz et al.[65] showed the risk of stroke following amaurosis to be about half that for patients experiencing a cerebral transient ischemic attack (TIA). A strength of this study is the use of arteriography in 90 of 93 patients with AF, but the study was not randomized and the mean follow-up was less than 5 years. This study may underestimate the risk of stroke for patients with atherosclerotic transient monocular blindness (TMB) because approximately 20% of the patients with AF did not have "significant" carotid disease, and surgery was performed on 52 of 59 patients. If surgery is beneficial, this would further reduce the apparent risk of stroke. Nonetheless, the risk of stroke for the *untreated* patients with AF is similar to that reported in another study, approximately 2% per year, although this latter study itself is open to question since it was retrospective and less than 25% of the patients underwent arteriography.[66]

Wray[67] has emphasized the heterogeneity of the AF patient population. The tendency to pool patients with AF weakens the conclusions of many reports. In some cases the demographic profile is insufficient and does not permit the reader to judge the adequacy of the study.[68] Low-risk patients with AF (e.g., migraine-related) are usually considered together with the high-risk atherosclerotic patients.[69-71] For instance, 13% of patients in a study by Poole and Ross Russell[70, 72] were under the age of 45; those with repeated attacks of AF underwent arteriography (64/110), and 60% of the results were normal. Poole et al.[73] performed cerebral angiography on patients with AF who were under the age of 40 years and found that 16 of 16 were normal, showing the bias that may affect studies that include younger patients. Clinical symptoms alone (i.e., duration of visual loss) do not dependably segregate the atherosclerotic patients. Five of 37 patients with AF and angiographically documented carotid artery disease experienced amaurosis longer than 15 minutes.[74]

High-risk AF patients with atherosclerosis were presumably selected out by Howard and Ross Russell.[75] Patients with visual loss who were observed to have retinal emboli had increased risks for stroke and early mortality when compared with reasonably well-matched controls. The 2.9% annual rate of stroke in this population is higher than the 1.8% annual rate found in the unsegregated population of patients with AF studied at the same hospital[70] and the 1.9% annual rate of the Hurwitz group[65] (calculations exclude strokes that occurred during the initial hospitalization). Poole and Ross Russell[70, 72] report a correlation between the degree of carotid stenosis and the subsequent risk of stroke in the AF population: the stroke rate increased from 2% (four times expected) to 5% per year if carotid stenosis or occlusion was present. The association between the risk of stroke and the degree of carotid stenosis is controversial.[57, 76, 77] As such, the annual rate of stroke for patients with AF with known atherosclerosis is slightly less than the 5% to 7% annual rate of stroke that follows a cerebral TIA.[64, 78]

Two other important risks for the AF population must be addressed: permanent visual loss and death. The risk of permanent visual loss following an episode of AF is estimated at 1% per year by Poole and Ross Russell,[70] although this figure includes some patients with retinal vein thrombosis as the cause of visual loss. This rate is similar to the 1.1% and 1.2% annual figures that can be derived from earlier publications.[66, 69] Patients who experience AF have reduced life expectancies. An annual mortality of 3.5% has been reported, which is 1.4 times the expected rate.[70] Ischemic cardiac disease was the leading cause of death. Patients with visual loss who had retinal emboli have an annual mortality of 5.2%, approximately twice the expected rate.[75]

The mechanisms underlying AF and cerebrovascular disease are complex, and any single theory is insufficient to explain the range of disease.[79] Older patients with AF have a high prevalence of atheromatous disease in the ipsilateral carotid artery[65, 71, 80–82] in comparison with an age-matched control population.[82] Nonstenotic ulceration of the carotid artery is also commonly found in patients with AF[80, 81] and is associated with an increased risk of hemispheric stroke. Risk of stroke may also be related to the degree of carotid artery ulceration.[83] Hemorrhage within carotid plaque is thought to play an important role in the initiation of neurologic symptoms.[84] Intracranial arterial occlusive disease is another etiologic consideration for AF,[85] an issue that is seldom addressed carefully. Reduced ophthalmic artery flow from internal carotid artery stenosis may be a factor in some cases.[86] Monocular visual loss coincident with cerebral infarction may be caused by optic nerve and not retinal infarction.[87] Proposed forms of treatment should take into account the multiple facets of this problem.

Angiography remains the "gold standard" for detection of carotid atherosclerotic disease, providing reliable anatomical correlation with a very high interobserver agreement rate.[88] A good review of angiographic findings in patients with AF is provided by Harrison.[82] Detection of carotid ulcers by angiography has a high false-negative rate.[89] Carotid ulcers can be detected noninvasively by combining

Doppler examination and high-resolution B-mode scanning, but the degree of accuracy is not yet sufficient for clinical purposes.[90]

Therapy

The wisdom of local repair (i.e., carotid endarterectomy) has been questioned by the recognition that most patients with carotid artery disease succumb to heart disease within 5 years.[57, 58, 70, 75] Since restoration of carotid flow has not been shown to improve a persistent neurologic deficit, carotid endarterectomy is a prophylactic operation.[64] Whatever long-term benefits may be obtained from carotid surgery must be weighed against the complications associated with the procedure.

The combined morbidity and mortality of carotid endarterectomy ranges from 2.5% to 25%.[57, 64, 91, 92] The tendency for more favorable data to be reported undoubtedly creates a bias.[93] Retrospective studies may be especially prone to underestimating complications. For instance, two neurologists performed a page-by-page chart review of patients who underwent carotid endarterectomy and discovered that a significant proportion of strokes was not listed in the discharge diagnosis.[94]

Therapeutic considerations for patients with carotid artery disease have been addressed repeatedly.[57–59, 61, 62, 95, 96] There are insufficient data to permit a definitive statement regarding treatment of AF and carotid artery disease in general; however, guidelines have been provided. Trobe[57] suggests that carotid endarterectomy be considered for patients with AF only if the surgical complication rate is 2% or less, assuming high risk factors for surgical complications are not present. Regarding cerebral TIAs, a complication rate of 3% or less is recommended, the higher figure apparently justified by the slightly higher risk of stroke for these patients (see previous section).[57, 96] A surgical complication rate of less than 1% would probably result in a 50% reduction in stroke at 5 years for patients who have had a cerebral TIA.[59] The consensus statement of the AF study group unfortunately provides only general guidelines regarding surgical intervention.[95]

From a medical standpoint, the Antiplatelet Trialists' Collaboration[97] (an analysis of 29,000 patients) describes a beneficial effect of aspirin in reducing vascular morbidity and mortality. The judicious use of aspirin is recommended. Scheinberg[61] has written an excellent review of this subject and tentatively concurs with the use of aspirin in low-risk patients. It is prudent to have all patients with the atherosclerotic form of TMB evaluated by an internist,[98] as well as young women with TMB because of the high incidence of mitral valve prolapse.

Other Retinal Vascular Diseases

Multiple Retinal Vascular Occlusive Disease

"Apparently healthy" persons may experience recurrent, multiple retinal arterial occlusions.[99] Risk factors were common among the nine patients with this "idiopathic" syndrome: one used intravenous cocaine, one had mitral valve prolapse, three patients had elevated serum lipids, and two had a history of migraine headaches. Focal retinal arteritis is suspected as an etiology. These patients retained good visual acuity despite multifocal retinal infarctions. One patient with this entity whom I have followed up also abused cocaine, and, interestingly, cocaine has been associated with central retinal artery occlusion and cerebral vasculitis.[100–102] Steroids were not of obvious benefit for these patients, and two of three patients who received anticoagulant therapy developed a serious complication (i.e., intracerebral hemorrhage, scrotal hemorrhage requiring orchiectomy). Three patients had auditory symptoms, which was a frequent finding among patients reported to have a similar syndrome of arterial occlusive retinopathy and encephalopathy.[103, 104] In this latter syndrome, the patients appeared to be steroid responsive.

A new hereditary syndrome, "cerebroretinal vasculopathy," has ben recognized in three generations of a single pedigree as well as in two other, unrelated patients.[105] This syndrome, apparently inherited in an autosomal dominant manner, includes perifoveal and peripheral capillary obliteration, with formation of microaneurysms, and central nervous system "pseudotumor." Patients experienced a reduction in central acuity, headache, loss of cognitive function, and seizures. The neuropathological findings, which are allegedly unique, are largely confined to the white matter of frontoparietal regions. Considering the markedly abnormal computed tomographic findings in these patients, I would hesitate to use the term *pseudotumor*.

"Acute, multifocal hemorrhagic retinal vasculitis" may be a distinct entity that can result in recurrent episodes of visual loss.[106]

Paraneoplastic Photoreceptor Degeneration

Paraneoplastic degeneration of photoreceptors was originally described in 1976 by Sawyer et al.,[107] and several recent reports elaborated on this interesting syndrome.[107–116] Loss of vision may be subacute or chronic, may be associated with positive visual phenomena, and not uncommonly occurred before the discovery of a neoplasm. Tumors of the lung (usually small cell), adenocarcinoma of the breast, undifferentiated cervical carcinoma, and malignant melanoma have been associated with a visual paraneoplastic syndrome. Loss of vision is thought to occur from the production of an antibody by a tumor or in response to a tumor.

This syndrome is rare, and only two groups of investigators have reported immunological data on their patients. Keltner et al.[108, 109] described a "total absence of photoreceptors and outer nuclear layers" and the presence of an antibody in the serum of an affected patient that stained the outer retinal layers. Electroretinograms were extinguished in all patients tested, which is consistent with the location of the pathology.

Kornguth et al.[110–113] described patients with neurofilament antibodies directed against ganglion cells, especially larger ganglion cells. Although interesting, I believe that additional evidence in support of their conclusions is needed for the following reasons. Their first patient had an abnormal electroretinogram with apparently no photoreceptor-generated waveforms (the waves are not presented), yet the abnormal retinal staining was concentrated in the ganglion cell layer.[110] Second, at least one of the immunohistochemical controls was inadequate. The controls should, among other things, eliminate the possibility that the observed staining pattern is related to nonspecific staining of the secondary antibody; the substitution of a mouse for the human secondary antibody does not accomplish this.[113] Further, in support of the hypothesis that the antibody is specific to the visual system, it would be useful to have evidence of negative immunohistochemical staining in other areas of the central nervous system, especially since positive Western blot staining is reported elsewhere.[112] Last, selective involvement of larger ganglion cells would not be expected to result in an early loss of central acuity, as occurred in their patients (see Ganglion Cells at the beginning of this chapter.)

Despite these unresolved issues, their results are interesting. It is certainly possible that the visual paraneoplastic syndrome may result from retinal lesions at various locations. In support of this is the description by Berson and Lessell[114] of a patient who developed night blindness secondary to a malignant melanoma. The electroretinogram was interpreted as showing a selective interruption of intraretinal rod signal transmission. To my knowledge, congenital stationary night blindness and Oguchi's disease are the only other retinal diseases in which the pathology is thought to involve sites other than the ganglion cells or photoreceptor cells.

A number of patients with cancer-associated retinopathy seem to be steroid responsive.[108, 116]

Leber's Hereditary Optic Neuropathy

The clinical and genealogic features of Leber's hereditary optic neuropathy (LHON) have been reiterated in several recent articles.[117, 118] Lopez and Smith[119] exemplified the importance of examining family members. They were able to diagnose LHON in a patient who did not have the characteristic retinal angiopathy by identifying the vascular pathology in asymptomatic family members. Charcot-Marie-Tooth disease and generalized dystonia have been added to the list of neurologic diseases that can be associated with LHON.[120, 121]

Working under the assumption that LHON is a mitochondrial disease, skeletal muscle biopsy specimens have been obtained from affected patients.[122] Subsarcolemmal deposits of enlarged mitochondria have been noted, with proliferation of cristae. The trichrome stain reveals a red subsarcolemmal pattern reminiscent of that seen in the well-characterized mitochondrial myopathies. Biochemical studies on the muscle tissue have demonstrated abnormal oxidative enzyme activity, but the respiratory chain enzymes and cytochrome enzyme systems appeared to be normal.[123]

The recent discovery of a mitochondrial DNA mutation in patients with LHON is significant.[124] This finding provides molecular evidence supporting the long-held suspicion that LHON is cytoplasmically inheritied. The abnormal DNA results from a single amino acid substitution. This mutation appears to be necessary but not sufficient for the overt expression of the disease. Two of the 11 pedigrees assumed to have LHON did not have the DNA abnormality, suggesting that there may be a spectrum of molecular abnormalities with a phenotypic expression similar or identical to LHON.

The pattern electroretinogram (PERG) is thought by some primarily to reflect retinal ganglion cell function.[125] The PERG may be of prognostic value for visual recovery in acquired optic nerve disorders, including LHON.[126] The authors report a correlation between "irreversible retinal damage" and abnormal PERG amplitudes that meet specified criteria. This conclusion should be cautiously applied to patients with LHON given that a small proportion of patients experience a late recovery of vision.[127] It is interesting to speculate whether patients with this "variation on a theme by Leber" have a molecular defect other than has been described.

Retinal Toxicity

Ocular tissue is generally not affected by visible light, but the retina is susceptible because it contains chromophores that absorb these wavelengths.[128–130] Characteristic retinal and retinal pigment abnormalities have been recognized following exposure to the sun (in the absence of an eclipse) and the bright light of an operating microscope.[128, 131, 132] In the latter case, the degree of retinal damage has been correlated with the duration of exposure.[131] There is growing suspicion that ultraviolet light is damaging to the retina, especially in aphakic patients.[128] A review of the protective value of sunglasses is provided in one article.[130]

The ocular toxicity of photosensitizing drugs has been reviewed by Lerman.[133] Indomethacin and canthaxanthin, a carotenoid available in health food stores as an oral tanning agent, are reported to be toxic to the retina.[134, 135] Low-dose tamoxifen (an antiestrogen used for breast cancer), and the chemotherapeutic agents cisplatin and carmustine, are also toxic to the retina.[136–138]

REFERENCES

1. Masland RH: The functional architecture of the retina. *Sci Am* 1986; 24:102–111.
2. Sterling P, Freed M, Smith RG: Microcircuitry and functional architecture of the cat retina. *Trends Neurosci* 1986; 9:186–192.
3. Kuljis RO, Karten HJ: Neuroactive peptides as markers of retinal ganglion cell populations that differ in anatomical organization and function. *Vis Neurosci* 1988; 1:73–81.
4. Barnstable CJ: A molecular view of vertebrate retinal development. *Mol Neurobiol* 1987; 1:9–46.
5. Kolb H, Nelson R, Mariani A: Amacrine cells, bipolar cells and ganglion cells of the cat retina: A Golgi study. *Vis Res* 1981; 21:1081–1114.
6. Rodiek RW: The primate retina, in: *Comparative Primate Biology*. New York, Alan R Liss, 1988, vol 4: *Neurosciences*, pp 203–278.
7. Rodiek RW, Binmoeller KF, Dineen J: Parasol and midget cells of the human retina. *J Comp Neurol* 1985; 233:115–132.
8. Connolly M, van Essen DC: The representation of the visual field in parvocellular and magnocel-

lular laminae of the lateral geniculate nucleus in the macaque monkey. *J Comp Neurol* 1984; 266:544–564.

9. Schein SJ, de Monasterio FM: Mapping of retinal and geniculate neurons onto striate cortex of macaque. *J Neurosci* 1987; 7:996–1009.

10. Ross JE: Clinical detection of abnormalities in central vision in chronic simple glaucoma using contrast sensitivity. *Int Ophthalmol* 1985; 8:167–177.

11. Motolko MA, Phelps CD: Contrast sensitivity in asymmetric glaucoma. *Int Ophthalmol* 1984; 7:45–50.

12. Regan D, Maxner C: Orientation-dependent loss of contrast sensitivity for pattern and flicker in multiple sclerosis. *Clin Vis Sci* 1986; 1:1–23.

13. Plant GT, Hess RF: Temporal frequency discrimination in optic neuritis and multiple sclerosis. *Brain* 1985; 108:647–676.

14. Wall M: Contrast sensitivity testing in pseudotumor cerebri. *Ophthalmology* 1986; 93:4–7.

15. Bulens C, Meerwaldt JD, Koudstaal PJ, et al: Spatial contrast sensitivity in benign intracranial hypertension. *J Neurol Neurosurg Psychiatry* 1988; 51:1323–1329.

16. Verplanck M, Kaufman DI, Parsons T, et al: Electrophysiology versus psychophysics in the detection of visual loss in pseudotumor cerebri. *Neurology* 1988; 38:1789–1792.

17. Kupersmith MJ, Siegal IM, Carr RE: Subtle disturbances of vision with compressive lesions of the anterior visual pathway measured by contrast sensitivity. *Ophthalmology* 1982; 89:68–72.

18. Nissen MJ, Corkin S, Buonanno FS, et al: Spatial vision in Alzheimer's disease: General findings and a case report. *Arch Neurol* 1985; 42:667–671.

19. Cronin-Golomb A, Corkin S, Growdon JH: Contrast sensitivity in Alzheimer's disease. *J Opt Soc Am A* 1987; 4:7.

20. Legge GE, Rubin GS: Contrast sensitivity function as a screening test: A critique. *Am J Optom Physiol Opt* 1986; 63:265–270.

21. Higgins KE, Jaffe MJ, Coletta NJ, et al: Spatial contrast sensitivity: Importance of controlling the patient's visibility criterion. *Arch Ophthalmol* 1984; 102:1035–1041.

22. King FA, Yarbrough CJ, Anderson DC, et al: Primates. *Science* 1988; 240:1475–1482.

23. Bito LZ: Species differences in the responses of the eye to irritation and trauma: A hypothesis of divergence in ocular defense mechanisms, and the choice of experimental animals for eye research. *Exp Eye Res* 1984; 39:807–829.

24. Shapley R, Perry VH: Cat and monkey retinal ganglion cells and their visual functional roles. *Trends Neurosci* 1986; 95:229–235.

25. Enroth-Cugell C, Robson JG: Functional characteristics and diversity of cat retinal ganglion cells: Basic characteristics and quantitative description. *Invest Ophthalmol Vis Sci* 1984; 25:250–267.

26. Derrington AM, Lennie P: Spatial and temporal contrast sensitivities of neurones in lateral geniculate nucleus of macaque. *J Physiol* 1984; 357:219–240.

27. de Monasterio FM: Properties of concentrically organized X and Y ganglion cells of macaque retina. *J Neurophysiol* 1978; 41:1394–1417.

28. Blakemore CB, Vital-Durand F: Distribution of X- and Y-cells in the monkey's lateral geniculate nucleus. *J Physiol* 1981; 320:17P–18P.

29. Shapley R, Kaplan E, Soodak R: Spatial summation and contrast sensitivity of X and Y cells in the lateral geniculate nucleus of the macaque. *Nature* 1981; 292:544–545.

30. Dacheux RF, Raviola E: The rod pathway in the rabbit retina: A depolarizing bipolar and amacrine cell. *J Neurosci* 1986; 6:331–345.

31. Masland RH: Amacrine cells. *Trends Neurosci* 1988; 11:405–410.

32. Dowling JE: Dopamine: A retinal neuromodulator? *Trends Neurosci* 1986; 9:236–240.

33. Masland RH, Tauchi M: A possible amacrine cell substrate for the detection of stimulus motion. *Neurosci Res* 1985; (suppl 2):S185–S199.

34. Mosinger JL, Yazulla S, Studholme KM: GABA-like immunoreactivity in the vertebrate retina: A species comparison. *Exp Eye Res* 1986; 42:631–644.

35. Masland RH, Mills HW, Cassidy C: The functions of acetylcholine in the rabbit retina. *Proc R Soc Lond* 1984; B223:121–139.

36. Hubel DH, Livingstone MS: Segregation of form, color, and stereopsis in primate area 18. *J Neurosci* 1987; 7:3378–3415.

37. Hendry SHC, Jones EG, Hockfield S, et al: Neuronal populations stained with the monoclonal antibody Cat-301 in the mammalian cerebral cortex and thalamus. *J Neurosci* 1988; 8:518–542.

38. Livingstone MS, Hubel DH: Psychophysical evidence for separate channels for the perception of form, color, movement, and depth. *J Neurosci* 1987; 7:3416–3468.

39. Carney T, Shadlen M, Switkes E: Parallel processing of motion and colour information. *Nature* 1987; 328:647–649.

40. Vaina L, LeMay M, Naili S, et al: Deficits of visual motion analysis after posterior right hemisphere lesions. *Soc Neurosci Abstr* 1988; no. 187.12. Part 1, p 458.

41. Masland RH, Ames A: Responses to acetylcholine of ganglion cells in an isolated mammalian retina. *J Neurophysiol* 1976; 39:1220–1235.

42. Ariel M, Daw NW: Pharmacological analysis of directionally selective rabbit retinal ganglion cells. *J Physiol* 1982; 324:161–185.

43. Bunt AH, Minckler DS: Foveal sparing: New anatomical evidence for bilateral representation of the central retina. *Arch Ophthalmol* 1977; 95:1445–1447.

44. Leventhal AG, Ault SJ, Vitek DJ: The nasotemporal division in primate retina: The neural bases of macular sparing and splitting. *Science* 1988; 40:66–67.

45. Schein SJ: Anatomy of macaque fovea and spatial densities of neurons in foveal representation. *J Comp Neurol* 1988; 269:479–505.

46. Sladek JR, Shoulson I: Neural transplantation: A call for patience rather than patients. *Science* 1988; 240:1386–1388.

47. Fishman PS: Neural transplantation: Scientific gains and clinical perspectives. *Neurology* 1986; 36:389–392.

48. Borges LF: Historical development of neural transplantation. *Appl Neurophysiol* 1988; 51:265–277.

49. del Cerro M, Gash DM, Rao GN, et al: Retinal transplants into the anterior chamber of the rat eye. *Neuroscience* 1987; 21:707–723.

50. Aramant R, Seller M, Turner JE: Donor age influences on the success of retinal grafts to adult rat retina. *Invest Ophthalmol Vis Sci* 1988; 29:498–503.

51. Turner JE, Blair JR: Newborn rat retina transplanted into a retinal lesion site in adult host eyes. *Dev Brain Res* 1986; 26:91–104.

52. Klassen H, Lund RD: Retinal transplants can drive a pupillary reflex in host rat brains. *Proc Natl Acad Sci USA* 1987; 84:6958–6960.

53. Balaban E, Teillet MA, Le Douarin N: Application of the quail-chick chimera system to the study of brain development and behavior. *Science* 1988; 241:1339–1342.

54. Villegas-Perez MP, Vidal-Sanz M, Bray GM, et al: Influences of peripheral nerve grafts on survival and regrowth of axotomized retinal ganglion cells in adult rats. *J Neurosci* 1988; 8:265–280.

55. Corwin JT, Cotanche DA: Regeneration of sensory hair cells after acoustic trauma. *Science* 1988; 240:1772–1774.

56. Ryals BM, Rubel EW: Hair cell regeneration after acoustic trauma in adult Coturnix quail. *Science* 1988; 240:1774–1776.

57. Trobe JD: Carotid endarterectomy: Who needs it? *Ophthalmology* 1987; 94:725–730.

58. Jones S: Can carotid endarterectomy be justified? No. *Arch Neurol* 1987; 44:652–654.

59. American Neurological Association Committee on Health Care Issues: Does carotid endarterectomy decrease stroke and death in patients with transient ischemic attacks? *Ann Neurol* 1987; 22:72–76.

60. Winslow CM, Solomon DH, Chassin MR, et al: The appropriateness of carotid endarterectomy. *N Engl J Med* 1988; 318:721–727.

61. Scheinberg P: Controversies in the management of cerebral vascular disease. *Neurology* 1988; 38:1609–1616.

62. Patterson RH: Can carotid endarterectomy be justified? Yes. *Arch Neurol* 1987; 44:651–652.

63. Hachinski V: Carotid endarterectomy. *Arch Neurol* 1987; 44:654.

64. Easton JD, Hart RG, Sherman DG, et al: Diagnosis and management of ischemic stroke: I. Threatened stroke and its management. *Curr Probl Cardiol* 1983; 8:1–76.

65. Hurwitz BJ, Heyman A, Wilkinson WE, et al: Comparison of amaurosis fugax and transient cerebral ischemia: A prospective clinical and arteriographic study. *Ann Neurol* 1985; 18:698–704.

66. Marshall J, Meadows S: The natural history of amaurosis fugax. *Brain* 1968; 91:419–434.

67. Wray SH: Visual aspects of extracranial internal carotid artery disease, in Bernstein EF (ed): *Amaurosis Fugax*. New York, Springer-Verlag New York, 1988, pp 81–89.

68. Gaul JJ, Marks SJ, Weinberger J: Visual disturbances and carotid artery disease: Five hundred symptomatic patients studied by non-invasive carotid artery testing including B-mode ultrasonography. *Stroke* 1986; 17:393–397.

69. Parkin PJ, Kendall BE, Marshall J, et al: Amaurosis fugax: Some aspects of management. *J Neurol Neurosurg Psychiatry* 1982; 45:1–6.

70. Poole CJM, Ross Russell RW: Mortality and stroke after amaurosis fugax. *J Neurol Neurosurg Psychiatry* 1985; 48:902–905.

71. Harrison MJG, Marshall J: Arteriographic comparison of amaurosis fugax and hemispheric transient ischemic attacks. *Stroke* 1985; 16:795–797.

72. Ross Russell RW: Natural history of amaurosis fugax, in Bernstein EF (ed): *Amaurosis Fugax*. New York, Springer-Verlag New York, 1988, pp 174–182.

73. Poole CJM, Ross Russell RW, Harrison P, et al: Amaurosis fugax under the age of 40 years. *J Neurol Neurosurg Psychiatry* 1987; 50:81–84.

74. Goodwin JA, Gorelick PB, Helgason CM: Symptoms of amaurosis fugax in atherosclerotic carotid artery disease. *Neurology* 1987; 37:829–832.

75. Howard RS, Ross Russell RW: Prognosis of patients with retinal embolism. *J Neurol Neurosurg Psychiatry* 1987; 50:1142–1147.

76. Grotta JC, Bigelow RH, Hu H, et al: The significance of stenosis or ulceration in symptomatic and asymptomatic carotid arteries. *Neurology* 1984; 34:437–442.

77. Harrison MJG, Marshall J: Prognostic significance of severity of carotid atheroma in early manifestations of cerebrovascular disease. *Stroke* 1982; 13:567–569.

78. Whisnant JP, Wiebers DO: Clinical epidemiology of transient cerebral ischemic attacks (TIA) in the anterior and posterior cerebral circulation, in Sundt TM Jr (ed): *Occlusive Cerebrovascular Disease: Diagnosis and Surgical Management*. Philadelphia, WB Saunders Co, 1987, pp 60–65.

79. Grady PA: Pathophysiology of extracranial cerebral arterial stenosis: A critical review. *Stroke* 1984; 15:224–236.

80. Adams HP, Putman SF, Corbett JJ, et al: Amaurosis fugax: The results of arteriography in 59 patients. *Stroke* 1983; 14:742–744.

81. Bernstein EF, Dilley RB: Late results after carotid endarterectomy for amaurosis fugax. *J Vasc Surg* 1987; 6:333–340.

82. Harrison MJG: Angiography in amaurosis fugax, in Bernstein EF (ed): *Amaurosis Fugax*. New York, Springer-Verlag New York, 1988, pp 227–235.

83. Dixon S, Pais O, Raviola C, et al: Natural history of nonstenotic, asymptomatic ulcerative lesions of the carotid artery. *Arch Surg* 1982; 117:1493–1498.

84. Fisher M, Blumenfeld AM, Smith TW: The importance of carotid artery plaque disruption and hemorrhage. *Arch Neurol* 1987; 44:1086–1089.

85. Weinberger J, Bender AN, Yang WC: Amaurosis fugax associated with ophthalmic artery stenosis: Clinical simulation of carotid artery disease. *Stroke* 1980; 11:290–293.

86. Ross RT, Morrow IM: Ocular and cerebral ischemic mechanisms in disease of the internal carotid artery. *Can J Neurol Sci* 1984; 11:262–268.

87. Bogousslavsky J, Regli F, Zografos L, et al: Opticocerebral syndrome: Simultaneous hemodynamic infarction of optic nerve and brain. *Neurology* 1987; 37:263–268.

88. Chikos PM, Fisher LD, Hirsch JH, et al: Observer variability in evaluating extracranial carotid artery stenosis. *Stroke* 1983; 14:885–892.

89. Eikelboom BC, Riles TR, Mintzer R, et al: Inaccuracy of angiography in the diagnosis of carotid ulceration. *Stroke* 1983; 14:882–885.

90. Otis SM: Noninvasive vascular examination in amaurosis fugax, in Bernstein EF (ed): *Amaurosis Fugax*. New York, Springer-Verlag New York, 1988, pp 183–199.

91. Stewart G, Ross-Russell RW, Browse NL: The long-term results of carotid endarterectomy for transient ischemic attacks. *J Vasc Surg* 1986; 4:600–605.

92. Browse NL, Ross-Russell R: Carotid endarterectomy and the Javid shunt: The early results of 215 consecutive operations for transient ischaemic attacks. *Br J Surg* 1984; 71:53–57.

93. Warlow C: Carotid endarterectomy: Does it work? *Stroke* 1984; 15:1068–1076.

94. Brott T, Thalinger K: The practice of carotid endarterectomy in a large metropolitan area. *Stroke* 1984; 5:950–955.

95. Amaurosis Fugax Study Group: Amaurosis fugax: A consensus statement, in Bernstein EF (ed): *Amaurosis Fugax*. New York, Springer-Verlag New York, 1988, pp 286–301.

96. Becker WL, Burde RM: Carotid artery disease: A therapeutic enigma. *Arch Ophthalmol* 1988; 106:34–39.

97. Antiplatelet Trialists' Collaboration: Secondary prevention of vascular disease by prolonged antiplatelet treatment. *Br Med J* 1988; 296:320–331.

98. Adams HP, Kassell NF, Mazuz H: The patient with transient ischemic attacks: Is this the time for a new therapeutic approach? *Stroke* 1984; 15:371–374.

99. Gass JDM, Tiedeman J, Thomas MA: Idiopathic recurrent branch retinal arterial occlusion. *Ophthalmology* 1986; 93:1148–1157.

100. Devenyl P, Schneiderman JF, Devenyl RG, et al: Cocaine-induced central retinal artery occlusion. *Can Med Assoc J* 1988; 138:129–130.

101. Mody CK, Miller BL, McIntyre HB, et al: Neurologic complications of cocaine abuse. *Neurology* 1988; 38:1189–1193.

102. Kaye BR, Fainstat M: Cerebral vasculitis associated with cocaine abuse. *JAMA* 1987; 258:2104–2106.

103. Coppeto JR, Currie JN, Monteiro MLR, et al: A syndrome of arterial-occlusive retinopathy and encephalopathy. *Am J Ophthalmol* 1984; 98:189–202.

104. Monteiro MLR, Swanson RA, Coppeto JR, et al: A microangiopathic syndrome of encephalopathy, hearing loss, and retinal arteriolar occlusions. *Neurology* 1985; 35:1113–1121.

105. Grand MG, Kaine J, Fulling K, et al: Cerebroretinal vasculopathy: A new hereditary syndrome. *Ophthalmology* 1988; 95:649–659.

106. Blumenkranz MS, Kaplan HJ, Clarkson JG, et al: Acute multifocal hemorrhagic retinal vasculitis. *Ophthalmology* 1988; 95:1663–1672.

107. Sawyer RA, Selhorst JB, Zimmerman LE, et al: Blindness caused by photoreceptor degeneration as a remote effect of cancer. *Am J Ophthalmol* 1976; 81:606–613.

108. Keltner JL, Roth AM, Chang S: Photoreceptor degeneration: Possible autoimmune disorder. *Arch Ophthalmol* 1983; 101:564–569.

109. Thirkill CE, Roth AM, Keltner JL: Cancer-associated retinopathy. *Arch Ophthalmol* 1987; 105:372–375.

110. Kornguth SE Klein R, Appen R, et al: Occurrence of anti-retinal ganglion cell antibodies in patients with small cell carcinoma of the lung. *Cancer* 1982; 50:1289–1293.

111. Grunwald GB, Simmonds MA, Klein R, et al: Autoimmune basis for visual paraneoplastic syndrome in patients with small-cell lung carcinoma. *Lancet* 1985; 1:658–661.

112. Kornguth SE, Kalinke T, Grunwald GB, et al: Anti-neurofilament antibodies in the sera of patients with small cell carcinoma of the lung and with visual paraneoplastic syndrome. *Cancer Res* 1986; 46:2588–2595.

113. Grunwald GB, Kornguth SE, Towfighi J, et al: Autoimmune basis for visual paraneoplastic syndrome in patients with small cell carcinoma. *Cancer* 1987; 60:780–786.

114. Berson EL, Lessell S: Paraneoplastic night blindness with malignant melanoma. *Am J Ophthalmol* 1988; 106:307–311.

115. Buchanan TAS, Gardiner M, Archer DB: An ultrastructural study of retinal photoreceptor degeneration associated with bronchial carcinoma. *Am J Ophthalmol* 1984; 97:277–287.

116. Klingele TG, Burde RM, Rappazzo JA, et al: Paraneoplastic retinopathy. *J Clin Neuro Ophthalmol* 1984; 4:239–245.

117. Nikoskelainen E: New aspects of the genetic, etiologic, and clinical puzzle of Leber's disease. *Neurology* 1984; 34:1482–1484.

118. Seedorff JT: The inheritance of Leber's disease. *Acta Ophthalmol* 1985; 63:135–145.

119. Lopez PF, Smith JL: Leber's optic neuropathy: New observations. *J Clin Neuro Ophthalmol* 1986; 6:144–152.

120. McCluskey DJ, O'Connor PS, Sheeney JT: Leber's optic neuropathy and Charcot-Marie-Tooth disease. *J Clin Neuro Ophthalmol* 1986; 6:76–81.

121. Novotny EJ, Singh G, Wallace DC, et al: Leber's disease and dystonia: A mitochondrial disease. *Neurology* 1986; 36:1053–1060.

122. Nikoskelainen E, Paljarvi L, Lang H, et al: Leber's hereditary optic neuroretinopathy: A mitochondrial disease? *Acta Neurol Scand* 1984; 69(suppl 98):172–173.

123. Uemura A, Osame M, Nakagawa M, et al: Leber's hereditary optic neuropathy: Mitochondrial and biochemical studies on muscle biopsies. *Br J Ophthalmol* 1987; 71:531–536.

124. Wallace DC, Singh G, Lott MT, et al: Mitochondrial DNA mutation associated with Leber's hereditary optic neuropathy. *Science* 1988; 242:1427–1430.

125. Maffei L, Fiorentini A, Bisti S, et al: Pattern ERG in the monkey after section of the optic nerve. *Exp Brain Res* 1985; 59:423–425.

126. Kaufman DI, Lorance RW, Woods M, et al: The pattern electroretinogram: A long-term study in acute optic neuropathy. *Neurology* 1988; 38:1767–1774.

127. Lessell S, Gise RL, Krohel GB: Bilateral optic neuropathy with remission in young men: Variation on a theme by Leber? *Arch Neurol* 1983; 40:2–6.

128. Young RW: Solar radiation and age-related macular degeneration. *Surv Ophthalmol* 1988; 32:252–269.

129. Lerman S: Ocular phototoxicity. *N Engl J Med* 1988; 319:1475–1477.

130. Sliney DH: Ocular injury due to light toxicity. *Int Ophthalmol Clin* 1988; 28:246–250.

131. Khwarg SG, Linstone FA, Daniels SA, et al: Incidence, risk factors, and morphology in operating microscope light retinopathy. *Am J Ophthalmol* 1987; 103:255–263.

132. Campo RV, Sipperley JO, Hall G, et al: Medjugorje maculopathy. *N Engl J Med* 1988; 318:1207.

133. Lerman S: Photosensitizing drugs and their possible role in enhancing ocular toxicity. *Ophthalmology* 1986; 93:304–318.

134. Lonn LI: Canthaxanthin retinopathy. *Arch Ophthalmol* 1987; 105:1590–1591.

135. Graham CM, Blanch RK: Indomethacin retinopathy: Case report and review. *Br J Ophthalmol* 1988; 72:434–438.

136. Griffiths MF: Tamoxifen retinopathy at low dosage. *Am J Ophthalmol* 1987; 104:185–186.

137. Kupersmith MJ, Frohman LP, Choi IS, et al: Visual system toxicity following intra-arterial chemotherapy. *Neurology* 1988; 38:284–289.

138. Miller DF, Bay JW, Lederman RJ, et al: Ocular and orbital toxicity following intracarotid injection of BCNU (Carmustine) and cisplatinum for malignant gliomas. *Ophthalmology* 1985; 92:402–406.

PART FIVE

THE ORBIT

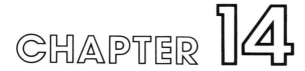

CHAPTER 14

The Orbit

Peter J. Savino, M.D.

Neuro-Ophthalmology Service, Wills Eye Hospital, Philadelphia, Pennsylvania

My chapter in the 1988 volume of *Current Neuro-ophthalmology*[1] dealt with two topics exclusively, magnetic resonance imaging (MRI) of the orbit and dysthyroid orbitopathy. This year, those topics will be given only brief mention and other aspects of orbital disease will be reviewed.

INFECTION

Cellulitis

Several articles have reviewed the etiologic agents and the predisposing factors of cellulitis, particularly in children. Much has been made about the distinction between periorbital (preseptal) cellulitis and true orbital cellulitis. Summaries of 179 cases of orbital infection (166 being preorbital cellulitis and only 12 being orbital cellulitis) occurring in patients under 19 years old were reviewed.[2] The time needed to collect this group of patients was 9 years, ending in 1984. In addition, these authors reviewed the literature and compared their results with a total of 1,010 cases of periorbital cellulitis and 606 cases of orbital cellulitis. They found that predisposing factors were skin infection and trauma in one quarter of the cases of preseptal cellulitis and that these were caused mainly by *Streptococcus* and *Staphylococcus* organisms. About half of the cases of preseptal cellulitis

© 1989, Year Book Medical Publishers, Inc.
0893–0147/89/02-241-254-$04.00

had otitis media, upper respiratory tract infections, and evidence of sinusitis, and the agent in these cases was mostly *Haemophilus influenzae*. Nine of their 12 patients with orbital cellulitis had sinus disease. This disease was an important factor in both preseptal and orbital cellulitis, with the ethmoid and maxillary sinuses being involved in both entities. A pathologic organism was isolated in only 33% of the patients with preseptal cellulitis, whereas 7 of 10 cultures were positive in the orbital cellulitis group. In the preseptal cellulitis group, 16 patients had negative cultures, but 15 of these had a positive urine antigen test for *H. influenzae*. Though there were no deaths in the group, central nervous system (CNS) complications occurred in 4 of 166 patients with preseptal cellulitis.

Another review in the otolaryngologic literature examined 226 patients with preseptal cellulitis and 11 with orbital cellulitis.[3] The findings were the same as in the previous study and emphasized that conjunctival cultures were not useful in this disorder. The authors recommend aggressive intravenous therapy for both preseptal and orbital cellulitis. No true distinction had to be made from a therapeutic standpoint between the two.

The types of etiologic agents seen in infants and children were reviewed in the pediatric infectious disease literature.[4] A suggestion was made that treatment for idiopathic preseptal cellulitis, not caused by sinusitis, consist of the same antibiotics directed against β-lactamase–producing strains of *H. influenzae* and *Staphylococcus aureus* as well as *Streptococcus pneumoniae*.

The most recent review studied 146 episodes of preseptal cellulitis in children with a specific aim to see if the ability to culture an organism changed the clinical profile of the disease.[5] Forty-four patients were pretreated with antibiotics before cultures were obtained; only 2 (5%) of these patients had positive cultures, and both of these were from purulent material. Blood cultures were negative in all of these pretreated patients. One hundred two episodes of cellulitis were not treated with antibiotics, and bacteria were isolated in 33 patients (32%), 31 from blood cultures. This article also examined countercurrent immunoelectrophoresis (CIE) on tears, urine, serum, and cerebrospinal fluid (CSF), particularly to look for *H. influenzae* type B capsular polysaccharide. Compared with blood cultures, the tear CIE for *H. influenzae* type B antigen had a sensitivity of 50% and a specificity of 93%. The authors suggest that antibiotic treatment of cellulitis not be dictated by predisposing factors such as upper respiratory infection or trauma but that all cellulitis be treated with broad-spectrum antibiotics until a specific organism is identified. They suggest culturing blood and purulent wound drainage as most useful. They suggest that CIE of tears may be useful to identify *H. influenzae* type B capsular antigen. They likewise recommend that all cellulitis be treated with antibiotics that have high CSF penetration and that specific *Staphylococcus* coverage be added if there is an infected wound near the involved eye.

An investigation was performed on 102 children specifically to address the role of spinal tap in periorbital cellulitis since CNS infection, though uncommon, is the most dreaded complication of this disease. One hundred two children at the Children's Hospital National Medical Center Washington, D.C., were studied; 2 children developed meningitis, and one developed bilateral subdural effusions. These authors recommend that routine spinal tap is therefore *not* needed in uncomplicated periorbital cellulitis in children 6 months of age or older.[6]

Slavin and Glaser[7] described three patients with a form of cellulitis that they termed "posterior" orbital cellulitis. These patients were initially misdiagnosed as having optic neuritis, ischemic optic neuropathy, and giant cell arteritis. Only computed tomographic (CT) scanning, which showed posterior sphenoethmoiditis, led to the correct diagnosis and appropriate treatment. Despite this, however, vision was not regained in any of the three eyes. The authors suggest that this type of abnormality is relatively rare, but this is another reason to argue in favor of imaging all cases of orbital cellulitis that appear the least bit atypical.

An article appears reviewing the role of subperiosteal abscesses in orbital cellulitis.[8] Seventeen patients with subperiosteal collections and sinusitis were reviewed, and 14 were drained surgically. In 11 of the 14, cultures yielded organisms, with 8 of these 11 showing viable bacteria in the subperiosteal space even though these patients had been treated for 3 or more days with antibiotics. Six of these patients had been treated for 6 days or more. This article shows that subperiosteal collections (abscesses) should be treated surgically and that they may contain viable organisms several days after institution of appropriate antibiotic therapy. Those that will respond to medical management do so quite rapidly. The authors suggest that surgery for a subperiosteal collection be performed if there is no improvement with medical therapy after 3 or 4 days. This appears to be a reasonable approach. This article also shows the changing investigation of orbital cellulitis. Skull and sinus roentgenograms are useless in this disease. The presence of a subperiosteal abscess that requires more aggressive surgical treatment is best documented by imaging of the orbit, and I would suggest that all patients with orbital infectious disease undergo CT scanning as the study of choice.

Mucormycosis

Rhino-orbital mucormycosis appears to be increasing either in frequency or in accuracy of diagnosis. Several articles reviewed this entity. The Johns Hopkins (Baltimore) experience was a 40-year review of 33 patients, but this review extended over such a long period that specific recommendations cannot be drawn from it.[9]

Kohn and Hepler[10] reviewed 44 patients with mucormycosis seen between 1972 and 1984 and described 8 in detail. These 8 are extremely interesting because they were successfully treated without orbital exenteration. This establishes an important point: mucormycosis does not necessarily need to be treated with aggressive, extensive, mutilating surgery. In the discussion of this important article, Dr. Andrew Ferry points out that it is difficult at times to tell if the clinical reaction that is visualized is due to a suppurative necrosis, in which case surgery would be indicated, or to an intense inflammatory reaction without necrosis, where medical treatment might be successful. He agrees that some patients with mucormycosis can and should be treated without radical surgery. Guidelines for treatment of mucormycosis are as follows:

1. Early definitive diagnosis.—This is one time when biopsy is critical at an early stage, often before the black eschars appear in the nose or on the face.
2. Correction of the underlying metabolic disorder.
3. Wide local excision and débridement of devitalized oral, nasal, sinus, and orbital tissue.
4. Adequate sinus and orbital drainage.
5. Local irrigation with a packing of the sinus and orbit with amphotericin B.—This is described by Kohn and Hepler[10] and seems to have a rationale, since many times the area involved by mucormycosis is ischemic and the intravenous amphotericin B may not reach this area.
6. Intravenous amphotericin B.

Another adjunct to the treatment of mucormycosis was described by Couch and colleagues,[11] who treated two patients who did not show clinical improvement with the standard treatment listed above but who did improve when hyperbaric oxygen (HBO) therapy was added to their systemic amphotericin B. These authors suggest that HBO works by improving oxygen tension in ischemic tissue, which may alleviate the acidosis in the infected tissue. Also, HBO augments the action of amphotericin B. Finally, hyperoxia also inhibits fungal growth in vitro, and this may play a role in its in vivo action. It seems that in desperate cases, and many of the patients with mucormycosis are desperate cases, HBO may be a useful adjunctive treatment.

A patient is described who had bilateral cavernous sinus thrombosis due to mucormycosis.[12] The patient had ethmoid sinus surgery, which showed no evidence of an organism. He died 5 days later, and autopsy showed mucormycosis with coagulant necrosis of "all ocular contents." The authors raise the issue of deferoxamine, which their patient was taking. This drug is a heavy metal chelator used in states of iron overload. For example, in patients on hemodialysis it is used to treated aluminum overload. This drug, however, has been shown to alter granulocyte and lymphocyte function and might have predisposed this patient to mucormycosis.

Deferoxamine is being used in dialysis units, so it would therefore be useful to keep this in mind. This case also illustrates to me the need for early biopsy, and the fact that biopsy may early in the course of the disease not yield the causative organism. The suspicion of mucormycosis, even with a negative biopsy, dictates that the patient should be treated with amphotericin B if there is any reasonable suspicion that mucormycosis is involved, despite an initially negative biopsy.

This is one disorder where CT scanning may not be helpful. Ten patients with mucormycosis were investigated with CT scanning.[13] Nine patients had abnormality of the nasal fossa and the paranasal sinuses. However, the abnormality was typically a rim of soft-tissue density of variable thickness along the bony walls. The authors state that this appearance could be distinguished from benign mucosal thickening *only* by the clinical symptoms of mucormycosis. Only two patients had bony erosion, indicating the less than benign nature of the process. Therefore, while all patients with suspected mucormycosis should have CT, the presence of "benign mucosal thickening" should not prevent aggressive diagnostic measures from being undertaken.

ORBITAL MASS LESIONS

Tumors

The diagnosis and management of orbital tumors has been simplified with the onset of high-resolution imaging of the orbit. Rarely do we need other than a CT and/or MRI scan in the investigation of a patient with proptosis. Appropriate surgical treatment may be directed toward total excision or biopsy depending on the imaging characteristics of the mass. One article reviewed the causes of space-occupying masses in children.[14] This article was from a general eye hospital and as such was not biased by the particular subspecialty or academic interest of the investigators. Between 1962 and 1983, 250 patients under age 18 had orbital tumors that were either biopsied or excised. Cysts were the most common, being seen in 130 patients (52%), with dermoid cysts numbering 115 of the 130 and representing 46% of all orbital lesions. Inflammatory lesions represented 16%, but the true incidence of inflammatory lesions is much higher because during this period not all orbital inflammatory processes were biopsied. Six percent of the orbital masses were primary malignant tumors, with most (10/14) being rhabdomyosarcomas. It is possible now with high-resolution imaging that many of these cysts will go unbiopsied, so this type of histopathologic information is worthwhile.

A host of case reports have appeared reporting various mass lesions in the orbit. Patients with schwannomas are described, and echography is touted as the best method of diagnosis.[15] However, echography did not change the outcome, and imaging with CT or MRI is still the one test to be done.

The first reported case of an angliolipoma in the orbit[16] and of six patients with nonocular (cutaneous) melanoma metastatic to the orbit[17] appeared. Thirty-five patients with orbital hydatid cysts were reviewed; these took 41 years to collect in Buenas Aires.[18] Prostate carcinoma metastatic to the orbit was described in eight patients,[19] which occurred over a 14-year period. The first report of a carcinoid tumor in the orbit seen with MRI scanning is also described.[20] Manor and Sira[21] described a patient with transient visual loss on downward gaze due to an orbital mass lesion. This symptom is important because it is atypical of orbital disease and might be confused with cardiac or carotid artery disease, for which the patient might have a totally inappropriate workup and treatment. Gaze-directed amaurosis is a symptom of orbital disease and should be recognized as such.

Hemorrhage

In the last few years, the presence of blood in the orbit has occupied chroniclers of orbital disease. There have been reports of orbital hemorrhage following anesthesia[22] that cleared with the patient being treated "conservatively with bedrest alone." A scuba diver had the onset of proptosis and pain and was found on CT and MRI to have bled into the orbit. This ability to detect blood is another benefit of high-resolution imaging.[23]

Two women developed proptosis during labor, but no optic nerve involvement was observed in either. Computed tomography and orbital echography were used to diagnose a hematoma, which resolved in both patients without complication. The authors state that orbital echography is superior to CT scan in following up these patients. This may be true in institutions where echography is readily available and done with a certain level of expertise, but I suspect in the general community, CT scanning will give better information more consistently. The authors also suggest that cerebral angiography be done to exclude an intracranial aneurysm if the CT or ultrasound fails to show an abnormality or if there is pupillary "involvement."[24] They do not state what involvement they mean, but I would of course agree with arteriography in a third-nerve palsy with a pupil involved. If the orbital signs alone are present, and the pupillary involvement is an afferent defect due to compression, cerebral angiography is not called for and should not be done.

Four patients were described with intraorbital hemorrhage following frontoethmoidectomy, anterior ethmoidal artery ligation, dacrycystorhinostomy, and a blowout fracture.[25] The authors report that immediate orbital decompression was undertaken and suggest that other methods, "medical, lateral canthotomy," are not useful. They suggest the ophthalmologist's role is "to measure ocular pressure and visual acuity and to assess the retina and optic discs."[25]

Chronic blood in the orbit was described in four patients, all of whom had progressive proptosis and a paucity of other signs.[26] The proptosis in these patients had progressed from 3 weeks to 4 years. Three of these hemorrhages were subperiosteal in the superior orbit and one was inferiorly located in the site of a previous repair of an orbital floor fracture. A CT scan showed the characteristic appearance of these lesions, and now that we have MRI, with its specificity for blood, this should be an easy diagnosis to arrive at preoperatively.

Hematic cysts of the orbit were reviewed[27] by describing two patients with expanding masses. The mechanism of expansion of these tumors was suggested to be due to an osmotic gradient, which draws fluid into the cyst once it is formed. In a letter in response to this article, an alternate mechanism for enlargement was proposed that consisted of fibrinolytic activity, which would cause expansion of these hematic cysts much like a subdural hematoma.[28] Again, the diagnosis of these lesions should be quite simple with CT and MRI.

ORBITAL INFLAMMATORY DISEASE

Pseudotumor/Lymphoma

The diagnosis of orbital inflammatory disease has become easier to make with the advent of high-resolution orbital imaging. Many times, however, there remains the problem of these lesions being truly benign or malignant or falling somewhere between, having malignant potential. Orbital inflammatory disease may present in many forms. An extensive review of posterior scleritis nicely places this entity firmly in the setting of orbital inflammatory disease.[29] This important review describes an entity that is often misdiagnosed because patients may present to a variety of ophthalmic subspecialists (uveitis, retinal, neuro-ophthalmic, or orbital). Computed tomographic scanning may be helpful in distinguishing the inflammatory scleritis from other, more invasive causes. Five patients with posterior scleritis underwent high-resolution CT scanning and they all showed diffuse scleral involvement, in contrast to other, more localized processes, which showed focal scleral alteration or extension of disease beyond the sclera. In all of these latter instances adjacent tissue was involved.[30]

A series of 38 patients with orbital lymphoproliferative and inflammatory diseases showed that the orbital findings in both these groups are clinically similar.[31] Inflammatory pseudotumor was diagnosed histopathologically in 12 of the 38 patients, and follow-up showed no systemic disease. Twenty-six patients had noninflammatory lymphoproliferative disorders (reactive lymphoid hyperplasia, malignant lymphoma, Hodgkin's disease, and atypical lymphoid hyperplasia). Histologically, these could be distinguished from inflammatory disease, and on long-term follow-up all these patients showed systemic involvement. This review seems to indicate that while histochemical techniques, electron microscopy, and immunologic studies are being proposed as effective ways to differentiate between orbital inflammatory and neoplastic disease, histopathologic determinations, when unequivocal, seem to be secure. The value of light microscopy should not be forgotten. When a lesion is inflammatory under light microscopy, it is inflammatory and not neoplastic. All other lesions should be investigated as if they were malignant or potentially malignant.

Several interesting forms of orbital inflammatory disease have been presented. Garrity et al.[32] described three patients with a particularly aggressive form of orbital inflammatory disease. These patients had a primary vasculitis, which was angiocentric as well as angiodestructive. Despite the inflammation being centered histopathologically within the walls of small blood vessels, no systemic vasculitis was ever identified. All of these patients had bilateral involvement, which was resistant to treatment with up to 100 mg of prednisone daily. Cyclophosphamide provided relief from inflammation and led to drug-free remission periods in all patients. One patient in addition had undergone orbital irradiation without benefit. Though this is a relatively uncommon form of orbital inflammatory disease, it does respond to aggressive treatment and therefore must be considered in the evaluation of these disorders.

Another patient was presented with "typical" orbital inflammatory disease diagnosed by CT scan that had a dramatic response to corticosteroids. Four months later, the patient was diagnosed as being human immunodeficiency virus (HIV) infected, although no recurrence of the orbital signs apparently ever occurred.[33] Although *orbital pseudotumor* is too all-inclusive a term, and frequently orbital inflammatory disease may look exactly like lymphoma, there is no evidence that this patient, or any other patient with HIV infection, is more prone to orbital inflammatory disease. Despite this isolated case report, patients with orbital inflammatory disease do not require HIV testing.

Finally, the most difficult distinction one faces in the patient with an acute orbital inflammatory syndrome is the distinction between inflammation and lymphoma. Jakobiec et al.,[34] in the Wendell Hughes lecture, described five patients with "benign reactive" lymphoid tumors on the basis of light microscopy and polyclonality by immunologic techniques. Using the technique of molecular genetic analysis, three of these patients had small monoclonal B-cell proliferation. This is an excellent review of recent methodology in the laboratory diagnosis of this disease, but even the authors conclude that "because both polyclonal and monoclonal ocular adnexal lesions can have associated nonocular disease . . . patients with all types of lymphoproliferative disorders have noninvasive workup and regular follow-up by an oncologist . . . during the first 3 years after orbital presentation." Obviously, the management of these patients remains in a constant state of flux.

Dysthyroid Orbitopathy

It would appear that it is relatively straightforward to diagnose dysthyroid orbitopathy. However, publications continue to appear describing mimickers of dysthyroidism. A patient was described with a sphenoid wing meningioma and ipsilateral extraocular muscle enlargement on CT scan, which was diagnosed as Graves' orbitopathy.[35] The patient went on to lose vision despite being treated with corticosteroids and orbital decompression. Finally, the correct diagnosis of a meningioma was made, and "subtotal" removal of the meningioma was done with "irradiation" afterward. The authors suggest that euthyroid Graves' disease should be viewed with suspicion and prompt a search for orbital tumors, especially when the abnormalities (presumably neuroradiologic abnormalities) are unilateral. The authors do not describe the patient in detail, and I suspect that typical lid signs of dysthyroidism were absent in this patient—the authors describe a "fullness of the right upper lid." The real lessons in this case are not to diagnose Graves' disease in less than typical presentations and not to rely on CT findings alone, since other disorders may cause eye muscle enlargement in the orbit. Another lesson is to review CT scans, since in this case the lesion was a slow growing one and almost assuredly was visible if complete high-resolution imaging had been done.

Dysthyroid optic neuropathy was described in a neuroradiologic report. The authors present a CT formula to calculate a predictive value for dysthyroid optic neuropathy.[36] I believe that dysthyroid optic neuropathy, like dysthyroid orbitopathy itself, remains largely a clinical diagnosis that may be supported or not by other findings, including neuroimaging.

The treatment of dysthyroid orbitopathy was addressed in several articles. An aggressive four-wall decompressive procedure was reported in 11 patients.[37] Eleven bilateral four-wall decompressions through a craniotomy approach were done on patients for the indications of dysthyroid optic neuropathy, but also for proptosis with corneal disease (class V) as well as some patients in class IV. The authors state that the results were satisfactory, but the range of decompression with this radical approach was only 1 to 14 mm, with a mean of 7 mm. The authors state that there were no deaths and no major morbidity. Despite this reassurance, the four-wall craniotomy approach to this disease appears to be overly aggressive. The transantral approach, if done correctly, will relieve the compression at the orbital apex in almost all of these patients. The complication rate in a transantral approach is less than in four-wall decompression with a craniotomy. This aggressive therapy might represent a form of overskill with regard to this disease.

As further proof that many different forms of decompression are successful in this disease, a 35-year-old woman with long-standing proptosis and subluxation of the globe was described.[38] She was struck in the right eye by her husband, which caused a sustained lessening in the proptosis and no further episodes of subluxation because of a blowout fracture. The patient then would taunt her husband in an effort to "fix" her left eye. Finally, he tried to oblige but fractured her nose instead of her orbit, and her proptosis on the fellow side remained unchanged. One can only hope that government officials do not read this report and realize the potential savings in operating room fees and hospitalization and propose this procedure as the primary reimbursable method for decompression in dysthyroid orbitopathy.

Sixty-three patients underwent 123 orbital decompressive procedures for dysthyroid orbitopathy.[39] One surgeon did all the procedures, 84 through a transantral ethmoidal approach, 6 as three-wall procedures, and 33 as transconjunctival orbital decompressions. There was a 16% (14 transantral patients) incidence of tearing due to nasal lacrimal duct obstruction postoperatively. This developed 11 to 18 months after the procedure, leading to the proposal of a "slow cicatricial process" causing a lacrimal obstruction from "damage to adjacent tissues." This 16% incidence is higher than the 2% incidence of a similar condition found in other comparable series.[40] The authors admit not knowing the cause of this apparent discrepancy. This should not cause abandonment of the transantral approach for dysthyroid orbitopathy with optic nerve involvement since it is, in my opinion, the surgical procedure of choice for this disorder.

Nonsurgical (radiation) therapy for Graves' disease was reviewed in two articles. Palmer et al.[41] reviewed 29 patients treated with radiotherapy, but only 1 did not have prior medical or surgical treatment. Their overall improvement was judged to be 48%, with soft-tissue changes resolving in 78% and proptosis being reduced in 52%. After radiotherapy, 26 (90%) of their 29 patients required no further therapy.

A review of patients from the Wills Eye Hospital and the University of Pennsylvania Radiation Therapy Department, Philadelphia, found 35 patients with dysthyroid orbitopathy treated with radiotherapy.[42] Seven patients were treated primarily with radiation. After radiotherapy, 25 patients (71%) did not require any further steroids or decompressive surgery, and 10 (29%) required further treatment, but none of these 10 patients progressed. This is an important review because the evaluations of success and treatment were done by ophthalmologists and not radiotherapists, something that has not been true in all previous studies of this type. Of equal importance is that the staging was done by a neuro-ophthalmologist familiar with the clinical spectrum of dysthyroid orbitopathy, so that chronic cicatricial Graves' orbitopathy was not treated. This article also presents what is possibly the largest series of dysthyroid optic neuropathy treated with radiotherapy and it shows convincingly that this modality of treatment is effective in the optic nerve compression of thyroid disease.

ORBITAL IMAGING

Many articles are beginning to appear describing MRI for orbital disease. One potential danger with this technology is the setting in movement of unsuspected ferromagnetic orbital foreign bodies, with subsequent ocular damage. Wilson et al.[43] placed 7-mm foreign bodies (Teflon, Lucite, and dry pine) in fresh, nonembalmed cadaver heads. The eyes were inflated with air and saline to simulate in vivo conditions. A variety of imaging techniques were then used (ultrasound, CT, MRI, and plain x-ray). Plain x-ray films failed to detect the foreign bodies consistently. Both CT and MRI detected and localized the foreign bodies well, but CT was better in delineating object size and characterizing its composition. The authors conclude that CT is better; however, they used a 0.35- and 0.5-tesla magnet. With stronger magnets, the advantage of CT over MRI may not be realized. However, because of the potential dangers with MRI scanning, CT must be recommended over MRI in any patient with known, suspected, or unknown but potential ferromagnetic foreign bodies in the orbit.

A comprehensive review of echography for intraocular and intraorbital disease suggests that this technology is competitive in some instances with CT or MRI.[44]

For orbital use, most institutions are unable to obtain studies of the high quality that appear in this article. The one test that might be useful is the 30 degree test, which can help distinguish fluid vs. solid tissue enlargement of the optic nerve profile. If the enlargement of the optic nerve is due to fluid, the sheath measurement on A-mode echography 30 degrees from primary position will show decreased sheath width. Optic nerve enlargement due to glioma, meningioma, etc. will not show this change of width with the 30 degree test.

Two articles from the Neuroradiology Department at the University of Pennsylvania advanced the experience of high-grade MRI with orbital disease.[45] Fifty-nine patients with a variety of orbital disorders underwent 1.5-tesla imaging with surface-coil receptors. The authors found that orbital MRI done in this way provided information not available on CT scanning in (1) identifying lesions in the orbital apex, superior orbital fissure, and optic canal; (2) differentiating inflammatory pseudotumor from malignant neoplasm in clinically similar patients; (3) characterizing lesions containing hemorrhage or other paramagnetic material; (4) defining the posterior extent of ophthalmic pathway gliomas; and (5) detecting abnormal flow in intraorbital vascular structures.

Part of the difficulty with orbital MRI results from artifacts produced by orbital fat. Utilizing proton spectroscopic phase-dependent contrast MRI, the visualization of orbital lesions can be enhanced. This technique actually eliminates fat as a possible cause of high-intensity signal and obviates the need for long TR–long TE sequences, which are often degraded by motion artifact in the orbit. The result, and essentially edge enhancement, provides better visualization of lesions. There are disadvantages with the technique, however, in that there is an intentional introduction of a prominent artifact into the image, and there may be a slight underestimation of the dimensions of a mass lesion. However, this technique appears to offer great advantages in delineating orbital apex masses, including lesions of the optic nerve and its sheath.[46]

Finally, an article appeared utilizing positron emission tomography (PET) in the evaluation of orbital lymphoid tumors.[47] Five patients, one with malignant lymphoma, three with lymphoid hyperplasia, and one with scar tissue secondary to chronic inflammation, underwent PET scanning. The malignant lesion showed the most activity, the hyperplasia showed medium radioactivity, and the chronic inflammation showed low radioactivity with rapid clearance. Until we have a foolproof way to distinguish between benign and malignant orbital lymphoid lesions, all methods of accomplishing this determination should be explored.

REFERENCES

1. Savino PJ: The orbit, in Lessell S, van Dalen JTW (eds): *Current Neuro-ophthalmology*, vol 1. Chicago, Year Book Medical Publishers, 1988, pp 219–230.

2. Israele V, Nelson JD: Periorbital and orbital cellulitis. *Pediatr Infect Dis J* 1987; 62:404–410.

3. Spires JR, Smith RJH: Bacterial infections of the orbital and periorbital soft-tissues in children. *Laryngoscope* 1986; 96:763–767.

4. Ginsburg CM: Aerobic microbiology of upper respiratory infections in infants and children. *Pediatr Infect Dis J* 1987; 6:843–847.

5. Powell KR, Kaplan SB, Hall CB, et al: Periorbital cellulitis. *Am J Dis Child* 1988; 142:853–857.

6. Antoine GA, Grundfast KM: Periorbital cellulitis. *Int J Pediatr Otorhinolaryngol* 1987; 13:273–278.

7. Slavin ML, Glaser JS: Acute severe irreversible visual loss with sphenoethmoiditis: "Posterior" orbital cellulitis. *Arch Ophthalmol* 1987; 105:345–348.

8. Harris GJ: Subperiosteal inflammation of the orbit: A bacteriological analysis of 17 cases. *Arch Ophthalmol* 1988; 106:947–952.

9. Parfrey NA: Improved diagnosis and prognosis of mucormycosis. *Medicine* 1986; 65:113–123.

10. Kohn R, Hepler R: Management of limited rhino-orbital mucormycosis without exenteration. *Ophthalmology* 1985; 92:1440–1444.

11. Couch L, Theilen F, Mader JT: Rhinocerebral mucormycosis with cerebral extension successfully treated with adjunctive hyperbaric oxygen therapy. *Arch Otolaryngol Head Neck Surg* 1988; 114:791–794.

12. Van Johnson E, Kline LB, Julian BA, et al: Bilateral cavernous sinus thrombosis due to mucormycosis. *Arch Ophthalmol* 1988; 106:1089–1092.

13. Gamba JL, Woodruff WW, Djang WT, et al: Craniofacial mucormycosis: Assessment with CT. *Radiology* 1986; 160:207–212.

14. Shields JA, Bakewell B, Augsburger JJ, et al: Space-occupying orbital masses in children: A review of 250 consecutive biopsies. *Ophthalmology* 1986; 93:379–384.

15. Byrne BM, van Heuven WAJ, Lawton AW: Echographic characteristics of benign orbital Schwannomas (neurolemomas). *Am J Ophthalmol* 1988; 106:194–198.

16. Feinfield RE, Hesse RJ, Scharfenberg JC: Orbital angiolipoma. *Arch Ophthalmol* 1988; 106:1093–1095.

17. Orcutt JC, Char DH: Melanoma metastatic to the orbit. *Ophthalmology* 1988; 95:1033–1037.

18. Morales AG, Croxatto JO, Crovetto L, et al: Hydatid cysts of the orbit. *Ophthalmology* 1988; 95:1027–1032.

19. Boldt HC, Nerad JA: Orbital metastases from prostate carcinoma. *Arch Ophthalmol* 1988; 106:1403–1408.

20. Braffman BH, Bilaniuk LT, Eagle RC Jr, et al: MR imaging of a carcinoid tumor metastatic to the orbit. *J Comput Assist Tomogr* 1987; 11:891–894.

21. Manor RS, Sira IB: Amaurosis fugax at downward gaze. *Surv Ophthalmol* 1987; 31:411–416.

22. Gunning KEJ, Collett BJ: Spontaneous retrobulbar hemorrhage following anaesthesia. *Anaesthesia* 1987; 42:875–876.

23. Chen JC, Kucharczyk W: Nontraumatic orbital subperiosteal hematoma in a scuba diver: CT and MR findings. *J Comput Assist Tomogr* 1988; 12:504–506.

24. Jacobson DM, Itani K, Digre KB, et al: Maternal orbital hematoma associated with labor. *Am J Ophthalmol* 1988; 105:547–553.

25. Sacks SH, Lawson W, Edelstein D, et al: Surgical treatment of blindness secondary to intraorbital hemorrhage. *Arch Otolaryngol Head Neck Surg* 1988; 114:801–803.

26. Milne HL III, Leone CR, Kincaid MC, et al: Chronic hematic cyst of the orbit. *Ophthalmology* 1987; 94:271–277.

27. Shapiro A, Tso MOM, Putterman AM, et al: A clinicopathologic study of hematic cysts of the orbit. *Am J Ophthalmol* 1986; 102:237–241.

28. Pearson PA, Rakes SM, Bullock JD: *Am J Ophthalmol* 1986; 102:804–805.

29. Benson WE: Posterior scleritis. *Surv Ophthalmol* 1988; 32:297–316.

30. Johnson MH, DeFilipp GJ, Zimmerman RA, et al: Scleral inflammatory disease. *Am J Neuroradiol* 1987; 8:861–865.

31. White V, Rootman J, Quenville N, et al: Orbital lymphoproliferative and inflammatory lesions. *Can J Ophthalmol* 1987; 22:362–373.

32. Garrity JA, Kennerdell JS, Johnson BL, et al: Cyclophosphamide in the treatment of orbital vasculitis. *Am J Ophthalmol* 1986; 102:97–103.

33. Benson WH, Linberg JV, Weinstein GW: Orbital pseudotumor in a patient with AIDS. *Am J Ophthalmol* 1988; 105:697–698.

34. Jakobiec FA, Neri A, Knowles DM II: Genotypic monoclonality in immunophenotypically polyclonal orbital lymphoid tumors. *Ophthalmology* 1987; 94:980–994.

35. Reifler DM, Holtzman JN, Ringel DM: Sphenoid ridge meningioma masquerading as Graves' orbitopathy. *Arch Ophthalmol* 1986; 104:1591.

36. Barrett L, Glatt HJ, Burde RM, et al: Optic nerve dysfunction in thyroid eye disease: CT. *Radiology* 1988; 167:503–507.

37. Stranc M, West M: A four-wall orbital decomprssion for dysthyroid orbitopathy. *J Neurosurg* 1988; 68:671–677.

38. Kersten RC, Kulwin DR: Truamatic orbital decompression. *Am J Ophthalmol* 1988; 105:699–700.

39. Seiff SR, Shorr N: Nasolacrimal drainage system obstruction after orbital decompression. *Am J Ophthalmol* 1988; 106:204–209.

40. DeSanto L: Transantral orbital decompression, in Gorman C, Waller RR, Dyer JA (eds): *The Eye and Orbit in Thyroid Disease*. New York, Raven Press, 1984, pp 231–251.

41. Palmer D, Greenberg P, Cornell P, et al: Radiation therapy for Graves' ophthalmology: A retrospective analysis. *Int J Radiat Oncol Biol Phys* 1987; 13:1815–1820.

42. Sandler H, Rubenstein J, Fowble B, et al: Results of radiation therapy for thyroid ophthalmopathy (abstract). *Int J Radiat Oncol Biol Phys* 1988; 15:209–210.

43. Wilson WB, Dreisbach JN, Lattin DE, et al: Magnetic resonance imaging of non-metallic orbital foreign bodies. *Am J Ophthalmol* 1988; 105:612–617.

44. Byrne SF: Standardized echography of the eye and orbit. *Neuroradiology* 1986; 28:618–640.

45. Atlas SW, Bilaniuk LT, Zimmerman RA, et al: Orbit: Initial experience with surface coil spin-echo MR imaging at 1.5 T. *Radiology* 1987; 164:501–509.

46. Atlas SW, Grossman RI, Axel L, et al: Orbital lesions: Proton spectroscopic phase-dependent contrast MR imaging. *Radiology* 1987; 164:510–514.

47. Kiyosawa M, Ohmura M, Mizuno K, et al: F-FGD positron emission tomography in orbital lymphoid tumor. *Acta Soc Ophthalmol Jpn* 1985; 89:1329–1333.

PART SIX

OCULAR MANIFESTATIONS OF NEUROLOGIC DISEASE

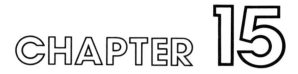

CHAPTER 15

Myasthenia Gravis

Dieter Schmidt, M.D.

Universitäts-Augenklinik, Freiburg, Federal Republic of Germany

In the last few years, an abundance of new publications has appeared on myasthenia gravis (MG). Papers by Balzereit et al.,[1] Haas,[2] Ravits[3] and Xian-Hao[4] give an overview of this disease.

Marsteller reported on the first American case of MG.[5] The illness of the Indian chief Opechankanough (d. 1644) was characteristic for MG. Historical accounts state that he was so weak he was unable to walk. There was improvement in his weakness after rest. His eyelids were so weak that they had to be raised by his attendants. Opechankanough's illness occurred 30 years before Thomas Willis' classic 1672 description of the disease.

OCULAR MYASTHENIA

The clinical findings of 43 patients with ocular signs among 60 patients with MG were compiled by Wade et al.[6] Twenty cases belonged to group I of the Osserman classification, 14 to group II, 5 to group III, and 3 to group IV. Ocular signs were found in 75% of all the patients. An isolated ptosis was seen in 16 out of 34 patients. Diplopia occurred in 21 patients (48.8%).

Saccadic eye movements of myasthenic eye muscle pareses were recorded by several scientists (Yee et al.,[7] Oohira et al.,[8] and Sollberger et al.[9]). It was the aim of the investigation by Yee et al. to differentiate myasthenic eye muscle pareses of 42 patients from other causes of ophthalmoplegia (26 patients with sixth

Curr Neuro Ophthalmol 2:257–292, 1989

cranial nerve palsy and 19 with chronic progressive external ophthalmoplegia, CPEO). It was striking that saccadic velocity measurements showed different characteristics in these groups: with the electro-oculographic (EOG) technique, significant decreases in mean velocities were found in MG patients compared with values in 28 normal subjects. The saccadic eye movement of 10 degrees in amplitude in normal subjects showed a velocity of 299 degrees/sec; in MG patients, 246 degrees/sec; in patients with sixth cranial nerve palsy, 184 degrees/sec; and in patients with CPEO, 168 degrees/sec. The authors demonstrated that measurement of peak velocity-amplitude relationships of saccades can be of diagnostic relevance in differentiating myasthenic eye muscle pareses from other causes of ophthalmoplegia. Myasthenic eye movement abnormalities can mimic cranial nerve palsies, CPEO, and internuclear ophthalmoplegia. The finding of normal velocity-amplitude relationships of saccades strongly suggests that MG is present. A total of 72% to 79% of MG patients had *saccadic velocities* within the normal range, whereas only 0% to 11% of cranial nerve palsy patients and 0% to 12% of CPEO patients had velocities within the normal range. However, the finding of abnormally low velocities does not help eliminate MG as a possible cause of ophthalmoplegia, since 21% to 28% of MG patients had velocities below the normal range.

Oohira et al. corroborated again, as shown in a previous publication by Yee et al.,[10] to show that myasthenic saccadic eye movements can demonstrate higher than normal velocities despite an ophthalmoplegia. A 38-year-old male with bilaterally restricted eye movements in all directions from MG—except for down gaze of the right eye—showed saccades of *supernormal velocity* in abduction and adduction of the right eye before treatment with prednisolone. Leftward saccades of both eyes were found to be much faster than normal after 10 days' treatment. At that time ptosis had improved and the ocular movement restriction had almost disappeared when the patient began to receive 80 mg of prednisolone on alternate days. The finding of persistent supernormal velocity of saccades means that the central adaptation mainly changed the pulse height during leftward saccades. Oohira et al. assume that the recovery of the conduction block may have been so fast in these gaze directions that the adaptation mechanism manifested itself at 10 days. However, after 1 year's treatment, the adaptation mechanism and the saccadic velocity had been decreased.

Sollberger et al. tried to determine which of the saccadic eye movement disorders can be detected in an early stage of the disease. Saccadic abnormalities were also found in clinically uninvolved eyes. The most frequent finding was *intersaccadic variation* (in 18 of 22 investigated patients with myasthenic eye muscle pareses). Two thirds of the patients showed intrasaccadic disorders as "decrescendo" of the velocity profiles. In addition, two thirds of the patients (had such postsaccadic abnormalities as an inability to hold steady eye position, called "waver" movements. Half of the cases demonstrated hypometric eye movements. It is emphasized that oculography led to the diagnosis in 4 of 9 patients with purely ocular myasthenia. "Stutter" was observed in 1 case and abnormally "slow" saccades in 3 cases. Suspected ocular myasthenia should be investigated in a questionable diagnosis by an edrophonium tonography test. Jacobson reported on a 33-year-old woman with 4 months of intermittent vertical diplopia.[11] She had a fluctuating right hypertropia and exotropia that increased with repeated measurements. There was no ptosis and she was able to fuse images intermittently for a few minutes. Results of edrophonium tonography were unequivocally positive.

Komiyama and Hirayama saw a *paradoxical reversal of ptosis* in MG caused by the administration of edrophonium to a 44-year-old woman and an 11-year-old girl.[12] The woman showed a severe left-sided ptosis, which developed approximately 1 year after thymectomy. Early in the morning, a transient ptotic right eyelid appeared, which decreased later in the day; however, a severe left persistent ptosis occurred. After the injection of 5 mg edrophonium, a paradoxical reversal of ptosis and, in addition, a reversed elevation of the eyebrows was obvious. The girl demonstrated an exacerbation of left ptosis which developed subsequent to physical exertion at the age of 11. In the morning she found a ptosis of her right eyelid. Shortly after, the ptosis shifted from right to left spontaneously. After the administration of 2 mg edrophonium, her left eyelid became retracted and her ptosis shifted from left to right. The authors explain this phenomenon (spontaneous shift of ptosis) by Hering's law of bilateral and equal levator muscle innervation. Fatigability of one eyelid was greater than that of the other. At this point edrophonium was more effective on the eyelid with the more pronounced defect.

Lid retraction in 4 of 150 patients with MG was the subject of another paper (Kansu and Subutay).[13] In a 26-year-old woman, right upper lid retraction was noted 1 month after thymectomy. It remained during the period of observation of the following 4 months. The right upper lid was 1 mm above the limbus, and her left eye was without ptosis (case 1). However, it is not mentioned if a motility disorder of the eyes, especially a paresis of elevation of the globe, also was present. Marked lid retraction of the left eye (3 mm above the limbus), which also occurred after thymectomy and again apparently without ptosis in the right eye, was noted in a 22-year-old man (case 4). The authors did not mention if there were continued restricted eye movements in all directions, which were present before thymectomy, in this patient; therefore, it is not clear if the lid retraction was due to an increased innervation of the upper eyelid coupled with an increased innervation of a paretic vertical eye muscle. It is a well-known phenomenon in patients with *unilateral ptosis* that, according to Hering's law of equal innervation of yoke muscles, the nervous system attempts to keep the eye open by increasing the level of innervation to the normal contralateral upper eyelid, leading to an upper lid retraction. This phenomenon might be an explanation for the unilateral ptosis and contralateral lid retraction in a 17-year-old woman (case 2) and a 24-year-old man (case 3). Smith, in discussing the paper by Kansu and Subutay, mentions patients who seemed to show unilateral lid retraction.[14] But modest ptosis of the contralateral upper lid was present, too. When the examiner's finger manually elevated the ptotic lid, the lid retraction of the other eye disappeared. Smith quoted the papers by Schechter[15] and Burde et al.,[16] who discussed these lid problems in their publications.

It is well known that approximately 90% of patients with MG eventually show involvement of extraocular muscles varying between an isolated eye muscle paresis and total external ophthalmoplegia. However, a rare sign of the motility disturbance in MG is represented by a *pseudointernuclear ophthalmoplegia* with downshoot of the adducting eye. This was observed in two patients with myasthenic eye muscle pareses, established by an edrophonium chloride test, and with an improvement of eye movements by treatment with pyridostigmine bromide or prednisone, respectively (Jay et al.[17]).

Not every patient complaining about intermittent diplopia suffers from MG, even if the Tensilon test seems to be positive. Rosenberg published case histories of two patients, a 55-year-old woman and a 28-year-old man, with *spasms of the near reflex* mimicking MG.[18] It was essential to ascertain that together with a marked esotropia the pupils became miotic. Particular attention must be paid to the observation of the pupil during episodes of diplopia.

DIAGNOSIS

Edrophonium Chloride Test

Quite often the Tensilon test is a useful office test for diagnosing MG. However, a mildly positive test result may occasionally be obtained from patients *without* MG. The conditions of patients with disorders of neuromuscular transmission such as Eaton Lambert Syndrome (ELS) or of some patients with amyotrophic lateral sclerosis can show improvement with Tensilon.[19] Daroff described his experience, together with Glaser, with positive Tensilon reactions in patients with cavernous sinus syndromes secondary to intracavernous aneurysms and lateral infiltrations by chromophobe adenomas, as well as in patients with cranial neuritis, and those with diabetic abducens paresis. In contrast, false-negative Tensilon responses were seen, too. It is emphasized that these occurred in patients with ocular motility problems without ptosis.

Younge and Bartley have stated that they are convinced that the Lancaster red-green test for diagnosing MG has almost never produced a false-positive response.[20] An aid in diagnosing MG, the well-known fatigue test of the upper eyelid ("test of enhanced ptosis"), was mentioned again by Gorelick.[21] This test should be combined with the edrophonium test. Edrophonium is of special importance in patients with neurotoxic poisoning from cobra stings.[22] Snake-venom neurotoxins binding to acetylcholine receptor (AChR) sites on the motor endplate produce effects similar to those of curare and MG. After the administration of edrophonium a significant improvement of symptoms, especially of the ptosis, occurred in ten investigated patients.

Icepack Test

Sethi et al. published a new test showing the improvement of ptosis by cold.[23] Ice wrapped in a towel was placed over the closed eye for 2 minutes. Eight of ten patients with MG demonstrated improvement of ptosis after local cooling.

Electromyogram

Double-step repetitive stimulation (RS) involves prolonged 3 Hz electrical stimulation to a peripheral nerve with and without limb ischemia. Gilchrist and Sanders investigated ten patients with MG.[24] They concluded that the double-step technique is slightly more sensitive than repetitive nerve stimulation to a proximal muscle. However, single-fiber electromyography showed an even greater sensitivity. Massey et al. demonstrated different *jitter measurements in single-fiber electromyography* in a 23-year-old woman with fluctuating ptosis and diplopia.[25] The disease severity throughout pregnancy and the postpartum period was paralleled by changes in single-fiber electromyography jitter measurements.

Neostigmine causes a postactivation repetition (PAR) that is generated by motor nerve endings. Roe et al. investigated ten patients, six with ocular MG and four with generalized MG.[26] They demonstrated that the PAR loss in patients with ocular myasthenia points to a motor-nerve-ending disorder. However, the reported changes in postjunctional structure were minimal and were correlated with small reductions in amplitude of microelectrode miniature endplate potentials (MEPPs).

CHILDHOOD MYASTHENIA

The follow-up observations of 23 children with childhood myasthenia were described by Descamps et al.[27] One patient had neonatal MG. The average age of the children (aged 0 to 15 years) was 11 years. Sixteen patients were 11 years or older. Fourteen patients had ptosis and 7 patients complained of diplopia; generalized muscular weakness occurred in 10 patients. Sixteen children underwent thymectomy. Only 56% of the children were improved 2 years after surgery. Thymus hyperplasia was found in 10 cases, and normal thymus tissue in 6. The authors advise against *routine* thymectomy in childhood myasthenia.

Congenital Myasthenia

Smit et al. published the cases of two boys with congenital myasthenia diagnosed in the first year of life.[28] Both patients showed similar clinical pictures: during pregnancy, decreased fetal movements and the appearance of congenital contractures were noted. Myasthenic crises occurred more often in the first 2 years of life than in later years. Pyridostigmine with ephedrine was beneficial during the exacerbations of the disease. Both boys showed a mild *fluctuating ptosis* and a regression of motor function, especially during febrile illnesses. In one patient, symptoms of ocular and generalized weakness recurred at the age of 3 years. Histopathologic studies from several muscle biopsies revealed no morphologic changes in the muscle fibers. In the first patient, 77% of the fibers were type I. In patient 2, 70% were type I. The ultrastructure of the endplates was investigated on the intercostal biopsy specimens, which revealed that the nerve terminals were grossly normal. A few terminals, however, were markedly elongated and extended over a distance of approximately 25 μm. The postsynaptic membrane had few if any infoldings. The postsynaptic membrane length was about half the control value. The reduced lengths were due to the paucity of secondary clefts. The *secondary synaptic cleft syndrome* is characterized by frequent circularly arranged clefts in cross-sections. This appearance is most likely explained by the existence of curved tubes and winding in the shallow postsynaptic sarcoplasm (Fig 1). The

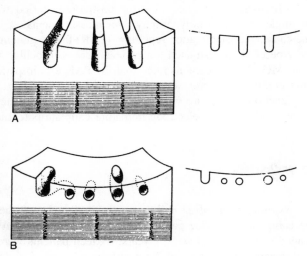

FIG 1.
Schematic drawings of postsynaptic cleft configuration in normal neuromuscular junction (**A**) and in neuromuscular junction of secondary synaptic cleft syndrome subject (**B**). (From Smit LME, et al: A myasthenic syndrome with congenital paucity of secondary synaptic clefts: CPSC syndrome. *Muscle Nerve* 1988; 11:337–438. Used by permission.)

synaptic defect in cleft development is likely to be expressed from the early stages of synapse formation. Microelectrode studies revealed that MEPPs were significantly reduced. Most probably a reduction in AChRs was mainly responsible for the decreased MEPPs amplitudes.

Neonatal MG

The development of neonatal MG was not related to the serum titer of maternal antiacetylcholine receptor antibodies (anti-AChR-abs), as shown in seven mothers with MG and their infants.[29] Serial serum determinations of total and "specific" anti-AChR IgG showed that (1) the decay in total IgG was within the normal range in all the babies, and (2) there was a shorter half-life of specific IgG in three of the cases, two of which were cases of neonatal MG. The amount of anti-AChR-abs transferred from mother to infant did not correlate with the development of neonatal MG.

Anti-AChR-ab titers in relation to the onset of neonatal MG in 30 children of myasthenic mothers were studied by Morel et al.[30] Affected newborns usually showed higher initial anti-AChR-ab titers than asymptomatic children, and among the former group the highest titers were usually observed in severely affected children. The mothers were classified into three groups according to anti-AChR-ab level at delivery. In the first group, comprising mothers with the highest antibody levels, eight of nine babies were affected. No baby had neonatal MG in the third group, which comprised mothers with the lowest antibody levels. In the group with high titers, *only one* baby was asymptomatic. In long-duration neonatal MG, anti-AChR-abs disappeared before clinical recovery. However, in short-duration neonatal MG, recovery sometimes preceded clearance of anti-AChR-abs. Two newborn infants with a severe form were treated by exchange transfusion. The anti-AChR-ab titer remained elevated after the first exchange in both cases, and then decreased rapidly.

It is important to point to the observation by Melber, who described a patient who became pregnant 3 months after the onset of MG.[31] Anti-AChR-ab were not detectable. The placental transfer of AChR-ab–negative serum produced transient neonatal MG. Her baby required intubation and mechanical ventilation for the first 27 days of life, and then recovered completely.

Familial Infantile MG

It has been shown in several publications that, unlike autoimmune MG, in familial infantile myasthenia (FIM) the ultrastructure of the neuromuscular junction is normal. Mora et al. looked for a morphologic correlate of the transmission failure in FIM, shown by abnormally decreased MEPP amplitudes when stimulated at 10 Hz.[32] In external intercostal muscles of three FIM patients, synaptic vesicles of nerve terminals were investigated before and after stimulation at 10 Hz for 10 minutes. The diameters of superficial and deep synaptic vesicles before stimulation were significantly smaller in the three FIM patients compared with the three normal controls. The abnormal decrease in quantal size in patients with FIM during prolonged 10-Hz stimulation could be caused by defects in (1) the facilitated uptake of choline by the nerve terminal, (2) acetylcholine resynthesis by choline acetyltransferase, or (3) the transport of acetylcholine molecules into the synaptic vesicles.

GENETICS

Thirteen of 44 patients with MG (30%) had positive family histories of autoimmune disease.[33] In all 13 families concerned, the affected relatives were related to the patients through the maternal line. A total of 12 unaffected relatives linked the affected relative to the MG patient. Investigation of human leukocyte antigens (HLA) coded for in the major histocompatibility systems revealed that HLA-B8 and HLA-DR3 were increased in patients with MG. This increase was highest among nonthymoma female patients with onset at less than 40 years of age. The authors reported a new finding of an increase in HLA-B5. This antigen was significantly increased in all younger-onset patients. In contrast, HLA-A3 was found in older-onset patients, including those with thymoma. None of the patients with thymoma were B8- or DR3-positive. Chiu et al. studied HLA phenotypes in 59 Chinese MG patients.[34] In comparison to 79 healthy control subjects, the patients showed increases of HLA-DRw9 (59.3%) and HLA-Bw 46 (47.5%), while HLA-DR3 was decreased (3.4%). Chiu et al.[35, 36] investigated 258 Chinese and 258 white patients with MG. They found that *ocular myasthenia* was approximately three times more common in Chinese patients, whereas the more severe forms were infrequent (grade IIb, 17%) or absent (grades III and IV). The predominant Gm haplotypes also differed greatly: in all Chinese patients G2m(n) allotypes were increased; this was also significant in patients with relatively high anti-AChR-titers. Zhi-Qiang described the findings of 7 patients with MG occurring in 3 families. All these patients showed ptosis and/or ophthalmoplegia of both eyes.[37] The good prognosis in long-term follow-up observation of familial MG is noted.

Murphy and Murphy published the case histories of identical twins with MG. Anti-AChR-abs were strongly positive in both twins.[38] Both patients showed bilateral ptosis and ophthalmoparesis as well as weakness of facial, oropharyngeal, and limb muscles. After thymectomy and steroid therapy a dramatic improvement occurred. Thymic histology showed follicular hyperplasia without thymoma.

Rosenberg[39] responded to the publication of Aoki et al.[40] concerning the viral etiology for MG in dependence of HLA-B8 phenotype. He emphasized that patients with HLA-B8 who have been exposed to the hepatitis B virus and develop antigenemia almost always clear the serologic evidence of infection and almost never develop chronic active hepatitis (CAH). Patients with a different HLA type, however, do not clear the antigen as well, and CAH occurs more frequently. The results of Wessel and Zitelli are worthy of note.[41] They raise the possibility of MG in a 15-year-old boy as the sole presenting clinical manifestation of human T-cell lymphotropic virus (HTLV-III) infection.

MYASTHENIA ASSOCIATED WITH OTHER DISEASES

The association of several autoimmune phenomena with MG has been described, such as heterozygous C2 deficiency associated with angioedema and systemic lupus erythematosus;[42] thymoma, multiple schwannomas, and monoclonal IgA gammopathy;[43] and multiple sclerosis and euthyroid restrictive Graves' ophthalmopathy.[44]

Ohno et al investigated the prevalence of MG in *Graves' disease* and found a low incidence of the diseases occurring in combination (0.14% out of 22,956 patients with Graves' disease).[45] Eight of 33 patients with both MG and Graves' disease developed MG first and 13 patients developed Graves' disease first. In 12 patients the two diseases occurred concurrently. Jimenez et al. found that 5% of 81 patients with MG had thyroid disease and 19.8% had subclinical hypothyroidism.[46] In 12.3% of the MG patients, antithyroid antibodies were positive without evidence of clinical thyroid disease.

Bowen and Kidd published the case of a 51-year-old woman complaining of diplopia and dysarthria due to MG.[47] At surgery, she showed a large mediastinal mass consisting of a malignant convoluted *lymphoblastic lymphoma*. This tumor had markers suggestive of an activated T helper/inducer cell phenotype. Treatment of the lymphoma led to resolution of MG. This case is further proof that immunoregulatory abnormalities may underlie the production of antibodies directed against AChR. Bramwell and Burns described a 36-year-old woman with an 8-year history of progressive muscular weakness of the arms and legs, who underwent thymectomy.[48] Histologic and electron microscopic examination of four "nodules" of the normally appearing thymus revealed proliferative clusters of Langerhans' cells, characteristic of *histiocytosis X*. In 5 patients, coexistent blepharospasm-oromandibular dystonia (Meige's disease) and MG were diagnosed (Kurlan et al. 1987).[49] Symptoms of Meige's disease preceded those of MG by several months in 1 patient, and symptoms of MG preceded those of Meige's disease in another. Three patients had simultaneous onsets. The authors emphasized that anti-AChR-ab titers were absent in 4 patients. The coexistence of two distinct neuromuscular diseases in one family is described by Maytal et al.[50] A 16-month-old baby girl presented with ptosis and bilateral ophthalmoparesis due to MG. Her mother and maternal grandmother showed definite signs of *myotonic dystrophy*.

The occurrence of MG after allogeneic *bone marrow transplantation* in 3 of 1,800 patients was reported by Bolger et al.[51] Symptoms of MG were observed after taper or discontinuation of immunosuppressive therapy. All patients developed anti-AChR-abs, and 1 patient had antibody formation to striated muscle.

ANTIBODIES

Seronegative MG

Soliven et al. found that the clinical characteristics of seronegative patients did not differ from patients with high antibody titer.[52] There are several possible explanations for seronegative cases, an important one being that the standard radioimmunoassay does not detect antibodies specifically directed against the toxin binding site. Of 221 patients with MG, 18.5% had no detectable antibodies to AChRs. Seven of 14 patients with ocular symptoms for more than 2 years, as well as 25 of 145 (17%) patients with generalized MG were seronegative.

However, special myasthenic congenital syndromes exist without detectable antibodies. Oosterhuis et al. reported two patients with the "slow channel syndrome," representing a congenital myasthenic syndrome with degeneration of junctional folds and diffusely thickened endplate basal lamina with a prolonged open time of the acetylcholine induced ion channel.[53] The clinical picture with absence of anti-AChR-abs, poor response to anticholinesterases, and the decrement at 3 Hz of stimulation in the EMG of the hand muscles is characteristic of this syndrome.

Three patients with *anti-AChR-ab–negative MG* were described by Hoogenraad and Meyling.[54] Antibodies directed to reticulin (A-Ret) were detected. It is probable that this form of MG is caused by an antibody to a *determinant at the neuromuscular junction (NMJ)* other than the AChR. The exact nature of the antigenic structure remains to be determined. Candidates for such an antigen would be proteins that have been found in the NMJ, such as vinculin, filamin, and α-actinin. Anti-AChR-ab titer does not always correlate with the severity of the clinical manifestations.[55] Filamin and vinculin exist in skeletal muscle; filamin is enriched on the Z-disk as well as at their peripheries, vinculin is concentrated in the subsarcolemmal region and at the peripheries of the Z-disks. Antifilamin and antivinculin antibody activities are significantly higher in MG patients compared with controls. The antifilamin antibody titer was highly positive (100%) in patients with ocular myasthenia.

Antibodies against saline-soluble components of skeletal muscle in MG were found by Komiyama et al.[56] In four of seven patients with ocular MG without anti-AChR-abs, low but appreciable levels of anti-saline-extract antibodies were detected.

Cerebral Disorders

Muscle anti-AChR-abs in the sera of patients with MG do not bind to human brain AChRs.[57] This finding means that the AChR in the brain is antigenically distinct from the AChR in skeletal muscle. Anti-CNS (central nervous system) antibodies in neurologic and psychiatric disorders were tested by Plioplys et al.[58] However, there were no significant differences in the numbers and locations of IgG immunoreactive bands between the various diagnostic groups and the controls. The investigation of immunoactivation in the CNS in patients with MG was performed by Müller et al.[59] The cerebrospinal fluid (CSF) of 44 MG patients was examined: altogether, 73% of the patients had some protein and/or cellular abnormality, 50% showed lymphoid reaction, and 37.5% showed an enrichment of anti-AChR-abs.

AChR

Cloning studies suggest there are at least five types of nicotinic acetylcholine receptors (n-AChRs) with different amino acid sequences. The difference between muscle and neuronal receptors is that most neuronal receptors are not blocked by α-bungarotoxin, which blocks the muscle type nearly irreversibly.[60] The n-AChR is a membrane-bound allosteric protein with two primary acetylcholine binding sites. The regions of the molecule that form the two major functional domains are the acetylcholine binding sites and the agonist-gated ion channel.[61]

Antibodies Against AchR

Oger et al. modified Lindstrom's and Tindall's techniques of measuring serum anti-AChR-abs.[62] With this new method they found that only 1 of 43 patients with generalized MG had no anti-AChR-abs. Toyka and Heininger confirmed that 99% of 340 patients with generalized MG had titers above 0.5 nmol/L.[63] The standard immunoprecipitation assay was used with detergent-extracted and ^{125}I-α-bungarotoxin (αBUTX) marked human AChRs as antibodies. Illa et al. found anti-AChR-abs in 84.4% of patients with MG.[64] Patients with MG and thymoma had higher levels of abs than patients without a tumor. This finding was confirmed by Penn et al.[65] The course of antibody titers of MG patients was investigated by Zeitlhofer et al.[66] Among 18 patients, two groups were differentiated: patients with relatively constant titers and those with fluctuating titers.[66] Patients with severe disease showed a slightly increased antibody titer. But Hinman et al.[67] and Lebrun-Grandie et al.[68] found no significant correlation between the titer of anti-AChR-abs and the patient's functional status.

Oda and Shibasaki used a new method to detect antibodies that react with extracellularly exposed antigenic determinants of AChR of cultured rat muscle.[69] The antibody titer did not correlate with clinical severity, but the ability of antibodies to bind to extracellularly exposed AChRs correlated well. The titer of autoantibodies does not correlate well with severity of symptoms. It is suggested that the α-BUTX assay may detect a mixture of pathogenic and nonpathogenic antibodies.[70] The antibodies in four of eight patients with MG were of a single light chain type; the others comprised different types. Studies by Lefvert and Holm have shown that the majority of antibodies of patients with MG were IgM; all of the antibodies had lambda light chains.[71]

DRUG-INDUCED MG

Penicillamine is an amino acid, named by Abraham et al., that was isolated from an acid hydrolysate of penicillin.[72] The clinical pharmacokinetics of penicillamine is summarized by Netter et al.[73] Two stereoisomers of penicillamine exist, but only the *D-isomer* is used therapeutically. D-Penicillamine (DPA) is rapidly but incompletely (40% to 70%) absorbed in the intestine. The peak plasma concentrations occur within 1 to 3 hours after ingestion. The concentration in plasma decreases rapidly then. More than 80% of plasma DPA is bound to proteins, particularly *albumin,* and to a lesser extent to α-globulins and ceruloplasmin. The rest is mainly in the free reduced form or as disulphides. Only a small portion of the dose is metabolized in the liver to S-methyl-DPA. The route of elimination is mainly renal. The plasma concentrations of DPA during long-term treatment show large individual variations for a given daily dose. Investigations have shown that there is no relationship between plasma concentrations and the appearance of side effects.

Kuncl et al. discussed the probable pathophysiology of DPA-induced *MG* (PMG).[74] A 57-year-old man who suffered from a disabling rheumatoid arthritis was treated with DPA (500 mg twice daily) for 20 months. He developed intermittent diplopia, a fatigue-dependent ptosis, and noted discomfort on swallowing. *Cogan's lid twitch sign* was present. After the administration of edrophonium chloride the ptosis resolved within 30 seconds. DPA was discontinued, and pyridostigmine treatment improved the patient's condition. After 6 months he was asymptomatic and required no pyridostigmine. The patient's initial serum showed a mild elevation of anti-AChR-ab level. However, after recovery there were no detectable anti-AChR-abs. The patient's initial serum produced significant blockade of AChR binding sites in vitro. Following recovery, blocking activity could not be detected anymore. The rate of degradation of AChRs in vitro was increased significantly by the initial serum of this patient. Yet, the "recovery" serum of the patient with PMG had no effect on AChR degradation. The deltoid muscles of the patient were biopsied at 2 weeks and at 8 months after cessation of treatment with

DPA. The first biopsy of the patient's muscle revealed that the junctional AChR count was significantly reduced. However, the second biopsy showed more than double the number of AChRs with a recovery into the normal range. The authors discuss several possible mechanisms causing the reduction of AChRs by DPA. They claim for the hypothesis that there is an *initiation of a new drug-induced autoimmune state* rather than an enhancement of ongoing subclinical MG. A direct toxic effect of DPA on the AChRs seems to be unlikely because the AChRs' turn-overs with halftimes of 5 to 13 days mean that AChRs will probably have largely recovered after discontinuance of therapy. It is assumed that the patient's normal number of AChRs reflects not only his state at recovery but also the premorbid state. Therefore, prior ongoing autoimmune MG seems to be unlikely.

Additional publications deal with PMG and with the patient's complete recovery after stopping treatment with DPA-therapy: Huaux and Delreux reported on 2 patients suffering from rheumatoid arthritis for many years.[75] Both patients developed such eye signs as ophthalmoparesis and ptosis after the administration of DPA. HLA-DR1-BW35 was present in both patients. Martin et al. published the cases of 4 patients with rheumatoid arthritis who showed myasthenic pareses after treatment with DPA.[76] The patients showed myasthenic eye muscle pareses appearing 12, 17, 19, and 13 months, respectively, after the initiation of therapy. Anti-aChR-abs were present in 2 patients. The authors mention that 156 rheumatoid patients with myasthenia following treatment with DPA have been reported since 1973 when Miehlke described his first observations. The case of a 57-year-old woman with rheumatoid arthritis and treatment with DPA for approximately 10 months showing no spontaneous ventilation after anesthesia for an ankle arthroplasty operation was published by Fried and Protheroe.[77] On the morning of the first day after surgery she had marked bilateral ptosis and ophthalmoplegia.

In a prospective study, Kolarz and Maida observed 13 patients with rheumatoid arthritis who received DPA for more than 1 year.[78] The anti-AChR-abs were tested in every patient. In two of these cases an elevated titer of antibodies was found without clinical signs or symptoms of MG. In addition, a 63-year-old woman with rheumatoid arthritis was described who received a daily dose of 250 to 500 mg of DPA from 1978 until 1982. Then she complained of diplopia, lasting only some days. However, in July 1983, she developed a myasthenic syndrome. Anti-AChR-abs have been found in the sera since 1981, i.e., 1½ years before the temporary diplopia. Therefore, the authors discuss the question whether anti-AChR-abs should be measured routinely in every patient receiving D-PA.

Chloroquine.—Sghirlanzoni et al. described a myasthenia-like syndrome after chloroquine therapy.[79] Examination revealed ptosis, bilateral facial weakness, nasal speech, difficulty in chewing, and dysphagia, as well as fatigability of all extremities. Ten days after chloroquine withdrawal the ocular symptoms improved. Over the following 6 months all myasthenic symptoms gradually receded. Ocular symptoms reappeared following a second, short course of chloroquine.

Antibiotics.—Antibiotics are most frequently implicated as causing MG or aggravating preexisting MG. Among the antibiotics, the most dangerous ones to patients with MG are aminoglycosides, but polypeptide antibiotics, tetracyclines, lincomycin, and clindamycine phosphate have also been reported to be harmful. Argov et al. published a report of two patients with MG who were treated with prednisone and pyridostigmine after thymectomy.[80] After treatment with ampicillin their myasthenic symptoms consistently worsened with treatments. When antibiotic therapy was discontinued, the symptoms improved within a few days.

Experimental Autoimmune MG.— Four rabbits and five rats showed that ampicillin increased the preexisting electrical decrement.[80] The animals developed general muscle weakness, disturbance in swallowing, and difficulties in breathing, and showed transitory improvement 30 to 60 seconds after the administration of edrophonium hydrochloride. None of the three healthy control rats showed any decrement after ampicillin administration.

Magnesium.— A report of a pre-eclamptic patient who was virtually quadriplegic after magnesium administration was published by Bashuk and Krendel.[81] Supramaximal repetitive 2-Hz median nerve stimulation revealed a decrement in amplitude. One month later there was no detectable weakness but single-fiber electromyography revealed markedly increased jitter and blocking. Her AChR-ab level was markedly elevated.

Trihexyphenidyl.— Ueno et al. discussed the occurrence of MG in a 55-year-old man with idiopathic Parkinson's disease shortly after the administration of 4 mg trihexyphenidyl (THP).[82]

One week after the start of this therapy, the patient noticed ptosis, diplopia, and weakness of shoulder and neck muscles. An increase of THP improved the tremor, although the weakness was worse and dysphagia occurred in addition. Two weeks' administration of pyridostigmine bromide showed no benefit. However, withdrawal of THP was followed by an improvement of myasthenic symptoms. Thymectomy resulted in transient improvement of the myasthenia. The thymus showed hyperplastic changes with few germinal centers. The severity of MG was closely correlated with the serum level of THP but not with that of anti-AChR-ab.

Contrast Agents.— Goldhammer et al. emphasized that the routine use of contrast enhancement in computed tomography of the mediastinum is not essential for the detection of a thymoma.[83] Three patients were described with myasthenic crisis after the intravenous administration of iodinated contrast agents. Hilton-Jones called attention to the administration of iothalamic acid (Conray) in myasthenic patients, too.[84] These three observations underline the caution necessary in using iodinated contrast agents in patients with MG. Contrary to that, Frank et al. reviewed the records of 136 patients with MG who had at least one radiologic procedure involving intravenously administered contrast media.[85] Contrast agents used included a combination of diatrizoate meglumine and diatrizoate sodium and a combination of iothalamate meglumine and iothalamate sodium. Seven of the 136 patients (5.1%) with MG showed contrast reactions. But the authors suggest that in five cases the increase of weakness could be explained by reasons *other* than contrast administration. Only one patient with increased respiratory muscle weakness showed frank respiratory arrest, which was most likely due to recurrent pulmonary embolism. Based on this experience the authors conclude that MG is not a contraindication to a contrast radiographic procedure.

Cardiovascular Agents.—Cardiovascular agents seemed to be responsible for myasthenic signs and symptoms in a 65-year-old man who developed severe eye muscle pareses 20 days after the administration of *etafenone* 2'-(2 diethylamino-ethoxy)-3-phenylpropiophenon, a calcium antagonistic agent, and *peruvoside* (a semisynthetic glycoside). After the administration of edrophonium chloride, no clinical improvement was observed. However, repetitive nerve stimulation at 3 cls of the ulnar nerve revealed a 30% decrement of the third response of the compound muscle action potential. Stimulation at 20 cls showed a progressive decrement of the response. Peruvoside and etafenone therapy was discontinued, and the patient's condition improved slowly. Within 1 week the patient gradually recovered, and completely normal ocular motility was observed.[85a]

Donnet et al. published the case of a 40-year-old woman who showed myasthenia-like signs after intoxication with ciguatera.[86]

EATON-LAMBERT SYNDROME

O'Neill et al. compiled the clinical findings of 50 consecutive patients with Eaton-Lambert syndrome (ELS).[87] Twenty-five patients had carcinomas, 21 had small cell lung cancers, which were poorly differentiated in 5 cases. The tumor was within the thoracic cavity in 24 of the 25 patients. One patient developed symptoms of ELS 4 years before discovery of a breast carcinoma. The other 25 cases had no carcinoma. The follow-up period in this group was over 5 years in 14 cases, and longer than 10 years in 2. Symptoms of ELS preceded diagnosis of the tumor by 5 months to 3.8 years in 17 of the 24 patients with an intrathoracic malignancy. In only 1 case did tumor diagnosis occur first, by an interval of 2 months. Eighteen patients (72%), all with thoracic cavity tumors, were regular smokers, with a mean consumption of 24 cigarettes per day. By contrast, only 9 (36%) of the noncarcinoma group of ELS were smokers, with a mean consumption of 18 cigarettes daily. The neurologic features were similar in the carcinoma group and in the noncarcinoma group. They consisted of proximal lower limb weakness, depressed tendon reflexes with post-tetanic potentiation, autonomic features, and mild to moderate ptosis. The presenting symptom was leg weakness in 62%, generalized weakness in 12%, and autonomic dysfunction in 6%. Cranial nerve symptoms, usually mild and transient, were experienced by 70% of patients, *diplopia* and *drooping of the eyelids* being the most common. Despite the frequency of transient diplopia as a complaint, clinical evidence of external ophthalmoplegia was not observed. Signs of autonomic dysfunction were seen in 6 cases with a sluggish pupillary reaction to light. Associated immunological disorders such as thyroid diseases, vitiligo, pernicious anemia, celiac disease, and juvenile-onset diabetes were seen more often in the noncarcinoma group of ELS patients than in the carcinoma group. Organ-specific autoantibodies (thyroid, stomach, skeletal muscle) were detected in 34% of all patients, and non–organ-specific antibodies were detected in 42%. Elevated serum anti-AChR-abs were detected in none. An intravenous edrophonium chloride test was performed in 21 patients. The results were negative in 5 patients, equivocal in 2, and positive in 14. The analysis indicates that a patient presenting with ELS has a 62% risk of an underlying small cell lung cancer. This risk declines sharply after 2 years, becoming very low at 4 to 5 years.

Heath et al.[88] described two patients, 59 and 72 years old, who had ELS for more than 10 years without evidence of underlying malignancy. *Autonomic function,* including the pupil cycle time, was severely abnormal in both patients. It is important to note that very rarely a *congenital ELS* can occur (Bady et al.[89]). A 4-year-old girl who had been hypotonic and areflexic since birth showed a delayed motor development. The incremental response at rapid rates of stimulation—noted at 3 years—was strongly suggestive of ELS. Guanidine hydrochloride induced a significant increase in muscle tone.

Very limited information exists with regard to *respiratory muscle involvement* in ELS. Wilcox et al. describe a 68-year-old woman who noted intermittent drooping of her eyelids and occasional double vision.[90] Biopsy of a mediastinal lymph node showed a poorly differentiated large cell bronchogenic carcinoma. Repetitive inspiratory pressure measurements and the electromyographic response to phrenic nerve stimulation established involvement of the diaphragm and the inspiratory muscles in general. The authors recommend regular screening using measurements of respiratory muscle strength in patients with ELS in order to determine the need for pharmacologic therapy.

Respiratory failure was also observed in a 63-year-old woman with ELS several hours after starting therapy with verapamil, a calcium channel blocking agent.[91] The temporal relationship to the deterioration of the patient's condition suggests that calcium channel blockers should be used cautiously in patients with ELS. Patients showing combined features of autoimmune MG and ELS were described by Oh et al.[92] and Taphoorn et al.[93] The combined occurrence of both diseases is called *overlap myasthenic syndrome.* Tannier et al. published a report of the rare combination of diseases in a 57-year-old man who showed an inappropriate secretion of antidiuretic hormone manifested by *hyponatremia* (Schwartz-Bartter syndrome) together with ELS.[94] Features included small-cell carcinoma of the lung and demyelinating peripheral neuropathy. Tendon reflexes were absent. Atrophy of proximal limb muscles was noticed. The repetitive nerve stimulation test showed a pattern consistent with ELS. The patient was successfully treated with guanidine.

The combined occurrence of two unusual diseases in a 56-year-old woman who showed systemic *lupus erythematosus* and ELS was described by Hughes and Katirji.[95] No systemic neoplasm was found. Treatment with plasmapheresis produced clinical and electrophysiologic improvement of ELS; however, symptoms of her systemic lupus erythematosus were not changed by this therapy.

The autoimmune etiology of ELS was documented by the responsiveness of ELS to plasmapheresis and immunosuppressive drug therapy, as well as by the association of non-neoplastic ELS with other autoimmune disorders and by the *passive transfer* of the electrophysiologic and morphologic features of the disease from humans to mice after ELS-IgG injection (Fukuoka et al.[96, 97]). The mouse passive-transfer model demonstrated a loss of active-zone particles at the freeze-fractured presynaptic membrane of the motor endplate. A paucity and disorganization of the active zones and clusters of 10 to 12 nm particles appeared. In mice treated with ELS-IgG, the initial alteration in the active zone was a decrease in the distance between particles in a given row and between adjacent rows of an array. The parallel orientation of the rows was disturbed and the arrays became clusters. The findings are consistent with the theory that ELS-IgG binds to the active-zone particles of the presynaptic membrane and modulates their density. The active zones are targets of the pathogenic ELS autoantibodies.

Furthermore, Login et al. found in rat anterior pituitary cells that IgG from patients with ELS inhibit calcium-dependent hormone secretion.[98] Pituitary cells may represent one among several "nonsynaptic" tissues with calcium channel activity susceptible to ELS-IgG. It is postulated that ELS-IgG modulates antigenic sites of anterior pituitary cells, which may share properties with similar presynaptic elements at the neuromuscular junction.

Kim and Neher showed that IgG antibodies from patients with ELS block calcium channels of test cells (bovine adrenal chromaffin cells).[99] This phenomenon can account for the presynaptic impairment characteristics of this disorder. An ultrastructural study of the motor endplate from patients with ELS revealed no changes in the presynaptic region.

In addition, no hypertrophy of the junctional folds of endplates was found.[100] Alterations of the motor endplate, decrease in membrane length and density, were restricted to the postsynaptic region.

THYMUS

Grody et al. emphasized the importance of finding germinal centers in thymectomy specimens from patients with MG or ELS.[101] This finding is highly dependent on the extent of sectioning of the gland. Isaacson detected a significant population of B lymphocytes in normal thymic tissue.[102] Therefore, the thymus can no longer be regarded as an organ exclusively concerned with T-cell function. *Myoid cells* of thymuses from 47 patients with MG were rare. They were located mainly in the medullary epithelial area.[103] Although myoid-cell AChRs appear antigenically similar to extrajunctional muscle AChRs, these cells did not appear to be foci of immunologic stimulation. Matsumoto et al.[104] investigated cultures of 19 thymuses with hyperplasia from patients with MG. They found no significant difference in the morphology of epithelial cells between thymuses from MG patients and those from 12 normal controls. In addition, there was no significant difference in the distribution of AChRs on the epithelial cells between the thymuses from MG patients and those from normal thymuses. Investigations of non-neoplastic thymus from 20 patients with MG revealed three types of histologic findings:[105]

1. Thymitis with lymphoid follicular hyperplasia (11 cases).
2. Thymitis with diffuse B-cell infiltration (5 cases).
3. Thymic atrophy (4 cases).

Morphologically the thymuses from ten consecutive patients with MG showed lymphofollicular hyperplasia in nine cases and benign thymoma in one case. The paramount feature was the intimate association of myoid cells with *interdigitating reticulum cells*. They were surrounded by T3+ lymphocytes in thymus medulla.[106] Morphometric studies confirmed that the great majority of myoid cells were in intimate contact with intramedullary interdigitating reticulum cells. This was less frequent in thymuses from nonmyasthenic subjects.[107] Tumor-free thymuses from MG patients and control patients contained cytoplasmic AChR epitopes and α-bungarotoxin binding sites on myoid cells and on some epithelial cells. Only myoid cells also expressed extracellular main immunogenic region (MIR) epitopes, suggesting that they bear complete AChRs, and that they are important targets for the autoimmune attack in tumor-free MG thymuses.[108]

The rare occurrence of a squamous cell carcinoma of the thymus in a 58-year-old patient with bilateral ptosis, facial diplegia, absence of palatal movement, and generalized muscle weakness was published by Di Mario et al.[109]

THYMOMA

Visualization of the anterior junction line on x-ray chest films renders unlikely the presence of a thymoma. This structure is found in approximately 40% of all high-quality posteroanterior chest films. It becomes visible as the thymus regresses after puberty.[110]

Thymoma and MG

Lewis et al. examined 283 patients with thymoma (aged 16 to 90): 46% had MG and 10% showed other paraneoplastic phenomena.[111] Twenty-two years is the longest reported interval for the appearance of metastatic thymoma and MG after the diagnosis and apparent cure of a primary thymoma.[112] A 62-year-old woman who presented in myasthenic crisis 22 years after radiation and chemotherapy of an invasive thymoma showed an isolated hepatic metastasis.

Bailey et al. published the case of an 81-year-old man with the combination of MG, thymoma, and *red blood cell aplasia*.[113] In contrast, two cases of a *neuromuscular hyperactivity* syndrome associated with a proliferative thymoma and high serum titers of AChR-abs showed no signs of MG. The electrodiagnostic findings indicated generalized cholinergic hyperactivity at the neuromuscular junction.[114] Sanders and Howard also reported three patients without MG who showed thymomas.[115] Single-fiber electromyography demonstrated abnormal neuromuscular transmission with increased jitter. The authors concluded that all patients with thymoma should be suspected of having MG.

The association of MG and ELS, an overlap syndrome, in a 42-year-old man with thymoma was described by Tabbaa et al.[116] High anti-AChR-ab titers were found.

Witt and Bolton published the case of a 41-year-old man showing symptoms of MG and additional changes consistent with an *asymmetrical motor neuropathy* as a cause of muscle atrophy.[117] At surgery, a lymphoepithelial, locally invasive thymoma was found.

Kawanami et al. isolated by affinity chromatography from human thymoma cobrotoxin-binding protein.[118] It is suggested that the cobrotoxin-binding protein has subunits similar to fish electric organs or mammalian muscles.

Antibodies

Aarli et al. detected that sera from 56 out of 66 patients (85%) with thymoma contained citric acid antibodies, while such antibodies were detected in only 6 of 75 (8%) of the nonthymoma patients.[119]

Three monoclonal antibodies that bind to the α-subunit of the AChR of Torpedo, Calif, were tested in patients with thymomas by Kirchner et al.[120] They found that the extent of a positive reaction with the anti-AChR monoclonal antibodies in the thymomas correlated with the manifestation of MG.

However, Willcox et al., who performed an immunohistologic study of thymomas from 23 patients with MG and 7 without, detected no major differences in 5 of 7 samples from nonmyasthenics.[121] They concluded that most thymoma patients risk development of MG. Chilosi et al. investigated 8 thymuses of patients with thymoma in order to assess the proportion of proliferating thymocytes.[122] It is suggested that intensive thymocyte proliferation in thymomas may represent one of the factors which lead to autoimmunity in MG and thymomas.

Lymphocyte subsets were examined using OKT series monoclonal antibodies and flow cytometry in the thymomas of 16 patients. These lymphocyte subsets showed three different types of thymomas: (1) thymus lymphocyte, (2) peripheral lymphocyte, and (3) intermediate. In thymus lymphocyte type the numbers of OKT-6$^+$ cells are more than 50%, in peripheral lymphocyte type, the numbers of OKT-6$^+$ cells are less than 10%.[123]

DRUG THERAPY

Immunosuppressive Therapy

1. Azathioprine.—A total of 104 patients with generalized MG treated with azathioprine (AZA) for a median period of 29 months (range, 1 month to 12 years) were surveyed for adverse reactions by Hohlfeld et al.[124] It was not always possible to differentiate between the complications of MG itself and those of AZA therapy and corticosteroids, sometimes given additionally. Adverse reactions occurred in 36 patients (35%): hematologic side effects in 18%, gastrointestinal side effects in 13%, major infectious diseases in 13%, and elevation of liver enzymes in 6%. The cause of death in the 9 patients who died during the follow-up period (up to 12 years) was related to myasthenic crisis in 2 patients. Malignant tumors were diagnosed in 5 cases.

Sixteen patients with MG who failed to improve 3 years after thymectomy or 6 months after prednisone therapy were treated with AZA.[125] Ten were considered definite responders, and six patients showed little or no response. The only laboratory value that correlated with clinical improvement was mean corpuscular volume (MCV) of the blood. A total of 81% of all patients revealed a rise in MCV while taking AZA. The development of macrocytosis, as opposed to leukopenia, may be due to the gradual increment of AZA dosage.

Kern and Stewart described two patients with MG, a 70-year-old woman and a 76-year-old man, who developed *Listeria monocytogenes meningitis* during therapy with AZA and prednisone.[126] It is emphasized that *L. monocytogenes* is the most frequent cause of meningitis in chronically immunosuppressed patients, in renal and cardiac transplant recipients, and in patients with malignancy.

A severe *pancytopenia* was caused by interaction of AZA and allopurinol in a 62-year-old man with MG and hyperuricemia. After both drugs had been discontinued, hematological side effects were mostly reversible. A tendency towards macrocytosis, however, remained. The occurrence of adverse effects after AZA therapy is the reason for Fischer's arguments: since either steroids or plasmapheresis can stabilize patients for surgery, there is little point in advocating long-term AZA therapy in the treatment of MG.[127] This drug should probably be used only in the most therapy-resistant cases.

2. Cyclosporin.—Twenty patients with progressively worsening generalized MG whose illnesses were not controlled by anticholinesterase therapy were randomly assigned either to cyclosporine therapy or placebo. The double-blind clinical trial of patients between the ages of 40 and 75 years, published by Tindall et al.,[128] showed that at 6 months and especially at 12 months after therapy patients in the cyclosporin group had had significantly more objective improvement in strength than patients in the control group. Nephrotoxicity occurred in three patients receiving cyclosporin and was reversible with discontinuation of the drug.

Nyberg-Hansen and Gjerstad reported on six patients with generalized MG who were treated with cyclosporin.[129] Three of these had previously used AZA without satisfactory improvement. In five patients cyclosporin therapy showed a moderate to marked improvement in muscle strength and fatigability. In one patient the effect was slight to moderate. The period of therapy was up to 34 months.

3. Combined Chemotherapy.—Combination chemotherapy with cyclophosphamide, Adriamycin, and vincristine in malignant thymoma and MG was used in five patients by Kosmidis et al.[130] Two patients with MG resistant to antimyasthenic drugs responded immediately to this regimen. The two patients with MG showed a thymoma with histologic characteristics of epithelial predominance.

4. Corticosteroid Therapy.—Ellis emphasized the importance of the adverse effects of corticosteroid therapy, especially during childhood: retardation of growth, development of cataract, osteoporosis, and avascular necrosis of the femoral head.[131]

Anticholinesterase Agents

The effectiveness of pyridostigmine therapy in ten patients with MG between the ages of 20 and 68 years was investigated by Milner-Brown et al.[132] In seven patients, a positive correlation between plasma pyridostigmine levels and the mean percent improvement of neuromuscular function was demonstrated. The acute effects of a single intravenous neostigmine injection (0.5 mg) on lung function before and during bicycle ergometry were measured in 15 patients with MG by Haber et al.[133] Lung function parameters of 15 patients showed a normal total lung capacity with an increase in functional residual capacity and residual volume, while vital capacity was diminished. There was a significant increase in airway resistance. The authors conclude that *dyspnea* in patients with MG can also be caused by therapy.

The treatment of myasthenic crises should be with continuously administered intravenous pyridostigmine infusion therapy, according to Janda and Brandstetter.[134] The side effects of pyridostigmine therapy in MG can be a major problem, consisting of diarrhea, excessive sweating, and salivation in some patients. Instead of the use of antidiarrheals and atropine sulfate, Grogan recommended another antimuscarinic agent, scopolamine hydrobromide, which has a slightly better effect on secretory glands than atropine.[135] Therefore, transdermal therapy is recommended. A 33-year-old man with MG who was treated with high-dose pyridostigmine (685 mg daily) together with atropine, prednisone, and AZA complained of abdominal colic. This was accompanied by nonbloody diarrhea and vomiting. Laparotomy revealed a 10-cm cecocolon-intussusception, which was easily reduced operatively. Pyridostigmine increases gastrointestinal motility. Murray and Baynes reasoned that the drug must have contributed to the formation of an intussusception in this case.[136]

Plasmapheresis

Three severely incapacitated patients with ocular myasthenia were treated with repeated plasmapheresis after unsatisfactory response to anticholinesterase and steroid therapy.[137] All three patients showed relief of symptoms within days, lasting weeks to months after plasmapheresis treatment.

Thorlacius et al. performed a plasma exchange (PE) in 20 patients with MG.[138] Detailed studies in 6 of these patients showed a considerable fall in the concentration of anti-AChR-ab after therapy. At the termination of the fifth PE, anti-AChR-abs were not detectable in the serums of 2 patients, while in 3 patients approximately 50% of the pre-PE values were still detectable. The clinical improvement was maximal during the week after PE, and correlated in time with increasing concentrations of anti-AChR-abs.

Gammaglobulin and Immunoglobulin Therapy

Arsura et al. administered high-dose intravenous immunoglobulin (400 mg/kg) to 12 patients with MG[139] and to 9 patients at the onset of an exacerbation of generalized MG.[140] The authors report in 1986 that 11 of 12 treated patients improved, beginning 3.6 ± 2.7 days after the start of treatment, with sustained improvement lasting 52 ± 37 days. There were no significant changes in anti-AChR-ab titers. Immunoglobulin seemed to produce a more rapid improvement than corticosteroids. The authors reported in 1988 that 20 of 23 courses resulted in satisfactory improvement, beginning 4.3 to 1.2 days after commencement of therapy, with sustained improvement lasting 106.6 ± 49.1 days. Side effects were minimal. Vital capacity increased significantly after therapy.

Bonaventura Ibars et al. treated a 14-year-old girl successfully with high-dose gamma-globulin.[141] In the beginning, anticholinesterase therapy led to no significant improvement of symptoms; however, the patient responded dramatically to intravenous gammaglobulin.

THYMECTOMY

In 1936 Alfred Blalock successfully removed a thymic tumor from a patient with MG. In 1941 he performed the first planned "trans-sternal" thymectomy in patients with nonthymomatous MG. By 1943 he had already performed 20 thymectomies.[142]

"Maximal" thymectomy for patients with MG and/or thymoma is necessary since, as surgical-anatomic studies have demonstrated, gross and microscopic thymus tissue is widely distributed in the neck and mediastinum. Therefore, it is a challenge for every surgeon to remove as much of this tissue as possible. In 8 patients with a relapse of myasthenic signs after thymectomy and with incapacitating weakness of their muscles, residual thymus was found in all surgical specimens after reexploration of the neck and the mediastinum.[143] Reoperation resulted in considerable improvement in 7 patients. During 1 year of observation, only 1 patient's state remained unchanged. The authors recommended an "en bloc transcervical–trans-sternal maximal thymectomy" in order to take out as much thymus tissue as possible, since a "total" thymectomy is not feasible. "Maximal" thymectomy revealed considerable improvement in 69 of 72 patients (96%) with MG without thymoma: 33 patients were in remission and 24 patients were symptom free when receiving low doses of pyridostigmine. In no patient did symptoms deteriorate (Table 1). The group of 15 patients suffering from MG and thymoma also showed unequivocal favorable results after this maximal surgical procedure.

The intention to perform a radical mediastinal dissection together with an extended thymectomy was realized in 27 patients suffering from generalized MG by Fischer et al.[144] The drug-free remission rate of these patients after this extended procedure was between 63% and 74%. The only patient showing no postoperative improvement had an invasive malignant thymoma. Evoli et al., too, emphasized radical excision of all anterior mediastinal fat and soft tissue after median sternotomies performed since 1980.[145] Follow-up observations after operation showed rapid progressive improvement in 30 of 84 patients with thymomas, and in 100 of 163 non-neoplastic myasthenic patients. Seventeen patients with *ocular or predominantly ocular symptoms* demonstrated no significant change of their clinical status after surgery. However, improvement occurred after steroid therapy. Therefore, the authors conclude that thymectomy should not be performed in patients with ocular myasthenia, unless a thymoma is diagnosed. Späth et al. (1987)[146] reported on 6 of 19 patients with *ocular MG* with unchanged clinical statuses postoperatively. It should be emphasized that clinical exacerbation was seen in 2 patients. However, 8 patients had marked clinical improvement, with reduced dosage of cholinesterase inhibitors.

Valli et al. compared thymectomized patients with ocular myasthenia with those without surgery.[147] Clinical remission occurred in 3 of 5 patients being operated on, but only in two of eight patients without surgery. A radical thymectomy was also feasible with a new surgical approach, the *small transverse sternotomy*.[148] The total remission rate and the overall improvements of myasthenic symptoms were high after the follow-up time of 18 to 24 months. It turned out that patients with short durations of the disease showed better long-term results from surgery than patients with long-standing MG. The clinical remission rate after thymectomy was better in young than in old patients.[147] According to Otto and Strugalska, the follow-up interval after thymectomy was 6 to 12 years in 100 patients. They revealed a total remission in 23%. Distinct improvement occurred in 48%, and some improvement in 10%. The relatively high frequency of complications after surgery, especially in patients with thymomas, is emphasized.[146, 149] Two patients with invasive thymomas showed irreversible pareses. Sixty-six patients with a thy-

TABLE 1.

Thymectomy

	Inderbitzi et al (1986)	Fischer et al (1987)	Fujimura et al (1987)	Otto & Strugalska (1987)
NUMBER OF CASES				
MG w/o thymoma	32	24 consec.	—	317
Encapsulated thymoma		2	31	12
Invasive thymoma	8	1	35	8
GENDER				
MG w/o and/or with thymoma				
Male	22	14	—	65
Female	18	13	—	252
Thymoma				
Male	—	—	33	—
Female	—	—	33	—
AGE (YEARS)				
MG (w/o and/or with thymoma)	16–69	6–75 (mean 36.5)	—	<20: 49 20–30: 131 31–40: 71 41–60: 53 >60: 13
Thymoma	—	—	13–76 (mean 50.9)	—
FOLLOW UP	5 mo. to 18 yrs (mean 4.7 yrs)	Approx 5 yr	—	100 patients: 6–12 yr
PREOPERATIVE STAGE (Osserman Classification)	I: 4 IIA: 14 IIB: 11 III: 5 IV: 6	I: 2 IIA: 10 IIB: 11 III: 4	5 out of 66 cases w/thymoma had MG	I: 8 IIA: 59 IIB: 250
OPERATIVE TECHNIQUE	Median sternotomy: 28 Transcervical 11; thoracal on the right side:1	Sternal split; extended thymectomy and radical mediastinal dissection	—	Transverse sternotomy:257; median sternotomy:80

Späth et al (1987)	Valli et al (1987)	Cooper et al (1988)	Evoli et al (1988)	Jaretzki et al (1988)
59	91	65 consec.	163 consec.	72 consec.
10	19	—	41 ⎫	15
6		—	43 ⎭	
35	49	15	48	27
40	61	50	115	45
—	—	—	41	7
—	—	—	43	8
<20: 10 20–29: 17 30–39: 17 40–59: 27 >60: 4	— —	14–55 (mean: 27)	7–67 (mean: 29.7)	9–66
—	—	—	15–69 (mean: 43)	25–73
"6 mo to 3 yr and longer"	2–12 yr	Min: 1 yr (median: 3.5 yr)	12–183 mo.	6–89 mo. (mean: 40 mo.)
I: 22 IIA: 19 IIB: 26 III: 7 IV: 1	I: 13 IIA: 28 IIB: 53 III: 13 IV: 3	Mild generalized weakness: 25 Moderate or severe weakness: 39	Severe forms of MG: 43%	MG: IIA:13 IIB:37 III and crisis:22 Thymoma: IIb:5 III and crisis: 9
Median sternotomy	Transcervical and transsternal (most)	Transcervical	Before 1980: transcervical and median sternotomy After 1980: median sternotomy	"En bloc transcervical transsternal maximal thymectomy"

(Continued.)

TABLE 1 (cont.).

	Inderbitzi et al (1986)	Fischer et al (1987)	Fujimura et al (1987)	Otto & Strugalska (1987)
COMPLICATIONS (Postoperative)	Respiratory insufficiency: 5; pneumothorax and pneumonia: 1; paresis of right arm: 1	Sterile sternal dehiscence: 1 reintubation: 1; ileus (aft. 4 days): 1; metabolic alkalosis (aft. 4 days): 1	—	Wound suppuration: 2 pneumothorax: 1; resuture of sternum: 1; bleeding of innominate vein: 1
MORTALITY RATE	3 yr postop: 1; 7 yr postop: 1	5 yr postop: 1 (unrelated to disease)	1.5 mo. to 10 yr postop: 15 cases with invasive thymoma	MG: no hosp. death; Thymoma: 2
CLINICAL REMISSION (no. of cases)	13	17	—	After 18-24 mo: 102
IMPROVEMENT (no. of cases)	MG: 14 Thymoma: 4	7	Survival rates: encapsul. thymoma: 74.3%; invasive thymoma: 49.4%	125
UNCHANGED	MG: 3 Thymoma: 2	3	—	5

moma were operated on by Fujimura et al.: 31 tumors were encapsulated and 35 invasive.[150] MG was diagnosed in only 5 cases. Three patients revealed pure red blood cell aplasia, and 1 an aplastic anemia.

Transcervical thymectomy was used only by Cooper et al.[151] A specially designed sternal retractor helped in accomplishing a complete thymectomy. With this new procedure, 65 consecutive patients had extremely good results postoperatively without major complications. However, the authors pointed to the difficulty of learning this method, which requires more experience than the sternotomy approach. But they conceded that a transcervical procedure does not allow a complete exenteration of the mediastinum similar to median sternotomy. In most of these published series (see Table 1) the long-term follow-up observations are not long enough to make a final judgment of the real results of different operative maneuvers. Rosenberg et al. (1986)[152] reported on a 23-year-old woman showing a

Späth et al (1987)	Valli et al (1987)	Cooper et al (1988)	Evoli et al (1988)	Jaretzki et al (1988)
Wound healing impairment: 6.7%; sternal instability: 1.3%; pneumonia: 5.3%; myasthenic crisis 9%; cholinergic crisis: 2.7%; paresis of phrenic nerve: 2.7%; paresis of recurrent laryngeal nerve: 1.3%	—	Postpericardiotomy syndrome: 1	—	Bilateral staphylococcal empyema: 1 deep sternal wound infection: 1; postpericardiotomy syndrome: 2; bilateral chylothorax: 1 sternal wound dehiscence: 1 pulmonary embolism: 1
No death	4	4 yr postop: 1; 5 yr postop: 1	MG: 9 Thymoma: 17	MG: 3 yr postop: 1 5 yr postop: 1; Thymoma: 2 yr postop: 1; 4 yr postop: 1
5	24	33	21	MG: 33 Thymoma: 2
36	—	≥1 grade: 95% ≤2 grades: 86%	MG: progressive improvement: 100 Thymoma: 30	MG: 24 Thymoma: 3
20	—	—	MG: 18 Thymoma: 7	MG: 4 Thymoma: 0

relapse of myasthenic symptoms 5 years after a trans-sternal–approach thymectomy. A remarkable improvement of symptoms occurred after the removal of hyperplastic thymus in the first surgical intervention. The reoperation by means of a second sternotomy revealed remnants of ectopic thymic tissue under the innominate vein and at a subthyroid cervical level. After the reexploration she experienced distinct improvement.

Thymectomy is a helpful and necessary procedure when steroids cannot be administered because of pregnancy and deterioration of myasthenic symptoms occurs because of failure to respond to increasing dosages of pyridostigmine. A 24-year-old pregnant woman was treated successfully by a trans-sternal thymectomy in the second trimester of pregnancy.[153]

However, thymectomy is effective not only in MG but also in autoimmune thrombocytopenic purpura, as shown in a 13-year-old girl with both diseases.[154]

This rare coexistence of two autoimmune diseases manifested by frequent epistaxis and easy bruising, as well as by diplopia, bilateral ptosis, and exercise-dependent inability to laugh. It is suggested that an altered T-cell function was one pathogenetic factor responsible for both affections. However, Cox et al. were not able to show a quantitative effect of thymectomy on peripheral blood mononuclear T-cell subsets in 6 patients with MG, studied before and after the operation.[155] In 23 patients a modest increase in the number of circulating T8$^+$ cells with a statistically significant increase in the T4/T8 ratio was found, compared with a control population of 20. These changes in T-cell subsets occurred both in patients with thymic hyperplasia and in those with normal thymic tissue. Nineteen patients had early onset MG and 4 patients late onsets. There was no patient with a thymoma. All but 1 patient's condition improved clinically postoperatively. Histologic investigation revealed hyperplasia of the thymus in 17 patients, and normal thymic tissue with absence of germinal center follicular hyperplasia in 6 patients.

Neau et al. discussed the cases of two patients, 53 and 54 years old, who developed myasthenic symptoms *after operative removal of the thymoma*.[156] One woman showed the first typical myasthenic symptoms 5 years after thymectomy, the other by 8 weeks after the operation.

Kam-Hansen studied the CSF in a young woman with MG 0.5 years prior to and 3.5 years after thymectomy.[157] Despite the fact that the patient became clinically healthy within at least 2 years after the operation, a pronounced *intrathecal immune response* was observed. A persistent mononuclear pleocytosis, high CSF IgG index, oligoclonal IgG bands, and increasing IgG synthesis rate were found in the CNS, reflecting a continuous humoral immune response. The proportion of total C-cells was slightly higher in CSF than in peripheral blood, while active T-cells were lower in the CSF.

Analgesics should be avoided in MG patients because of possible deterioration of pareses. After thymectomy, pain interferes with the myasthenic respiratory insufficiency. Therefore, a high thoracal epidural anesthesia (C7-Th1/Th1-Th2/Th2-Th3) with a solution of bupivacaine and 10% morphine means an improved procedure in order to save drugs. With this type of analgesia early mobilization and good postoperative cooperation was possible in three patients.[158]

Brearley et al. performed immunologic investigations in the blood of thymectomized children, aged 3 months or less at the time of operation.[159] Thymectomy was not avoidable in these 18 very young children during cardiac bypass operations in order to facilitate cannulation of the great vessels. These thymectomized children demonstrated significantly lower numbers of T-cells and T-cell subsets than age-matched control children who had surgical operations without thymus operations. The findings of significantly lower numbers of helper, suppressor, and total T-cells in patients after thymectomy within the first 3 months of life supports the importance of the thymus in the normal development of the immune system.

REFERENCES

1. Balzereit F, Fateh-Moghadam A, Besinger KA, et al: Myasthenia gravis: Humorale Diagnostik und Therapie einer Autoimmunkrankheit. *Münch Med Wochenschr* 1986; 128:654–657.

2. Haas J: Myasthenia gravis: Aktuelle Therapie unter pathophysiologischen Aspekten. *Dtsch Ärzteblatt* 1988; 85:126–130.

3. Ravits J: Myasthenia gravis: A well-understood neuromuscular disorder. *Postgrad Med* 1988; 83:219–223.

4. Xian-Hao X: Myasthenia gravis: Laboratory and clinical analysis of 120 cases. *Chin Med J* 1986; 99:555–560.

5. Marsteller HB: The first American case of myasthenia gravis. *Arch Neurol* 1988; 45:185–187.

6. Wade A, Kassir M, Ndiaye IP: Les manifestations oculaires de la myasthénie: A propos de 60 cas de myasthénie observés au C.H.U. de Dakar. *J Fr Ophtalmol* 1986; 9:653–656.

7. Yee RD, Whitcup SM, Williams IM, et al: Saccadic eye movements in myasthenia gravis. *Ophthalmology* 1987; 94:219–225.

8. Oohira A, Goto K, Sato Y, et al: Saccades of supernormal velocity: Adaptive response to ophthalmoplegia in a patient with myasthenia gravis. *Neuro-Ophthalmol* 1987; 7:203–209.

9. Sollberger CE, Meienberg O, Ludin H-P: The contribution of oculography to early diagnosis of myasthenia gravis: A study of saccadic eye movements using the infrared reflection method in 22 cases. *Eur Arch Psychiatr Neurol Sci* 1986; 236:102–108.

10. Yee RD, Cogan DG, Zee DS, et al: Rapid eye movements in myasthenia gravis: II. Electroculographic analysis. *Arch Ophthalmol* 1976; 94:1465–1472.

11. Jacobson DM: Edrophonium tonography in suspected ocular myasthenia. *Arch Ophthalmol* 1987; 105:1174–1175.

12. Komiyama A, Hirayama K: Paradoxical reversal of ptosis in myasthenia gravis by edrophonium administration. *J Neurol Neurosurg Psychiatry* 1988; 51:315.

13. Kansu T, Subutay N: Lid retraction in myasthenia gravis. *J Clin Neuro Ophthalmol* 1987; 7:145–148.

14. Smith JL: Lid position in neuro-ophthalmology. Editorial comment. *J Clin Neuro Ophthalmol* 1987; 7:149–150.

15. Schechter RJ: Ptosis with contralateral lid retraction due to excessive innervation of the levator palpebrae superioris. *Ann Ophthalmol* 1978; 10:1324–1328.

16. Burde RM, Savino P, Trobe J (eds): *Clinical Decisions in Neuro Ophthalmology.* St. Louis, Mo: CV Mosby, 1985: 246–274.

17. Jay WM, Nazarian SM, Underwood DW: Pseudo-internuclear ophthalmoplegia with downshoot in myasthenia gravis. *J Clin Neuro Ophthalmol* 1987; 7:74–76.

18. Rosenberg ML: Spasm of the near reflex mimicking myasthenia gravis. *J Clin Neuro Ophthalmol* 1986; 6:106–108.

19. Seybold ME: The office tensilon test for ocular myasthenia gravis. *Arch Neurol* 1986; 43:842–843.

20. Younge BR, Bartley GB: Lancaster test with tensilon for myasthenia. *Arch Neurol* 1987; 44:472–473.

21. Gorelick PB: Office tensilon test. *Arch Neurol* 1987; 44:689–690.

22. Watt G, Theakston RDG, Hayes CG, et al: Positive response to edrophonium in patients with neurotoxic envenoming by cobras *(Naja philippinensis). N Engl J Med* 1986; 315:1444–1448.

23. Sethi KD, Rivner MH, Swift TR: Ice pack test for myasthenia gravis. *Neurology* 1987; 37:1383–1385.

24. Gilchrist JM, Sanders DB: Double-step repetitive stimulation in myasthenia gravis. *Muscle Nerve* 1987; 10:233–237.

25. Massey JM, Grandis AS, Sanders DB: Single fiber electromyography in myasthenia gravis during pregnancy. *Muscle Nerve* 1987; 10:667A.

26. Roe RD, Riker WF, Standaert FG: Motor nerve ending disorder in myasthenia gravis. *Neurology* 1988; 38:293–297.

27. Descamps H, Bataille, J, Estournet B, et al: La myasthénie de l'enfant: Evolution à long terme. *Ann Med Interne* 1987; 138:615–619.

28. Smit LME, Hageman G, Veldman H, et al: A myasthenic syndrome with congenital paucity of secondary synaptic clefts: CPSC syndrome. *Muscle Nerve* 1988; 11:337–348.

29. Bartoccioni E, Evoli A, Casali C, et al: Neonatal myasthenia gravis: Clinical and immunological study of seven mothers and their newborn infants. *J Neuroimmunol* 1986; 12:155–161.

30. Morel E, Eymard B, Vernet-Der Garabedian B, et al: Neonatal myasthenia gravis: A new clinical and immunologic appraisal on 30 cases. *Neurology* 1988; 38:138–142.

31. Melber D: Maternal-fetal transmission of myasthenia gravis with acetylcholine-receptor antibody. *N Engl J Med* 1988; 318:996.

32. Mora M, Lambert EH, Engel AG: Synaptic vesicle abnormality in familial infantile myasthenia. *Neurology* 1987; 37:206–214.

33. Kerzin-Storrar L, Metcalfe RA, Dyer PA, et al: Genetic factors in myasthenia gravis: A family study. *Neurology* 1988; 38:38–42.

34. Chiu HC, Hsieh R-P, Hsieh K-H, et al: Association of HLA-DRw9 with myasthenia gravis in Chinese. *J Immunogenet* 1987; 14:203–207.

35. Chiu HC, Vincent A, Newsom-Davis J, et al: Myasthenia gravis: Population differences in disease expression and acetylcholine receptor antibody titres between Chinese and Caucasians. *Neurology* 1987; 37:1854–1857.

36. Chiu HC, De Lange GG, Willcox N, et al: Immunoglobulin allotypes in caucasian and Chinese myasthenia gravis: Differences from Japanese patients. *J Neurol Neurosurg Psychiatry* 1988; 51:214–217.

37. Zhi-Qiang C: Familial myasthenia gravis: Report of 7 cases in 3 families. *Chin Med J* 1986; 99:749–750.

38. Murphy J, Murphy SF: Myasthenia gravis in identical twins. *Neurology* 1986; 36:78–80.

39. Rosenberg ML: Viral etiology for MG and the HLA-B8 phenotype. *Neurology* 1986; 36:1275.

40. Aoki T, Drachman DB, Asher DM, et al: Attempts to implicate viruses in myasthenia gravis. *Neurology* 1985; 35:185–192.

41. Wessel HB, Zitelli BJ: Myasthenia gravis associated with human T-cell lymphotropic virus type III infection *Pediatr Neurol* 1987; 3:238–239.

42. Efthimiou J, D'Cruz D, Kaplan P, et al: Heterozygous C2 deficiency associated with angioedema, myasthenia gravis, and systemic lupus erythematosus. *Ann Rheumat Dis* 1986; 45:428–430.

43. Oda K, Miyasaki K, Ohta M, et al: A case of myasthenia gravis associated with thymoma, multiple Schwannomas and monoclonal IgA gammopathy. *Jpn J Med* 1987; 26:223–225.

44. Bixenman WW, Buchsbaum HW: Multiple sclerosis, euthyroid restrictive Graves' ophthalmopathy, and myasthenia gravis. *Graefes Arch Clin Exp Ophthalmol* 1988; 226:168–171.

45. Ohno M, Hamada N, Yamakawa J, et al: Myasthenia gravis associated with Graves' disease in Japan. *Jpn J Med* 1987; 26:2–6.

46. Jimenez MD, Yusta A, Liano M: Asociación de miastenia grave con trastornos tiroideos. *Med Clin (Barc)* 1987; 89:675–677.

47. Bowen JD, Kidd P: Myasthenia gravis associated with T helper cell lymphoma. *Neurology* 1987; 37:1405–1408.

48. Bramwell NH, Burns BF: Histiocytosis X of the thymus in association with myasthenia gravis. *Am J Clin Pathol* 1986; 86:224–227.

49. Kurlan R, Jankovic J, Rubin A, et al: Coexistent Meige's syndrome and myasthenia gravis: A relationship between blinking and extraocular muscle fatigue? *Arch Neurol* 1987; 44:1057–1060.

50. Maytal J, Spiro AJ, Sinnar S, et al: The coexistence of myasthenia gravis and myotonic dystrophy in one family. *Neuropediatrics* 1987; 18:8–10.

51. Bolger GB, Sullivan KM, Spence AM, et al: Myasthenia gravis after allogeneic bone marrow transplantation: Relationship to chronic graft-versus-host disease. *Neurology* 1986; 36:1087–1091.

52. Soliven BC, Lange DJ, Penn AS: Seronegative myasthenia gravis. *Neurology* 1988; 38:514–517.

53. Oosterhuis HJGH, Newsom-Davis J, Wokke JHJ, et al: The slow channel syndrome: Two new cases. *Brain* 1987; 110:1061–1079.

54. Hoogenraad TU, Gmelig Meyling FHJ: Putative role of antireticulin antibody in antiacetylcholine-receptor-antibody negative myasthenia gravis. *Arch Neurol* 1987; 44:536–538.

55. Yamamoto T, Sato T, Sugita H: Antifilamin, antivinculin, and antitropomyosin antibodies in myasthenia gravis. *Neurology* 1987; 37:1329–1333.

56. Komiyama A, Kamo I, Furukawa S, et al: Antibodies against saline-soluble components of skeletal muscle in myasthenia gravis. *J Neurol* 1988; 235:207–213.

57. Whiting PJ, Cooper J, Lindstrom JM: Antibodies in sera from patients with myasthenia gravis do not bind to nicotinic acetylcholine receptors from human brain. *J Neuroimmunol* 1987; 16:205–213.

58. Plioplys AV, Thibault J, Bouchard J-P, et al: Anti-CNS antibodies in neurological and psychiatric disorders. *J Neurol Neurosurg Psychiatry* 1987; 50:1514–1521.

59. Müller KMI, Taskinen E, Lefvert AK, et al: Immunoactivation in the central nervous system in myasthenia gravis. *J Neurol Sci* 1987; 80:13–23.

60. Colquhoun D, Ogden DC, Mathie A: Nicotinic acetylcholine receptors of nerve and muscle: Functional aspects. *Trends Pharmacol Sci* 1987; 8:465–472.

61. Changeux J-P, Giraudat J, Dennis M: The nicotinic acetylcholine receptor: Molecular architecture of a ligand-regulated ion channel. *Trends Pharmacol Sci* 1987; 8:459–465.

62. Oger J, Kaufman R, Berry K: Acetylcholine receptor antibodies in myasthenia gravis: Use of a qualitative assay for diagnostic purposes. *Can J Neurol Sci* 1987; 14:297–302.

63. Toyka KV, Heininger K: Acetylcholin-Rezeptor-Antikörper in der Diagnostik der Myasthenia gravis: Untersuchungen bei 406 gesicherten Fällen. *Dtsch Med Wochenschr* 1986; 111:1435–1439.

64. Illa I, Rodriguez JL, Grau JM, et al: Anticuerpos antirreceptor de acetilcolina en miastenia grave. *Immunologia* 1988; 7:41–46 (21–26).

65. Penn AS, Schotland DL, Lamme S: Antimuscle and antiacetylcholine receptor antibodies in myasthenia gravis. *Muscle Nerve* 1986; 9:407–415.

66. Zeitlhofer J, Maida EM, Mamoli B, et al: Wertigkeit der Acetylcholin-Rezeptor-Antikörper bei Myasthenia gravis. *Wien Med Wochenschr* 1986; 13:329–332.

67. Hinman CL, Ernstoff RM, Montgomery N, et al: Clinical correlates of enzyme-immunoassay versus radioimmunoassay measurements of antibody against acetylcholine receptor in patients with myasthenia gravis. *J Neurol Sci* 1986; 75:305–316.

68. Lebrun-Grandie P, Souan ML, Geffard M, et al: Anticorps anti-acétylcholine et anti-récepteur dans la myasthénie. *Presse Med* 1987; 16:1577–1580.

69. Oda K, Shibasaki H: Myasthenia gravis: Antibodies to extracellularly exposed antigenic determinants of acetylcholine receptor. *Neurology* 1986; 36:1374–1377.

70. Knight JG, Laing P, Adams DD, et al: Autoantibodies to acetylcholine receptor in myasthenia gravis: Light chains. *Neurology* 1986; 36:1531–1533.

71. Lefvert AK, Holm G: Idiotypic network in myasthenia gravis demonstrated by human monoclonal B-cell lines. *Scand J Immunol* 1987; 26:573–578.

72. Abraham EP, Chain E, Baker W, et al: Penicillamine, a characteristic degradation product of penicillin. *Nature* 1943; 151:107.

73. Netter P, Bannwarth B, Pere P, et al: Clinical pharmacokinetics of D-penicillamine. *Clin Pharmacokinet* 1987; 13:317–333.

74. Kuncl RW, Pestronk A, Drachman DB, et al: The pathophysiology of penicillamine-induced myasthenia gravis. *Ann Neurol* 1986; 20:740–744.

75. Huaux JP, Delreux V: Penicillamine-induced myasthenia. *Acta Neurol Belg* 1986; 86:297–303.

76. Martin C, Kuntz JL, Asch L: Myasthénie lors du traitement de la polyarthrite rhumatoide par la D-pénicillamine. A propos de quatre observations. *Semin Hop Paris* 1988; 64:961–965.

77. Fried MJ, Protheroe DT: D-Penicillamine induced myasthenia gravis. *Br J Anaesth* 1986; 58:1191–1193.

78. Kolarz G, Maida EM: Azetylcholin-Rezeptorantkörper unter D-Penicillamintherapie. *Z Rheumatol* 1986; 45:118–121.

79. Sghirlanzoni A, Mantegazza R, Mora M, et al: Chloroquine myopathy and myasthenia-like syndrome. *Muscle Nerve* 1988; 11:114–119.

80. Argov Z, Brenner T, Abramsky O: Ampicillin may aggravate clinical and experimental myasthenia gravis. *Arch Neurol* 1986; 43:255.

81. Bashuk RG, Krendel DA: Myasthenia gravis presenting as weakness after magnesium administration. *Muscle Nerve* 1987; 10:666A.

82. Ueno S, Takahashi M, Kajiyama K, et al: Parkinson's disease and myasthenia gravis: Adverse effect of trihexyphenidyl on neuromuscular transmission. *Neurology* 1987; 37:832–833.

83. Goldhammer Y, Chagnac Y, Hadani M: Myasthenic crisis precipitated by iodinated contrast agents. Reply from the authors. *Neurology* 1986; 36:444.

84. Hilton-Jones D: Myasthenic crisis precipitated by iodinated contrast agents. To the editor. *Neurology* 1986; 36:444.

85. Frank JH, Cooper GW, Black WC, et al: Iodinated contrast agents in myasthenia gravis. *Neurology* 1987; 37:1400–1402.

85a. Fierro B, Castiglione MG, Salemi G et al: Myasthenia-like syndrome induced by cardiovascular agents. Report of a case. *J Neurol Sci* 1987; 8:167–170.

86. Donnet A, Habib M, Vigouroux RA: Manifestations myasthéniformes persistantes après intoxication ciguatérique. Effet favorable des anticholinestérasiques. *Presse Med* 1987; 16:734.

87. O'Neill JH, Murray NMF, Newsom-Davis J: The Lambert-Eaton myasthenic syndrome. *Brain* 1988; 111:577–596.

88. Heath JP, Ewing DJ, Cull RE: Abnormalities of autonomic function in the Lambert Eaton myasthenic syndrome. *J Neurol Neurosurg Psychiatry* 1988; 436–439.

89. Bady B, Chauplannaz G, Carrier H: Congenital Lambert-Eaton myasthenic syndrome. *J Neurol Neurosurg Psychiatry* 1987; 50:476–478.

90. Wilcox PG, Morrison NJ, Anzarut ARA, et al: Lambert-Eaton myasthenic syndrome involving the diaphragm. *Chest* 1988; 93:604–606.

91. Krendel DA, Hopkins LC: Adverse effect of verapamil in a patient with the Lambert-Eaton syndrome. *Muscle Nerve* 1986; 9:519–522.

92. Oh SJ, Dwyer DS, Bradley RJ: Overlap myasthenic syndrome: Combined myasthenia gravis and Eaton-Lambert syndrome. *Neurology* 1987; 37:1411–1414.

93. Taphoorn MJB, Van Duijn H, Wolters ECH: A neuromuscular transmission disorder: Combined myasthenia gravis and Lambert-Eaton syndrome in one patient. *J Neurol Neurosurg Psychiatry* 1988; 51:880–882.

94. Tannier C, Hamidou M, Morlock G, et al: L'association syndrome de Lambert et Eaton syndrome de Schwartz-Bartter est-elle pathognomonique d'un carcinome bronchique? Revue de la littérature à propos d'un case. Association à une neuropathie périphérique. *Semin Hop Paris* 1988; 64:1181–1185.

95. Hughes RL, Katirji MB: The Eaton-Lambert (myasthenic) syndrome in association with systemic lupus erythematosus. *Arch Neurol* 1986; 43:1186–1187.

96. Fukuoka T, Engel AG, Lang B, et al: Lambert-Eaton myasthenic syndrome: I. Early morphological effects of IgG on the presynaptic membrane active zones. *Ann Neurol* 1987; 22:193–199.

97. Fukuoka T, Engel AG, Lang B, et al: Lambert-Eaton myasthenic syndrome: II. Immunoelectron microscopy localization of IgG at the mouse end-plate. *Ann Neurol* 1987; 22:200–211.

98. Login IS, Kim YI, Judd AM, et al: Immunoglobulins of Lambert-Eaton myasthenic syndrome inhibit rat pituitary hormone release. *Ann Neurol* 1987; 22:610–614.

99. Kim YI, Neher E: IgG from patients with Lambert-Eaton syndrome blocks voltage-dependent calcium channels. *Science* 1988; 239:405–408.

100. Tsujihata M, Kinoshita I, Mori M, et al: Ultrastructural study of the motor end-plate in botulism and Lambert-Eaton myasthenic syndrome. *J Neurol Sci* 1987; 81:197–213.

101. Grody WW, Jobst S, Keesey J, et al: Pathologic evaluation of thymic hyperplasia in myasthenia gravis and Lambert-Eaton syndrome. *Arch Pathol Lab Med* 1986; 110:843–846.

102. Isaacson PG, Norton AJ, Addis BJ: The human thymus contains a novel population of B lymphocytes. *Lancet* 1987; 2:1488–1490.

103. Schluep M, Willcox N, Vincenta A, et al: Acetylcholine receptors in human thymic myoid cells in situ: An immunohistological study. *Ann Neurol* 1987; 22:212–222.

104. Matsumoto Y, Furuya A, Kobayashi T: Primary cultures of human myasthenia gravis thymus and normal thymus: Studies of cell morphology, cell proliferative pattern and localization of α-bungarotoxin binding sites on cultured thymic cells. *J Neurol Sci* 1986; 75:121–133.

105. Kirchner T, Schalke B, Melms A, et al: Immunohistological patterns of non-neoplastic changes in the thymus in myasthenia gravis. *Virchows Arch (Cell Pathol)* 1986; 52:237–257.

106. Melms A, Schalke BCG, Kirchner T, et al: Thymus in myasthenia gravis: Isolation of T-lymphocyte lines specific for the nicotinic acetylcholine receptor from thymuses of myasthenic patients. *J Clin Invest* 1988; 81:902–908.

107. Kirchner T, Hoppe F, Schalke B, et al: Microenvironment of thymic myoid cells in myasthenia gravis. *Virchows Arch (Cell Pathol)* 1988; 54:295–302.

108. Kirchner T, Tzartos S, Hoppe F, et al: Pathogenesis of myasthenia gravis acetylcholine receptor-related antigenic determinants in tumor-free thymuses and thymus epithelial tumors. *Am J Pathol* 1988; 130:268–280.

109. Di Mario FJ, Lisak RP, Kornstein MJ, et al: Myasthenia gravis and primary squamous cell carcinoma of the thymus: A case report. *Neurology* 1988; 38:580–582.

110. Sweeney PJ, O'Donovan PB: Myasthenia gravis, thymoma, and the anterior junction line, in Smith JL (ed): *Neuro-Ophthalmology Now!* New York, Springer-Verlag, 1986; 23:239–244.

111. Lewis JE, Wick MR, Scheithauer BW, et al: Thymoma: A clinicopathologic review. *Cancer* 60:2727–2743.

112. Denayer M-A, Rao KR, Wirz D, et al: Hepatic metastatic thymoma and myasthenia gravis twenty-two years after the apparent cure of an invasive thymoma: A case report and review of the literature. *J Neurol Sci* 1986; 76:23–30.

113. Bailey RO, Dunn HG, Rubin AM, et al: Myasthenia gravis with thymoma and pure red blood cell aplasia. *Am J Clin Pathol* 1988; 89:687–693.

114. Halbach M, Hömberg V, Freund H-J: Neuromuscular, autonomic and central cholinergic hyperactivity associated with thymoma and acetylcholine receptor-binding antibody. *J Neurol* 1987; 234:433–436.

115. Sanders DB, Howard JF: Thymoma without myasthenia gravis: Electrophysiological study after thymectomy. *J Neurol Neurosurg Psychiatry* 1988; 51:160–161.

116. Tabbaa MA, Leshner RT, Campbell WW: Malignant thymoma with dysautonomia and disordered neuromuscular transmission. *Arch Neurol* 1986; 43:955–957.

117. Witt NJ, Bolton CF: Neuromuscular disorders and thymoma. *Muscle Nerve* 1988; 11:398–405.

118. Kawanami S, Kamei H, Oita J, et al: Acetylcholine-receptor-like protein from human thymoma associated with myasthenia gravis. *J Neurol* 1987; 234:207–210.

119. Aarli JA, Gilhus NE, Hofstad H: CA-antibody: An immunological marker of thymic neoplasia in myasthenia gravis? *Acta Neurol Scand* 1987; 76:55–57.

120. Kirchner T, Hoppe F, Müller-Hermelink HK, et al: Acetylcholine receptor epitopes on epithelial cells of thymoma in myasthenia gravis. *Lancet* 1987; 1:218.

121. Willcox N, Schluep M, Ritter MA, et al: Myasthenic and nonmyasthenic thymoma: An expansion of minor cortical epithelial cell subset? *Am J Pathol* 1987; 127:447–460.

122. Chilosi M, Iannucci A, Menestrina F, et al: Immunohistochemical evidence of active thymocyte proliferation in thymoma. *Am J Pathol* 1987; 128:464–470.

123. Ito M, Taki T, Miyake M, et al: Lymphocyte subsets in human thymoma studied with monoclonal antibodies. *Cancer* 1988; 61:284–287.

124. Hohlfeld R, Michels M, Heininger K, et al: Azathioprine toxicity during long-term immunosuppression of generalized myasthenia gravis. *Neurology* 1988; 38:258–261.

125. Witte AS, Cornblath DR, Schatz NJ, et al: Monitoring azathioprine therapy in myasthenia gravis. *Neurology* 1986; 36:1533–1534.

126. Kern RZ, Stewart JD: Listeria meningitis complicating treatment of myasthenia gravis with azathioprine and steroids. *Neurology* 1986; 36:1011–1012.

127. Fischer JE: Azathioprine and myasthenia gravis. *Lancet* 1987; 2:1020.

128. Tindall RSA, Rollins JA, Phillips JT, et al: Preliminary results of a double-blind, randomized, placebo-controlled trial of cyclosporine in myasthenia gravis. *N Engl J Med* 1987; 316:719–729.

129. Nyberg-Hansen R, Gjerstad L: Myasthenia gravis treated with cyclosporin. *Acta Neurol Scand* 1988; 77:307–313.

130. Kosmidis PA, Iliopoulos E, Pentea S: Combination chemotherapy with cyclophosphamide, adriamycin, and vincristine in malignant thymoma and myasthenia gravis. *Cancer* 1988; 61:1736–1740.

131. Ellis EF: Adverse effects of corticosteroid therapy. *J Allergy Clin Immunol* 1987; 80:515–517.

132. Milner-Brown HS, Mellenthin M, Sharma ML, et al: Quantitative correlation between plasma pyridostigmine levels and neuromuscular function in myasthenia gravis. *Neurology* 1987; 37:800–803.

133. Haber P, Harmuth P, Wolf C, et al: Akute Effekte von Prostigmin auf Lungenfunktion und Atmung von Patienten mit Myasthenia Gravis in Ruhe und bei dosierter Ergometerbelastung. *Respiration* 1987; 52:59–68.

134. Janda Ä, Brandstetter A: Therapie der Myasthenia gravis. *Dtsch Med Wochenschr* 1986; 111:1081–1082.

135. Grogan WA: Treatment of myasthenia gravis with pyridostigmine. *Arch Neurol* 1987; 44:995–996.

136. Murray N, Baynes C: Caeco-colic intussusception in a patient with myasthenia gravis. *J Neurol Neurosurg Psychiatry* 1986; 49:219.

137. Bowen JW, Daltner CJ, Troost BT: The treatment of ocular myasthenia with plasmapheresis: Three case reports. *Neuro-Ophthalmol* 1986; 6:109–112.

138. Thorlacius S, Lefvert AK, Aarli JA, et al: Plasma exchange in myasthenia gravis: Effect on anti-AChR antibodies and other autoantibodies. *Acta Neurol Scand* 1986; 74:486–490.

139. Arsura EL, Bick A, Brunner NG, et al: High-dose intravenous immunoglobulin in the management of myasthenia gravis. *Arch Intern Med* 1986; 146:1365–1368.

140. Arsura EL, Bick A, Brunner NG, et al: Effects of repeated doses of intravenous immunoglobulin in myasthenia gravis. *Am J Med Sci* 1988; 295:438–443.

141. Bonaventura Ibars I, Ponseti J, Espanol T, et al: High-dose intravenous gamma-globulin therapy for myasthenia gravis. *J Neurol* 1987; 234:363.

142. Kirschner PA: Alfred Blalock and thymectomy for myasthenia gravis. *Ann Thorac Surg* 1987; 43:348–349.

143. Jaretzki A, Penn AS, Younger DS, et al: "Maximal" thymectomy for myasthenia gravis. *J Thorac Cardiovasc Surg* 1988; 95:747–757.

144. Fischer JE, Grinvalski HT, Nussbaum MS, et al: Aggressive surgical approach for drug-free remission from myasthenai gravis. *Ann Surg* 1987; 205:496–503.

145. Evoli A, Batocchi AP, Provenzano C, et al: Thymectomy in the treatment of myasthenia gravis; Report of 247 patients. *J Neurol* 1988; 235:272–276.

146. Späth G, Brinkmann A, Huth C, et al: Complications and efficacy of transsternal thymectomy in myasthenia gravis. *Thorac Cardiovasc Surgeon* 1987; 35:283–289.

147. Valli G, Jann S, Premoselli S, et al: Myasthenia gravis treatment: Twelve years' experience on 110 patients. *Ital J Neurol Sci* 1987; 8:593–601.

148. Otto TJ, Strugalska H: Surgical treatment for myasthenia gravis. *Thorax* 1987; 42:199–204.

149. Inderbitzi R, Glutz L, Nachbur B: Die Bedeutung der Thymektomie in der Behendlung der Myasthenia gravis pseudoparalytica im Berner Krankengut. *Schweiz Med Wochenschr* 1986; 116:1297–1302.

150. Fujimura S, Kondo T, Handa M, et al: Results of surgical treatment for thymoma based on 66 patients. *J Thorac Cardiovasc Surg* 1987; 93:708–714.

151. Cooper JC, Al-Jilaihawa AN, Pearson FG, et al: An improved technique to facilitate transcervical thymectomy for myasthenia gravis. *Ann Thorac Surg* 1988; 45:242–247.

152. Rosenberg M, Jaúrgni WO, Herrera MR: Recurrence of thymic hyperplasia after trans-sternal thymectomy in myasthenia gravis. *Chest* 1986; 89:888–889.

153. Ip MSM, So SY, Lam WK, et al: Thymectomy in myasthenia gravis during pregnancy. *Postgrad Med J* 1986; 62:473–474.

154. Jansen PHP, Renier WO, De Vaan G, et al: Effect of thymectomy on myasthenia gravis and autoimmune thrombocytopenic purpura in a 13-year-old girl. *Eur J Pediatr* 1987; 146:587–589.

155. Cox A, Lisak RP, Skolnik P, et al: Effect of thymectomy on blood T-cell subsets in myasthenia gravis. *Ann Neurol* 1986; 19:297–298.

156. Neau J-P, Robert R, Pourrat O, et al: Myasthénie survenant après ablation d'un thymome. *Presse Med* 1988; 17:391–392.

157. Kam-Hansen S: Asymptomatic oligoclonal CSF IgG and progressive increase of intrathecal IgG synthesis in a patient with myasthenia gravis treated with thymectomy—A 4-year follow-up. *J Neurol Sci* 1986; 75:285–292.

158. Ferretti F, Crestani S, Rodriguez NJ: Peut-on employer l'analgésie épidurale thoracale haut dans les soins intensifs postopératoires du myasténique après thymectomie transsternale. *Schweiz Med Wochenschr* 1987; 117:438–441.

159. Brearley S, Gentle TA, Baynham MID, et al: Immunodeficiency following neonatal thymectomy in man. *Clin Exp Immunol* 1987; 70:322–327.

CHAPTER 16

Stroke

Jonathan D. Trobe, M.D.

Departments of Ophthalmology and Neurology, University of Michigan Medical Center, Ann Arbor, Michigan

Effective treatment for ischemic stroke remains more a wish than a consummation. Many drugs have come and gone in the search for a way to protect the "ischemic penumbra," the viable edges of an infarct. Much hope now rides on finding a safe and effective thrombolytic agent. Tissue plasminogen activator, so helpful in coronary occlusion, may be the answer. It shows promise in experimental stroke and is being tested now on patients.

The value of carotid endarterectomy remains an unresolved issue. Fortunately, some progress has been made to bring science into the discussion, as the North American Symptomatic Carotid Endarterectomy Trial gets underway.*

In the meantime, good data about stroke risk factors and natural history are being gathered. Magnetic resonance imaging (MRI) is making diagnosis much easier, and positron emission tomography (PET), single photon emission computed tomography (SPECT), MR spectroscopy, and transcranial Doppler ultrasound are exciting advances.

EPIDEMIOLOGY

Cigarette smoking was again strongly linked to stroke. Among 118,539 women aged between 35 and 50 years and followed up for 10 years, those who smoked up

---

*London, Ontario, Canada, (519) 663-3693.

Curr Neuro Ophthalmol 2:293–306, 1989
© 1989, Year Book Medical Publishers, Inc.
0893–0147/89/02-293-306-$04.00

to 14 cigarettes per day had a 2.2 relative risk of stroke.[1] For those who smoked 25 or more cigarettes, the relative risk climbed to 3.7. In this group, the relative risk of subarachnoid hemorrhage was 9.8. In the Framingham Study, stroke risk was twice as high for heavy (>40 cigarettes per day) as for light (<10 per day) smokers.[2] Interestingly, stroke risk fell rapidly in lapsed smokers—it was at the level of nonsmokers after 5 years—a finding previously reported.[3] This suggests that smoking promotes stroke by an exquisitely reversible mechanism, perhaps by elevating fibrinogen or enhancing platelet aggregation.[4]

The profile of the stroke-prone individual is filling out. In Sweden, the four main stroke risk factors for 789 men followed up from age 54 for 18.5 years were high blood pressure, obesity, elevated fibrinogen level, and a maternal history of stroke.[5] The authors point out that smoking causes elevated fibrinogen levels. In the Framingham Study, three risk factors were identified: high blood pressure, electrocardiographic signs of left ventricular hypertrophy, and glucose intolerance.[6] A Japanese study named elevated diastolic (but not systolic) blood pressure, atrial fibrillation, and proteinuria.[7] In Hawaii, the risk factors were elevated diastolic blood pressure, increased serum glucose level, left ventricular hypertrophy, proteinuria, and cigarette smoking.[8]

The skillful tracking of patients in Rochester, Minn. has again turned up some valuable facts. Among 1,804 people 50 years or older and free of stroke, as determined by a Mayo Clinic examination in 1960, the following relative risks for ischemic stroke were determined: 1.6 for age (each 10 years), 2.0 for male sex, 4.0 for hypertension, 3.9 for transient ischemic attacks (TIAs), 2.2 for hypertensive or coronary heart disease, and 1.7 for congestive heart failure or diabetes mellitus.[9]

Although not perfectly consistent, these studies reveal a pattern of risk for stroke similar but not identical to that for myocardial infarction, where elevated lipids and cholesterol may play a greater causative role.[10] In risk factor analysis, stroke is now being divided into three groups: cerebral infarction, intracerebral hemorrhage, and subarachnoid hemorrhage. The risk profiles for these three groups are not identical.[10]

The role of oral contraceptives in stroke is still controversial.[11] Most of the information relates to the old high-dose estrogen formulations. Nevertheless, the results of a long-term retrospective study in Denmark are striking. Lidegaard[12] compared stroke mortality between 1954 to 1966 and 1967 to 1981, the precontraceptive and postcontraceptive eras, and found that the incidence of thromboembolic stroke death in women climbed 33% while the incidence in men fell by 14%. The best explanation is a relative risk of 3.3 to 4.5 for oral contraceptive users. Current wisdom is that oral contraceptives are especially likely to increase thromboembolism in women aged more than 35 years who smoke and who have arteriosclerotic risk factors.[13]

The availability of sensitive noninvasive tests has taught us more about the natural history of extracranial carotid artery atherostenosis. In a serial ultrasound study in Düsseldorf, West Germany, of 339 asymptomatic patients (mean follow-up, 29 months), Hennerici et al.[14] found that the risk of developing a stroke without a prior TIA was only 0.4% per year. They concluded that this low probability of stroke did not justify carotid endarterectomy in asymptomatic patients with ultrasound-documented carotid stenosis. In a similar study, Chambers and Norris[15] showed only a 1.7% annual stroke rate, but the incidence jumped to 5.5% in patients with more than 75% stenosis. Still, most of those strokes were heralded by TIAs. Meissner et al.[16] found a higher annual stroke rate of 3.4% in patients with hemodynamically significant carotid stenosis, but only half the strokes were on the side of the abnormal hemodynamics. Some observers are now looking at the morphologic structure rather than the size of the carotid plaque. O'Holleran et al.[17] found that ultrasonically defined "softness" is an added risk factor for stroke, and Seeger and Klingman[18] found that plaques removed from symptomatic patients contained more lipid than those removed from asymptomatic patients. These points are being considered in the current randomized trial of endarterectomy in asymptomatic patients.*

A duplex study of the cervical carotid in patients with amaurosis fugax and retinal arterial occlusions showed that only 16% had greater than 60% stenosis.[19] Even among those with retinal arterial occlusions, fewer than a quarter had such a degree of stenosis. One should conclude that amaurosis fugax occurs in many patients without atheromatous disease, and that many retinal vascular occlusions must be caused either by emboli or by distal vascular disease.

The prognosis for patients with retinal emboli is not a happy one. In a series of 85 patients from London,[20] the chance of stroke was 12 times greater than expected for an age-matched population, and the chance of death 2.3 times greater. Most of those deaths were from stroke, an unexpected finding since a previous series[21] had found a higher number of deaths from heart attacks. This report does confirm previous studies[21, 22] in showing that retinal emboli are a worse omen than amaurosis fugax. In fact, in a previous series of 110 patients with amaurosis fugax from the same London hospital, the stroke rate was 4 times expected, and the death rate 1.5 times expected.[23]

DIAGNOSIS

Imaging

If most strokes cannot be fixed, at least they can now be located. Progress in neuroimaging is spectacular along several fronts. With the addition of gadolinium, MRI is threatening to supplant computed tomography (CT) except in patients with head trauma, pacemakers and other life-support systems, or claustrophobia.

However, MRI is not perfect. A recent study[24] reminds us that in acute brainstem hemorrhage, the lesion may be missed within the first week because its in-

---

*Asymptomatic Carotid Atherosclerosis Study, Winston-Salem, N.C., (919) 748-2757.

tensity is equal to brain substance. On the other hand, for visualizing arteriovenous malformations, MRI is certainly better than CT and may even be better than angiography.[25, 26] Magnetic resonance imaging outdid CT and angiography in defining the nidus, feeding and draining vessels, and associated parenchymal hemorrhage as well as other abnormalities. Still, MRI could not distinguish calcium from rapid blood flow or hemosiderin, so the authors[25] cautioned that angiography would still be necessary before planning treatment.

In ischemic stroke, MRI—even without gadolinium—appears to be more sensitive (though less specific) than CT, especially within the first 72 hours after onset.[27] Gadolinium does for MRI what intravenous contrast material does for CT: it lights up lesions where the blood-brain barrier is broken. Magnetic resonance imaging enhancement begins 24 hours or more after stroke onset and may be greater and cover a broader time span than CT enhancement.[28]

The sensitivity of T_2-weighted MRI to brain lesions of any kind has created a major diagnostic quandary. In over 30% of patients aged greater than 60 years, hemispheric periventricular high-intensity signals have been turning up that look like frosting on a cake (the lateral ventricles). These signals, which are often found in entirely asymptomatic patients, may or may not be distinct from high-intensity signals located in the deep white matter near the ventricular walls, and sometimes are associated with long-tract signs, dementia, and a history of hypertension.[29] Because patchy demyelination of deep hemispheric white matter in hypertensive patients had first been described by Binswanger[30] in 1894, some radiologists initially interpreted these new MRI findings as "compatible with Binswanger's disease." When it became clear that many patients did not fit that diagnosis clinically, the frosted signals came to be called "unidentified bright objects" or UBOs.[28] Hachinski et al.[31] prefer the more erudite term *leuko-araiosis,* or white matter thinning. Whatever they are called, in a recent MRI-autopsy correlation study of 14 brains, Marshall et al.[32] traced the periventricular high signals to pathologic signs of infarction. Does this mean that all these nonhypertensive, asymptomatic patients over age 60 with MRI UBOs have occult infarcts? More work is needed in careful neurologic and neuropsychometric examination and MRI-pathologic correlation.

Duplex (B-mode and Doppler) ultrasound examination of the extracranial carotid[33] has now been perfected to the point that some users consider it superior to angiography. In one series,[34] duplex and angiography were equally sensitive to degree of luminal narrowing (94% to 97%), but duplex was twice as accurate as angiography in gauging ulceration and plaque morphology, features vascular surgeons now consider important in determining the need for endarterectomy. Although few surgeons will perform endarterectomy without an angiogram, many now believe that duplex findings are reliable enough to dismiss noncandidates for surgery. Computed tomography may add a dimension not offered by duplex by allowing visualization of the entire vessel wall, a helpful point in diagnosing fibromuscular dysplasia and arterial dissections.[35]

Doppler ultrasound has also been modified to measure intracranial blood flow in major arteries.[36] It is being used to monitor patients undergoing clamping during endarterectomy and to decide if heparinization would be useful in acute stroke.[37] Perhaps most exciting for neuro-ophthalmologists is the possibility that transcranial Doppler might be used to measure intracranial pressure (ICP). Reporting on this new development, Klingelhofer et al.[38] found good correlation between middle cerebral artery flow parameters measured by Doppler and epidural ICP monitoring in 26 patients with elevated ICP. Wouldn't this be useful in managing pseudotumor cerebri?

Positron emission tomography permits evaluation of CNS metabolic functioning by tagging radioactive isotopes to substrates such as glucose. Its drawbacks are enormous expense (it requires a cyclotron) and poor resolution. Given the complexities of the medium, few dazzling contributions have yet been made in stroke. An example is a recent report by Bosley et al.[39] that showed that glucose metabolism was appropriately depressed in the occipital lobe in five patients with acute ischemic homonymous hemianopia. Hemispheric asymmetries were sometimes larger on PET than on CT, but PET will have to do more than that to justify its high cost. A less predictable PET finding came in a study of amblyopia[40] that showed reduced activation of primary and accessory visual cortex by stimuli shown to the amblyopic as compared with the normal fellow eye.

Although PET can image regional cerebral blood flow, it is expensive and time-consuming. A simpler method, SPECT, uses commercially available isotopes that generate gamma rays. In one report,[41] technetium 99m was complexed with hexamethylpropyleneamine so it would cross the blood-brain barrier and be immediately trapped by one-step degradation; imaging by gamma camera revealed cerebellar hemispheric hypoperfusion in a patient with chronic lateral medullary syndrome. The usefulness of this intriguing diagnostic test is yet to be determined.

Another space-age technique for sampling brain metabolic function is MR phosphorus spectroscopy. Levine et al.[42] found that persistent hyperglycemia was associated with failure of high-energy phosphate metabolism to recover in a patient with a large ischemic hemispheric stroke. This technique should be especially useful in monitoring the effects of drugs used to treated acute infarction.

Even the now-traditional imaging techniques have undergone improvement. Using rapid-sequence 1.5-mm CT slices and bolus injection ("angio-CT"), it was possible to identify 74 of 76 intracranial aneurysms.[43] Can MRI beat that record? At the same time, transfemoral cerebral angiography may be getting safer. Not a single permanent neurologic deficit was documented in 159 patients studied for possible carotid endarterectomy.[44] Although this is an excellent record, the authors caution that a 7.7% rate of transient neurologic deficits in patients with ongoing TIAs has frightened them away from studying this group. Intravenous digital angiography, once viewed as a low-risk, low-cost alternative, has been largely abandoned because of poor image quality and unexpectedly high complications from high dye loads. The digital instrumentation has, however, been applied to arterial injection, where the advent of nonionic agents and smaller catheters is expected to reduce morbidity further.

Clinical Entities

Our understanding of stroke in young adults has been enriched by the careful work of Adams and colleagues[45] at the University of Iowa. Of 144 patients between 15 and 45 years old with cerebral infarction, nearly one third (27%) had atherosclerosis. Cardiac lesions that could have sprung emboli accounted for another 24% of cases. The authors attributed 27% to "other vasculopathies," including dissection, moya moya, migraine, connective tissue disease, and miscellaneous vasculitides. Another 15% of strokes were associated with hematologic abnormalities, broadly including oral contraceptive use, acute alcohol ingestion, postpartum state, pregnancy, malignant neoplasia, lupus anticoagulant (LA), thrombocytosis, severe anemia, and antithrombin III deficiency. The authors urged that stroke in young patients not be written off to mitral valve prolapse, birth control pills, or migraine until some of these other entities have been excluded.

Six of the patients in the Iowa series had right-to-left cardiac shunts demonstrated by contrast echocardiography.[46] Presumably, their strokes occurred when venous or right-sided heart clots got into the left side of the heart and arterial circulation without clearing the pulmonary capillary bed ("paradoxical emboli"). One of these patients had an isolated occipital infarct. None had evidence of deep vein thrombosis, and conventional echocardiography was always normal. Lechat et al.[47] found a 54% prevalence of patent foramen ovale in 26 patients without other identifiable causes of stroke—double the prevalence in 19 patients with identifiable causes. There are two points: (1) consider paradoxical emboli if no other reasonable cause appears, even without predisposing conditions, and (2) contrast (not conventional M-mode or two-dimensional) echocardiography is the proper screening test.

Lupus anticoagulant has replaced mitral valve prolapse as the favorite cause of stroke when traditional risk factors have been excluded. It is an antiphospholipid immunoglobulin first discovered in patients with systemic lupus erythematosus (SLE) in 1952 and subsequently found in patients with idiopathic thrombocytopenia, Behçet's disease, cancer, and acquired immunodeficiency syndrome (AIDS) and in otherwise healthy individuals who suffer spontaneous abortions.[48] Patients bearing LA often have false-positive Venereal Disease Research Laboratory tests (VDRLs) without having SLE. The LA is believed to promote thrombosis by reacting with phospholipid moieties of platelets, clotting factors, and vascular endothelium. Its presence is detected by finding a prolonged tissue partial thromboplastin time (PTT) that does not correct when the patient's serum is mixed 1:1 with normal plasma. Lupus anticoagulant is now being blamed for unaccountable ischemic stroke, including retinal infarction and ischemic optic neuropathy.[49] Is there a cause-and-effect case for LA and these strokes? Unlike with mitral valve prolapse, where the problem was common occurrence in unaffected patients, the problem with invoking LA is that other risk factors are often present. Much more solid epidemiologic work will be needed before LA can be accepted as actor rather than bystander. Nevertheless, where no risk factors are evident in young patients, they had best undergo a test battery of PTT, VDRL, and antiphospholipid antibodies.[50]

The pathogenesis of neurologic symptoms and signs in SLE has been a mystery. Although "vasculitis" is colloquially mentioned, there is little evidence for it pathologically. Instead, arteriolar thromboses are typically found. In a recent clinicopathologic study of 50 patients with CNS lupus, the best pathologic correlation was with nonvasculitic thromboses caused by emboli (Libman-Sacks endocarditis) and thrombotic thrombocytopenic purpura.[51] On the other hand, Bonfa et al.[52] have confirmed previous evidence that autoimmune cytotoxic reaction may be responsible for exacerbations of lupus psychosis. They found that the levels of antibodies to ribosomal P proteins were highly correlated with episodes of psychosis. Another marker for active CNS lupus is reduced cerebral blood flow.[53]

What exactly is granulomatous angiitis of the brain and what is its relation to temporal (or cranial) arteritis? A superlative review of 74 reported cases and 4 new ones[54] disclosed that most patients presented with headache and disturbances of cognition or consciousness and later developed focal deficits. In many cases, imaging and cerebrospinal fluid studies were normal and diagnosis was made either on brain-leptomeningeal biopsy or on autopsy. About half the cases had no associated illness; the others had herpes zoster, lymphoma, sarcoidosis, or temporal arteritis. Pathologically it looked exactly like temporal arteritis. Another report emphasized the value of prompt and intensive corticosteroid-cyclophosphamide treatment.[55] Although the prevalence of positive temporal biopsies was not discussed, that may be a good first step in these patients. A review of 166 consecutive patients with biopsy-proved temporal arteritis[56] revealed a panoply of neurologic findings unrelated to vision, reminding us either that the vasculopathy of this disease is widespread or that Mayo-style retrospective reviews sometimes give misleading information. For example, were the five neuropsychiatric syndromes, eight cases of vertigo, and 23 peripheral neuropathies really due to the arteritis?

Two reports remind us that herpes zoster ophthalmicus can wreak devastation, not just in the eye but behind it. One patient developed a classic ipsilateral middle cerebral artery stroke ("zoster hemiplegia"),[57] and two others had ruptured mycotic aneurysms.[58] The presumption is that the zoster gets to the basal vessels by way of trigeminal branches that innervate them. It would appear that intravenous acyclovir is indicated when zoster ophthalmicus develops in immunosuppressed patients, although there is no evidence that it forestalls CNS complications.

Deficiencies of natural anticoagulants protein S, protein C, and antithrombin III have been implicated in venous thrombosis. Now comes a report[59] that single patients with each of these deficiencies have had extensive arterial thromboses. Presumably, a search for these factors will have to be added to the workup of unexplained stroke.

Stroke in migraineurs is evidently quite uncommon. Of nearly 5,000 patients diagnosed as having migraine or vascular headache at the Mayo Clinic from 1976 to 1980, only 20 (0.4%) had migraine-associated brain infarctions, mostly in the occipital lobe.[60] Eighteen of 20 had minimal functional impairment. On the other hand, during the same period, these strokes accounted for one quarter of the total in patients aged 50 years or less. Why do these few unlucky migraineurs have a stroke? Bogousslavsky et al.[61] studied 22 such victims and could determine only that they had particularly long classic migraine attacks. In a similar study of 22 patients, Rothrock et al.[62] found no special features but noted that only one patient developed a second stroke in a mean of 22 months' follow-up. Whether these strokes are caused by vasospasm, heightened coagulation, or sluggish blood flow is a pressing issue to which no new information has been forthcoming. Goodwin et al.[63] found that, when it comes to monocular amaurosis fugax, you cannot tell migraine from presumed carotid thromboembolism based on the description of the attack. Scintillations and vision loss lasting longer than 6 minutes occurred frequently in patients who had good evidence of thromboembolism.

The distribution of strokes in patients with sickle cell disease has been clarified with MRI. In two recent studies,[64, 65] lesions were found mostly in the large cerebral border-zone regions. Both reports concluded that large-vessel stenosis, as well as distal sludging in cortical arterioles, was responsible. Current thinking is that repeated exchange transfusion to maintain hemoglobin S levels below 20% is helpful in preventing progression of large-artery disease.[66]

There is good news that in spite of an occasional but spectacular stroke syndrome, cardiac catheterization[67] and balloon valvuloplasty[68] appear to have an acceptably low risk of major permanent neurologic deficits.

TREATMENT

Grotta[69] has admirably summarized matters as they stood at the close of 1987. I have updated his report and emphasized areas of special interest to neuro-ophthalmologists.

Prevention of Stroke

Based on a magnificent review[70] of the 25 completed aspirin-in-stroke-prevention trials, the authors conclude that aspirin reduces nonfatal stroke by 30%. Doses of 300 mg/day are as effective as higher doses and less gastrotoxic. However, not all studies show such a beneficial effect. The United Kingdom TIA aspirin trial, with 2,435 randomized patients, found only a 7% reduction in stroke.[71]

As for other effective antiplatelet drugs, the landscape is barren. Sulfinpyrazone is already in oblivion, and, after an authoritative review, dipyridamole was recently dismissed with the following words: "the evidence that . . . dipyridamole exerts antithrombotic action in humans is very limited . . . the emerging consensus does not support its use as an antiplatelet drug."[72]

The efficacy of anticoagulants such as heparin and warfarin is supported more by anecdote and intuition than by controlled study. Neither a retrospective study of heparin after first TIA[73] nor a prospective randomized study of heparin in acute partial stable stroke[74] showed any benefit. Adherents of anticoagulant therapy for TIA generally restrict its use to patients who have "breakthrough" TIAs while taking aspirin, and then limit treatment duration to 3 to 6 months. Other accepted indications for anticoagulants are cardioembolic and progressing stroke and nonhemorrhagic infarct associated with proximal large cerebral artery occlusion. None of these customs is fortified with sound data. In view of this, and because of the high long-term risk of hemorrhage when coagulation times are prolonged to twice normal, it is recommended that 1.5 times (rather than twice) control values be sought; they are much safer and may be just as effective.[75]

The past 2 years saw the debate about the advisability of carotid endarterectomy heat up in the medical literature, the newspapers, and even the television talk shows. With mounting reports of relatively high surgical morbidity, a demonstrated efficacy of aspirin, the downward revision of the untreated stroke risk (especially for patients with ocular, as opposed to hemispheric, ischemia), and the failure of temporal–middle cerebral artery bypass, proponents of endarterectomy fell on the defensive.[76-83] An authoritative decision analysis[84] disclosed that surgery should not be considered at all for patients with an annual risk of stroke of 3% or less. That would exclude patients with amaurosis fugax, retinal artery occlusions, Hollenhorst plaques, and asymptomatic carotid bruits or stenosis. The only exceptions in those groups might be patients with progressing or greater than 90% stenosis who, in some studies, appear to have a higher stroke risk.

Then came the Rand Corporation study,[85] in which a national panel of experts was asked to determine the "appropriateness" of 1,302 endarterectomies performed in 1981 in three geographic areas in the United States. The panel found only 35% of the procedures indicated. Most of the nonindicated procedures occurred in patients with less than 50% stenosis or without TIAs in the carotid distribution. There was a 9.8% major complication rate.

The safety of this procedure remains a serious question. The University of Alabama group[86] reported a combined morbidity and mortality of only 2.1% among 142 consecutive cases, but another study[15] revealed 3 serious strokes (10%) among 30 patients operated on, 19 of whom had never had a single TIA before surgery.

With an enrollment of 44 North American surgical centers, the North American Symptomatic Carotid Endarterectomy Trial should resolve some of these issues. However, getting patients to accept randomization in such a critical matter has been difficult, and data from the study will not surface for several years. In the meantime, this observer believes that patients should not have surgery except as part of the study.

Treatment of Acute Infarction

The treatment of acute brain or spinal cord infarction is based on two approaches: (1) to open closed arteries quickly to reestablish perfusion to viable tissue, and (2) to interrupt the cytotoxic cascade of ischemia by blocking excitatory neurotransmitters, calcium channels, or opiates. Neither approach has yet yielded bankable clinical results, but there is still room for optimism.

Hemodilution with low-molecular-weight dextran is a means of improving cerebral blood flow by lowering hematocrit to an optimal 30% to 33%. Unfortunately, the definitive Italian trial of 1,267 patients with acute hemispheric stroke showed no benefit.[87] Pentoxifylline (Trental), a drug that makes red blood cells more pliable, has been touted for ischemic peripheral vascular disease but has failed in cerebral infarction.[88] Prostacyclin held promise as a vasodilator and antiplatelet agent but fell short in two controlled trials.[89, 90]

By inducing a hibernatory low metabolic state and by blocking calcium channels, barbiturates were expected to help abort the cytotoxic cascade but evidently did not.[69] Naloxone, an opiate antagonist, was moderately effective in a small trial.[91] MK-801 is the long-sought glutamate antagonist at the *N*-methyl-D-aspartate (NMDA) receptor that easily penetrates the blood-brain barrier after intravenous injection. By interfering with glutamate binding at the NMDA receptor, this agent could interrupt glutamate's "excitotoxic" actions—persistent depolarization leading to cell death. In two rat cerebral ischemia models, MK-801, injected 5 minutes after injury, reduced neurologic deficits.[92] Nimopidine, a member of the dihydropyridine family of neuronal calcium channel blockers, has improved outcome in acute stroke in males in a large clinical trial.[93]

Despite these more or less encouraging reports, the hot item this year is thrombolysis, probably because of the extravagant success of tissue plasminogen activator (TPA) in treating myocardial infarction. The advantage of TPA is that it can be given intravenously and will break up clots without causing systemic fibrinolysis and hemorrhage. Two experimental studies[94, 95] have shown its effectiveness in accelerating reperfusion without unwanted hemorrhage. Clinical trials are expected to get under way.

If TPA does not catch fire in stroke management, perhaps transluminal balloon angioplasty for inoperable stenosis will. Higashida et al.[96] reported that in 16 of 17 patients, narrowed vertebrobasilar vessels were opened and stayed open for a mean of 15 months. One patient suffered a brain-stem infarct; the others were asymptomatic at last visits. At this writing, can there be many "interventional neuroradiologists" so skilled or so bold? Will their success continue, and can they pass on their tricks?

REFERENCES

1. Colditz GA, Bonita R, Stampfer MJ, et al: Cigarette smoking and risk of stroke in middle-aged women. *N Engl J Med* 1988; 318:937–941.

2. Wolf PA, D'Agostino RB, Kannel WB, et al: Cigarette smoking as a risk factor for stroke, the Framingham Study. *JAMA* 1988; 259:1025–1029.

3. Abbott RD, Yin Y, Reed DM, et al: Risk of stroke in male cigarette smokers. *N Engl J Med* 1986; 315:717–720.

4. Wilhelmsen L, Svardsudd K, Korsan-Bengsten K, et al: Fibrinogen as a risk factor for stroke and myocardial infarction. *N Engl J Med* 1984; 311:501–505.

5. Welin L, Svardsudd K, Wilhelmsen L, et al: Analysis of risk factors for stroke in a cohort of men born in 1913. *N Engl J Med* 1987; 317:521–526.

6. Kannel WB, Wolf PA, Verter J: Manifestations of coronary disease predisposing to stroke: The Framingham Study. *JAMA* 1983; 250:2942–2946.

7. Tanaka H, Hayashi M, Date C, et al: Epidemiologic studies of Shibata, a Japanese provincial city: Preliminary report on risk factors for cerebral infarction. *Stroke* 1985; 16:773–780.

8. Kagan A, Popper JS, Rhoads GG, et al: Dietary and other risk factors for stroke in Hawaiian Japanese men. *Stroke* 1985; 16:390–396.

9. Davis PH, Dambrosia JM, Schoenberg BS, et al: Risk factors for ischemic stroke: A prospective study in Rochester, Minnesota. *Ann Neurol* 1987; 22:319–327.

10. Wolf PA, Kannel WB, McGee DL: Epidemiology of strokes in North America, in Barnett HJM, Mohr JP, Stein BM, et al (eds): *Stroke: Pathophysiology, Diagnosis, and Management.* New York, Churchill Livingstone, Inc, 1986, pp 19–29.

11. Benson MD, Rebar RW: Relationship of migraine headache and stroke to oral contraceptive use. *J Reprod Med* 1986; 31:1082–1088.

12. Lidegaard O: Cerebrovascular deaths before and after the appearance of oral contraceptives. *Acta Neurol Scand* 1987; 75:427–433.

13. Longstreth W, Koepsell T, Yerby M, et al: Risk factors for subarachnoid hemorrhage. *Stroke* 1985; 16:377–385.

14. Hennerici M, Hulsbomer HB, Hefter H, et al: Natural history of asymptomatic extracranial arterial disease: Results of a long-term prospective study. *Brain* 1987; 110:777–791.

15. Chambers BR, Norris JW: Outcome in patients with asymptomatic neck bruits. *N Engl J Med* 1986; 315:860–865.

16. Meissner I, Wiebers DO, Whisnant JP, et al: The natural history of asymptomatic carotid artery occlusive lesions. *JAMA* 1987; 258:2704–2707.

17. O'Halleran LW, Kennelly MM, McClurken M, et al: Natural history of asymptomatic carotid plaque. *Am J Surg* 1987; 154:659–662.

18. Seeger JM, Klingman N: The relationship between plaque composition and neurologic symptoms. *J Surg Res* 1987; 43:78–85.

19. Chawluk JB, Kushner MJ, Bank WJ, et al: Atherosclerotic carotid artery disease in patients with retinal ischemic syndromes. *Neurology* 1988; 38:858–863.

20. Howard RS, Ross Russell RW: Prognosis of patients with retinal embolism. *J Neurol Neurosurg Psychiatry* 1987; 50:1142–1147.

21. Pfaffenbach DD, Hollenhorst RW: Morbidity and survivorship of patients with embolic cholesterol crystals in the ocular fundus. *Am J Ophthalmol* 1966; 61:1159–1165.

22. Savino PJ, Glaser JS, Casady J: Retinal stroke: Is the patient at risk? *Arch Ophthalmol* 1982; 89:1336–1347.

23. Poole CJM, Ross Russell RW: Mortality and stroke after amaurosis fugax. *J Neurol Neurosurg Psychiatry* 1985; 48:902–905.

24. Komiyama M, Baba M, Hakuba A, et al: MR imaging of brainstem hemorrhage. *AJNR* 1988; 9:261–268.

25. Smith JH, Strother CM, Kikuchi Y, et al: MR imaging in the management of supratentorial intracranial AVMs. *AJNR* 1988; 9:225–235.

26. Leblanc R, Levesque M, Comair Y, et al: Magnetic resonance imaging of cerebral arteriovenous malformations. *Neurosurgery* 1987; 21:15–20.

27. Kertesz A, Black SE, Nicholson L, et al: The sensitivity and specificity of MRI in stroke. *Neurology* 1987; 37:1580–1585.

28. Imakita S, Nishimura T, Naito H, et al: Magnetic resonance imaging of human cerebral infarction: Enhancement with Gd-DTPA. *Neuroradiology* 1987; 29:422–429.

29. Kertesz A, Black S, Takar G, et al: Periventricular and subcortical hyperintensities on magnetic resonance imaging: "Rims, caps, and unidentified bright objects." *Arch Neurol* 1988; 45:404–408.

30. Binswanger O: Die Abgrenzung der allgemeinen progressiven Paralyse. *Berl Klin Wochenschr* 1894; 31:1103–1105, 1137–1139, 1180–1186.

31. Hachinski VC, Potter P, Merskey H: Leuko-araiosis. *Arch Neurol* 1987; 44:21–23.

32. Marshall VG, Bradley WG Jr, Marshall CE, et al: Deep white matter infarction: Correlation of MR imaging and histopathologic findings. *Radiology* 1988; 167:517–522.

33. Taylor DC, Strandness DE Jr: Carotid artery Duplex scanning. *J Clin Ultrasound* 1987; 15:635–644.

34. Rubin JR, Bondi JA, Rhodes RS: Duplex scanning versus conventional arteriography for the evaluation of carotid artery plaque morphology. *Surgery* 1987; 102:749–755.

35. Hodge CJ Jr, Lesson M, Cacayorin E, et al: Computed tomographic evaluation of extracranial carotid artery disease. *Neurosurgery* 1987; 21:167–176.

36. Mattle H, Grolimund P, Huber P, et al: Transcranial Doppler sonographic findings in middle cerebral artery disease. *Arch Neurol* 1988; 45:289–295.

37. Caplan LR, Stein R: *Stroke: A Clinical Approach.* Stoneham, Mass, Butterworth Publishers Inc, 1986.

38. Klingelhofer J, Conrad B, Benecke R, et al: Evaluation of intracranial pressure from transcranial Doppler studies in cerebral disease. *J Neurol* 1988; 235:159–162.

39. Bosley TM, Dunn R, Silver FL, et al: Recovery of vision after ischemic lesions: Positron emission tomography. *Ann Neurol* 1987; 21:444–450.

40. Demer JL, von Noorden GK, Gould KL: Imaging of cerebral blood flow and metabolism in amblyopia by positron emission tomography. *Am J Ophthalmol* 1988; 105:337–347.

41. Foster NL, Mountz JM, Bluemlein MS, et al: Blood flow imaging of a posterior circulation stroke: Use of technetium Tc 99m hexamethylpropyleneamine oxime and single photon emission computed tomography. *Arch Neurol* 1988; 45:687–690.

42. Levine SR, Welch KMA, Helpern JA, et al: Prolonged deterioration of ischemic brain energy metabolism and acidosis associated with hyperglycemia: Human cerebral infarction studied by serial 31P NMR spectroscopy. *Ann Neurol* 1988; 23:416–418.

43. Schmidt VD, Steiger HJ, Huber P: Accuracy of high resolution computed tomography in direct diagnosis of cerebral aneurysms. *Neuroradiology* 1987; 29:152–159.

44. Theodotou BC, Whaley R, Mahaley MS: Complications following transfemoral cerebral angiography for cerebral ischemia. *Surg Neurol* 1987; 28:90–92.

45. Adams HP, Butler MJ, Biller J, et al: Nonhemorrhagic cerebral infarction in young adults. *Arch Neurol* 1986; 43:793–796.

46. Biller J, Adams HP, Johnson MR, et al: Paradoxical cerebral embolism: Eight cases. *Neurology* 1986; 36:1356–1360.

47. Lechat PH, Mas JL, Lascault G, et al: Prevalence of patent foramen ovale in patients with stroke. *N Engl J Med* 1988; 318:1148–1152.

48. Gastineau DA, Kazmier FJ, Nichols WL, et al: Lupus anticoagulant: An analysis of the clinical and laboratory features of 219 cases. *Am J Hematol* 1985; 19:265–275.

49. Levine SR, Crofts JW, Lesser GR, et al: Visual symptoms associated with the presence of a lupus anticoagulant. *Ophthalmology* 1988; 95:686–692.

50. Triplett DA, Brandt JT, Musgrave KA, et al: The relationship between lupus anticoagulants and antibodies to phospholipid. *JAMA* 1988; 259:550–554.

51. Devinsky O, Petito CK, Alonso DR: Clinical and neuropathological findings in systemic thrombocytopenic purpura. *Ann Neurol* 1988; 23:380–384.

52. Bonfa E, Golombek SJ, Kaufman LD, et al: Association between lupus psychosis and anti-ribosomal P protein antibodies. *N Engl J Med* 1987; 317:265–271.

53. Kushner MJ, Chawluk J, Fazekas F, et al: Cerebral blood flow in systemic lupus erythematosus with or without cerebral complications. *Neurology* 1987; 37:1596–1598.

54. Younger DS, Hays AP, Brust JCM, et al: Granulomatous angiitis of the brain: An inflammatory reaction of diverse etiology. *Arch Neurol* 1988; 45:514–518.

55. Vanderzant C, Bromberg M, MacGuire A, et al: Isolated small-vessel angiitis of the central nervous system. *Arch Neurol* 1988; 45:683–687.

56. Caselli RJ, Huder GC, Whisnant JP: Neurologic disease in biopsy-proven giant cell (temporal) arteritis. *Neurology* 1988; 38:352–359.

57. Freedman MS, MacDonald RD: Herpes zoster ophthalmicus with delayed cerebral infarction and meningoencephalitis. *Can J Neurol Sci* 1987; 14:312–314.

58. O'Donohue JM, Enzmann DR: Mycotic aneurysm in angiitis associated with herpes zoster ophthalmicus. *AJNR* 1987; 8:615–619.

59. Coller BS, Owen J, Jesty J, et al: Deficiency of plasma protein S, protein C or antithrombin III and arterial thrombosis. *Arteriosclerosis* 1987; 7:456–462.

60. Broderick JP, Swanson JW: Migraine-related strokes. *Arch Neurol* 1987; 44:868–871.

61. Bogousslavsky J, Regli F, Van Melle G, et al: Migraine stroke. *Neurology* 1988; 38:223–226.

62. Rothrock JF, Walicke P, Swenson MR, et al: Migrainous stroke. *Arch Neurol* 1988; 45:63–67.

63. Goodwin JA, Gorelick PB, Helgason CM: Symptoms of amaurosis fugax in atherosclerotic carotid artery disease. *Neurology* 1987; 37:829–832.

64. Adams RJ, Nichols FT, McKie V, et al: Cerebral infarction in sickle cell anemia: Mechanism based on CT and MRI. *Neurology* 1988; 38:1012–1017.

65. Pavlakis SG, Bello J, Prohovnik I, et al: Brain infarction in sickle cell anemia: Magnetic resonance imaging correlates. *Ann Neurol* 1988; 23:125–130.

66. Russell MO, Goldberg HI, Hodson A et al: Effect of transfusion therapy on arteriographic abnormalities and on recurrence of stroke in sickle cell disease. *Blood* 1984; 63:162–169.

67. Kosmorsky G, Hanson MR, Tomsak RL: Neuro-ophthalmologic complications of cardiac catheterization. *Neurology* 1988; 38:483–485.

68. Davidson CJ, Skelton TN, Kisslo KB, et al: The risk for systemic embolization associated with percutaneous balloon valvuloplasty in adults. *Ann Intern Med* 1988; 108:557–560.

69. Grotta JC: Current medical and surgical therapy for cerebrovascular disease. *N Engl J Med* 1987; 317:1505–1516.

70. Antiplatelet Trialists' Collaboration: Secondary prevention of vascular disease by prolonged antiplatelet treatment. *Br Med J* 1988; 296:320–331.

71. United Kingdom Transient Ischaemic Attack Study Group: United Kingdom transient ischaemic attack (UK-TIA) aspirin trial: Interim results. *Br Med J* 1988; 296:316–320.

72. Fitzgerald GA: Dipyridamole. *N Engl J Med* 1987; 316:1247–1256.

73. Keith DS, Phillips SJ, Whisnant JP, et al: Heparin therapy for recent transient focal cerebral ischemia. *Mayo Clin Proc* 1987; 62:1101–1106.

74. Duke RJ, Bloch RF, Turpie AGG, et al: Intravenous heparin for the prevention of stroke progression in acute partial stable stroke: A randomized controlled trial. *Ann Intern Med* 1986; 105:825–828.

75. Hirsh J, Levine M: Therapeutic range for the control of oral anticoagulant therapy. *Arch Neurol* 1986; 43:1162–1164.

76. North American Symptomatic Carotid Endarterectomy Study Group: Carotid endarterectomy: Three critical evaluations. *Stroke* 1987; 18:987–989.

77. American Neurological Association Committee on Health Care Issues: Does carotid endarterectomy decrease stroke and death in patients with transient ischemic attacks? *Ann Neurol* 1987; 22:72–76.

78. Sandercock P: Asymptomatic carotid stenosis: Spare the knife. *Br Med J* 1987; 294:1368.

79. Patterson RH: Can carotid endarterectomy be justified? Yes. *Arch Neurol* 1987; 44:651–652.

80. Jonas S: Can carotid endarterectomy be justified? No. *Arch Neurol* 1987; 44:652–654.

81. Trobe JD: Carotid endarterectomy: Who needs it? *Ophthalmology* 1987; 94:725–730.

82. Becker WL, Burde RM: Carotid artery disease: A therapeutic dilemma. *Arch Ophthalmol* 1988; 106:34–39.

83. Loftus CM, Quest DO: Technical controversies in carotid artery surgery. *Neurosurgery* 1987; 20:490–495.

84. Matchar DB, Pauker SG: Endarterectomy in carotid artery disease: A decision analysis. *JAMA* 1987; 258:793–798.

85. Winslow CM, Solomon DH, Chassin MR, et al: The appropriateness of carotid endarterectomy. *N Engl J Med* 1988; 318:721–727.

86. Zeiger HE, Zampella EJ, Naftel DC, et al: A prospective analysis of 142 carotid endarterectomies for occlusive vascular disease, 1979–1985. *J Neurosurg* 1987; 67:540–544.

87. Italian Acute Stroke Study Group: Haemodilution in acute stroke: Results of the Italian Haemodilution Trial. *Lancet* 1988; 1:318–321.

88. Pentoxifylline Study Group: Pentoxifylline (PTX) in acute ischemic stroke, abstracted. *Stroke* 1987; 18:298.

89. Hsu CY, Faught RE Jr, Furlan AJ, et al: Intravenous prostacyclin in acute nonhemorrhagic stroke: A placebo-controlled double-blind trial. *Stroke* 1987; 18:352–358.

90. Martin JF, Hamdy N, Nicholl J, et al: Double-blind controlled trial of prostacyclin in cerebral infarction. *Stroke* 1985; 16:386–390.

91. Adams HP Jr, Olinger CP, Barsan WB, et al: A dose-escalation study of large doses of naloxone for treatment of patients with acute cerebral ischemia. *Stroke* 1986; 17:404–409.

92. Kochhar A, Zivin JA, Lyden PD, et al: Glutamate antagonist therapy reduces neurologic deficits produced by focal central nervous system ischemia. *Arch Neurol* 1988; 45:148–153.

93. Gelmers HJ, Gorter K, DeWeerdt CJ, et al: A controlled trial of nimodipine in acute ischemic stroke. *N Engl J Med* 1988; 318:203–207.

94. Papadopoulos SM, Chandler WF, Salamat MS, et al: Recombinant human tissue-type plasminogen activator therapy in acute thromboembolic stroke. *J Neurosurg* 1987; 67:394–398.

95. Zivin JA, Lyden PD, DeGirolami U, et al: Tissue plasminogen activator. *Arch Neurol* 1988; 45:387–391.

96. Higashida RT, Hieshima GB, Tsai FY, et al: Transluminal angioplasty of the vertebral and basilar artery. *AJNR* 1987; 8:745–749.

CHAPTER 17

Migraine and Facial Pain

B. Todd Troost, M.D.

Department of Neurology, Bowman Gray School of Medicine, Wake Forest University, Winston-Salem, North Carolina

George M. McCormick, M.D.

Department of Neurology, Bowman Gray School of Medicine, Wake Forest University, Winston-Salem, North Carolina

Migraine has been estimated to affect nearly 10% of the population. It may be manifested by focal neurologic as well as neuro-ophthalmologic symptoms and signs. Most patients experience infrequent and benign transient problems, while a few may have significant permanent sequelae. There are a number of migraine "equivalents" that may have the common stereotyped visual and neurologic symptoms but lack unilateral throbbing headache. In this chapter we will discuss some of the contributions made in the last 2 years to the understanding of migraine and its treatment. Several excellent reviews have been published recently.[1-3]

PATHOPHYSIOLOGY

There is still much debate over the mechanisms and underlying causes of migraine. Theories for the pathogenesis of migraine include a primary vascular disorder with dysregulation of the arteries supplying the brain (a "spreading oligemia"), a systemic origin due to platelet abnormalities, and a dysfunction of central nervous system regulatory mechanisms that modulate pain systems as well

Curr Neuro Ophthalmol 2:307–330, 1989
© 1989, Year Book Medical Publishers, Inc.
0893–0147/89/02-307-330-$04.00

as central control of the cerebral vasculature.[2, 4] Olesen[5] believes the controversy revolves around whether cortical arteriolar spasm plays a primary role or whether the spreading wave of reduced cerebral blood flow is secondary to metabolic depression from reduced neuronal function.

Asymmetric differences in regional cerebral blood flow (rCBF) have been found in migraineurs between attacks.[6] Reduced rCBF during classic migraine attacks may last for up to 3 hours after the prodrome resolves and the headache begins, making it unlikely that the headache is triggered by the subsequent hyperemic stage.[7] In a study[8] of patients with classic or hemiplegic migraine during the prodromal phase of the migraine, there were no detected arterial occlusions or spasms of the larger arteries by angiography, and on rCBF studies there was the appearance of focal ischemic hypoperfusion associated with transient neurologic deficits and the development of severe headache. There were unstable washout rates with 12- to 60-second intervals of very low ischemic blood flow alternating with periods of normal or hyperemic blood flow, termed *cerebrovascular tone instability,* and this was thought to be transient vasospasm of the small-resistance vessels in the brain.[8-10] In a small study, 2 of 3 patients had focal hyperperfusion preceding hypoperfusion, associated with unstable vascular tone.[11] Solomon et al.,[12] reviewing angiograms obtained during migraine attacks, noted that segmental narrowing could be unrelated to the timing of the attack and did not always correlate with the side of headache, neurologic deficits, or duration. Vasospasm, edema, or inflammation would give the same picture. Thie and associates[13] noted prolonged diffuse vasospasm in migraineurs even while asymptomatic.

Two studies found reduced rCBF only in classic migraine and not other types, though many of the latter had hyperemic stages.[5, 14] The reduction was not limited to one arterial territory. Olesen[15] noted differences in autoregulation of rCBF between classic and common migraineurs, suggesting they may be distinct in pathophysiology and supporting a neurogenic etiology.

Several studies have been conducted recently concerning the spreading depression of Leão.[16-18] Cerebral glucose metabolism is decreased during the initial and later events of migrainous headache. The spreading depression can be provoked in animals by localized electrical or mechanical stimulation as well as potassium chloride and amino acid injections to the cortex,[18] and the depression wave is associated with a brief initial vasodilation and followed by a longer phase of reduced local blood circulation, as has been noted in patients with migraine. During the cortical spreading depression activity, other structures of the brain, especially deeper structures, can be affected and may explain some of the vegetative effects accompanying migraine, perhaps by liberation of thalamic and hypothalamic centers from cortical inhibition. This could cause a temporary deafferentation between cranial nerve nuclei and thalamus and cortex. The initial depolarization wave of the spreading depression has been suggested to give rise to the scotomata of migraine and the neurophysiologic phenomena. In contrast to this, Gloor[19] noted that, in his experience of 30 years of recording electroactivity on the exposed cortex of some 1,000 humans who were locally anesthetized, he had never encountered activity resembling spreading depression. He noted that spreading depression was more difficult to elicit in highly evolved cortex and he doubted that spreading depression played a role in human cerebropathophysiology such as migraine. However, De Noordhout et al.[20] described a slow cerebral potential recorded over the scalp, called contingent negative variation, which reflects simple reaction time to tasks when a warning stimulus is given. The amplitude variation was increased in migraineurs between attacks and was thought to reflect central catecholaminergic hyperactivity since norepinephrine and dopamine facilitate this system.

Many of the prophylactic antimigraine agents, used because of their vasoconstrictive properties, have been shown to have high affinity for serotonin receptors in brain.[21] Methysergide, cyproheptadine, pizotyline, propranolol, amitriptyline, and calcium channel blockers show growing evidence of having central neuronal effects. The interaction of the serotonergic and catecholaminergic pathways in the raphe nuclei, hypothalamus, and forebrain with substance P and biogenic amines in the limbic and cortical areas could offer explanations of the autonomic, emotional, and pain states of migraineurs.[21-29] Raskin[26] notes that drugs may act as agonists in ascending systems and antagonists in descending systems and that an inherited serotoninergic instability could cause dysmodulation. Potentiating factors, such as sex, age, and chronic stress, and activating factors, such as trauma, vasodilators, and diet, may also affect this system.[30] Fasting may result in a chronic stress reaction with heightened sympathetic activity, affecting carbohydrate and fatty acid metabolism and increasing turnover of brain serotonin, possibly initiating headache.[1]

The relationship between migraine and platelets continues to be controversial. Hanington[31, 32] reviewed evidence that the platelets of migraineurs show a significant increase in the release of serotonin between attacks and that this culminates in a very large release at the onset of a migraine. It has been shown that reserpine, exertion, and trauma can increase platelet aggregation and lead to significant increases of serotonin release, as can vasoactive amines such as tyramine and β-phenylethylamine (found in cheese and chocolate). However, a study with flunarizine, a calcium antagonist, showed that the therapeutic effect of the drug did not correlate with platelet activation, indicating that platelet activation may be an epiphenomenon only.[33] Others also believe that the platelet activities are epiphenomena.[34, 35] D'Andrea et al.[36] believe high serotonin levels in platelets of patients with classic migraine are indicative of a low serotonin turnover. They believe this may similarly occur in presynaptic terminals in the brain and cause postsynaptic supersensitivity to serotonin.

Mitral valve prolapse was more prevalent in complicated migraine in one study,[37] but another[38] found no differences among migraine types. Neither group found differences in platelet function in patients with mitral valve prolapse or migraine or in controls.

In immunologic studies, dysfunctional regulation of immunoglobulin isotype expression,[39] and an increased association with antiphospholipid antibodies (lupus anticoagulant and autocardiolipin antibodies), antinuclear antibodies, and anti–smooth-muscle antibodies,[40–42] have been seen in migraineurs. No differences in complement levels or immune complex titers were found between migraineurs and control patients.[43] Levine et al.[44] suggested that these antibodies could alter prostaglandins or neuronal phospholipids, thereby altering release of neurotransmitters. Leukotrienes, which are inflammatory mediators and pain modulators, are elevated during migraine and cluster headaches.[45, 46]

Further evidence for central nervous system dysfunction in migraineurs comes from studies of altered autonomic function in cardiovascular reflexes[47–49] and of pupillary asymmetry[50–52] in migraineurs.

Common Migraine

In considering the diagnosis of common migraine, Solomon et al.[53] have considered features of patients with common migraine that could help differentiate them from patients with chronic daily headaches. Features associated more often with the common migraine diagnosis included nausea, vomiting, unilateral site, throbbing quality, photophobia, and the association with menstruation and family history of migraine.

Classic Migraine

Peatfield[54] noted that headache is frequent in transient ischemic attacks (TIA) and that classic migraine may have focal neurologic symptoms. Both can result in infarctions and are associated with platelet abnormalities and mitral valve prolapse. He suggested that TIA and migraines originate from "similar, if not identical, mechanisms and that a predisposition to spreading depression" in migraineurs may cause the symptoms.

Magnetic resonance imaging (MRI) was compared with computed tomography (CT) in evaluating patients with migraine.[55] Magnetic resonance imaging found additional lesions in one third of patients, including cerebral infarctions, multiple white matter infarcts, and a malignant medullary astrocytoma.

In reviewing symptoms of classic migraineurs, Andersen et al.[56] found visual aura symptoms were frequent (86% overall) both before (exclusively in 43%) and during the headache phase (22%). Nonvisual symptoms (aphasia, paresis, paresthesias) were noted in 75% of patients. Paresis (29%) and speech disturbances (33%) were observed during the headache. They noted that visual auras usually occurred before and nonvisual auras usually during headache. Many of the visual auras continued into the headache phase.

Ophthalmoplegic Migraine

Coppeto and Greco[57] described a 29-year-old woman with migraines and a family history of migraine, including ophthalmic migraine, who complained of lightheadedness and horizontal diplopia on left gaze. Examination was normal except for slow and limited adduction in the right eye and end-gaze nystagmus on left gaze in the left eye. Convergence was normal, and the ocular motility abnormalities cleared within 1 week. Cranial MRI was performed and showed a frontal arteriovenous malformation, confirmed on arteriography. At surgery, the malformation appeared stained from recent bleeding and was removed completely. The authors suggested that this was an internuclear ophthalmoplegia due to vascular steal by an arteriovenous malformation, but could not rule out the possibility of vasospasm in a pontine penetrating artery due to subarachnoid hemorrhage from the arteriovenous malformation.

Amit and Benezra[58] described a 14-month-old infant with paroxysmal episodes of vomiting followed by oculomotor nerve palsy that persisted for several weeks, then completely resolved. They believed this to be ophthalmoplegic migraine.

Anterior Visual Pathway (Retinal) Migraine

Under the heading of Retinal Migraine, articles will be reviewed dealing with monocular visual symptoms in migraine. "Anterior visual pathway" migraine is a more accurate but less used term. Tomsak and Jergens[59] discussed 24 patients with recurrent transient monocular blindness who were felt to have variants of acephalgic migraine. The suggested mechanism of visual loss was hypoperfusion of the retina or optic nerve due to vasospasm of the central retinal artery or ophthalmic artery. They felt that 19 (79%) of the patients had visual disturbances most consistent with a generalized ocular hypoperfusion with concentric contraction of vision, and only five of their patients had an altitudinal or quadrantic visual change that was thought to be more consistent with an embolic event or possibly vasospasm of the retinal artery branch. There was no change in perfusion of the blood vessels of the choroidal circulation. A personal history of migraine was found in one third of their patients.

In an editorial by Edmeads,[60] theories of monocular migraine were discussed in relation to the Tomsak and Jergens article.[59] He noted that one third of their patients had a history of migraine, and though the outcome appeared benign, the investigation was not exhaustive in many of their patients, as only seven had CT scans, only three had carotid angiography, and only two had echocardiograms. Though 20% of the population had migraine, these same people were still at risk for atherosclerosis, heart disease, and clotting diatheses. Also, the follow-up period averaged less than 2 years. Edmeads still felt that monocular migraine is a diagnosis of exclusion.

Goodwin et al.[61] studied 37 patients with amaurosis fugax and angiography-proved carotid atherosclerosis ipsilateral to the symptomatic eye. One third of the patients had prolonged attacks or positive visual phenomena, symptoms that were believed in the past to be more typical of monocular migraine. None of their patients showed slow progression or change in size of the scotomata, and one of their patients had severe ipsilateral pain that occurred several hours after the onset of visual symptoms. They therefore felt that amaurosis fugax and retinal migraine had symptoms of such overlap that clinical differentiation would be difficult based on clinical symptoms alone.

Cerebral Migraine

Twenty percent of migraineurs may experience acephalgic attacks of migraine, as noted in a review by Kunkel.[62] Recurrent symptoms, such as transient paresthesias, slurring of words, expressive aphasias, monoparesis or hemiparesis, benign recurrent vertigo, transient global amnesia, dysphrenic migraine with mood lability, and personality changes can occur as equivalents or auras. Acute confusional states in children and adolescents, without headache, may be migrainous.[63] Abdominal migraine may be due to alterations in the autonomic pathways to the gastrointestinal tract. Acephalgic migraine may respond to standard antimigraine drugs, prophylactically and at the onset of the aura.

Broderick and Swanson[64] reviewed 20 patients who had migraine-associated brain infarctions at age 50 years or younger who were diagnosed with migraine, migraine equivalent, or vascular headache. The neurologic deficit occurred with an attack of the typical migraine for the patient, and no other mechanisms of brain infarction could be found. Two of the 20 patients had a history of classic migraine and 2 had a history of common migraine. Seven had no clear history of migraine attacks. However, these 7 patients and the 2 patients who had had common migraines before developed classic migraine attacks, with auras that were similar to the symptoms of the infarction. Four events were associated with more than one arterial distribution. In contrast to patients with thrombotic or embolic strokes, their patients were predominantly women and had infarctions in the posterior circulation. The angiographic findings consisted of small-branch involvement with spasm and occlusions especially in the posterior cerebral and posterior branches of the middle cerebral arteries. They concluded that stroke related to migraine was rare in migraineurs but that a significant proportion of people younger than 40 years of age who had a stroke had migraine. Most of the patients had mild residual deficits.[64]

Featherstone[65] reviewed cases of stroke in migraine in the English and French literature between 1950 and 1983. Many predated cranial CT scanning and many did not have adequate workups for cardioembolic disease or abnormal clotting factors. The typical patient was a young adult who had prior classic or complicated migraine and had deficits of a homonymous hemianopia and/or hemiplegia. Mortality was about 5%, but prognosis for these patients was good. Complicated migraine was felt to be a serious risk factor for stroke. Two cases were associated with heavy use of ergot preparations and two cases with starting propranolol therapy. In another study,[66] of 41 patients with ischemic stroke who were less than 30 years old, 15% were felt to have migrainous infarction, whereas 29% were felt to have stroke related to mitral valve prolapse and 22% to arterial dissection.

Rothrock et al.,[67] in a study of 22 patients with acute migraine-associated stroke, found 36% had a history of complicated migraine, 41% had a history of classic migraine, and 23% had common migraine. Thirty percent were active smokers, 18% had chronic hypertension, and 14% were taking oral contraceptives or estrogen replacement. Three patients were taking ergotamine acutely during the stroke, and four had been receiving chronic prophylactic agents such as propranolol, nifedipine, cyproheptadine, or amitriptyline. Ninety-five percent of the patients developed headache acutely in association with the stroke, and 73% suffered permanent neurologic deficit. Radionuclide scanning or MRI was performed in 11 patients and demonstrated ischemic or hemorrhagic infarction in 55%. No single process was thought responsible for the majority of the permanent neurologic deficits caused by migraine. Cerebral arteriography showed abnormalities in 5 (42%) of the 12 patients studied, revealing internal carotid artery stenosis, distal carotid artery occlusion, posterior cerebral artery beading, bilateral anterior cerebral artery, middle cerebral artery, or vertebral spasm (in 3 cases), and luxury perfusion in 1 case. However, they noted that headache could be seen with atherothrombotic or embolic strokes, intracranial neoplasms, arteriovenous malformations, and arterial dissections.

There have been several reports of stroke in patients started on propranolol therapy for migraine.[65, 68] But, as discussed in the last review, the evidence for a true causal link is meager and only anecdotal. We believe the association is coincidental. Strokes may occur in patients with migraine not taking propranolol. Propranolol may, in fact, prevent strokes by eliminating migraine attacks.

Several reports have shown neuropsychological alterations in patients with migraine during attacks, some returning to baseline after rCBF returned to normal and others with continued abnormal testing between attacks.[14, 69, 70]

Shuaib and Hachinski[71] reviewed the charts of 142 patients with migraine who had had a total of 149 angiograms performed, the majority for either headache or new focal neurologic symptoms. Transient events were seen in 6 patients consisting of amnesia, hemisensory changes, hemiparesis, global confusion, or angina. Focal cerebral events occurred in 2.6% of cases. This was contrasted to a 2.8% rate of complications of angiography in a prospective study of 1,002 patients.[72] They felt that a history of migraine did not increase risk of complications of angiography and that angiography during an acute headache episode would appear to be a safe procedure, though transient focal neurologic symptoms could occur, especially in patients with classic migraine.

Van den Bergh et al.[73] found that the main headache precipitators in migraineurs were menstruation in 48% (or ovulation in 8.5%) in women, certain foods in 44.7%, alcoholic beverages in 51.6%, stress in 48.8%, and fatigue in 16.1%. The most common foods were cheese and dairy products at 18.5%, chocolate, 22.5%, and fatty foods, 17%. Weather was reported as a triggering factor in 6.9%, and 2.7% reported visual stimuli as a trigger. Certain smells were a frequent trigger in 4.6%. Smoking was a trigger in 4.1%.

Basilar Migraine

Electroencephalographic (EEG) abnormalities were found in 18% of patients with basilar artery migraine not known to be epileptics. Most were nonspecific paroxysmal changes, only one patient having spike and wave discharges.[1, 29, 74] Cyproheptadine or propranolol relieved the headaches. Drake and associates,[75] using computerized EEG spectral measures in patients with common migraine, tension headaches, and complicated migraine and in normal controls, found that patients with complicated migraine had lower maximal alpha frequencies than controls or patients with common migraine. Narbone et al.[76] described a patient with migraine and epilepsy whose headaches were controlled by adding flunarizine to her anticonvulsant medications. Sacquegna et al.[77] reviewed the impairment of consciousness and memory in migraine and felt there were four separate patterns that could be recognized during a migraine attack. The first was syncope, the second was a transient global amnesia, the third was a confusional state, and the fourth was an epileptic seizure. Terzano et al.[78] described a 12-year-old girl whose classic migraine attacks had seizures intercalated between the visual prodrome and headache. It was felt that the spreading depression of the migraine could possibly activate an epileptic focus. Flunarizine treatment controlled both the migraine and the seizure components. Wauquier[79] felt that flunarizine could increase the threshold for spreading depression and reduce epileptogenic bursts from the hippocampus. However, Miller et al.[80] in a study of transient global amnesia believed that EEG abnormalities were only seen in patients with seizure disorders.

Cluster Headaches

Some excellent reviews have been published in the last 2 years on cluster headache.[2, 81-83] Kudrow[81] gave an especially graphic first-hand account of an episode of cluster attack. In a review of 60 patients with chronic cluster headache, Watson and Evans[82] found that 17% of pain sites were outside of the trigeminal territory, including some in the chest or arm. Overall, 50% of patients benefitted from operations on the trigeminal nerve or greater superficial petrosal nerve. Sacquegna et al.[83] studied the natural history of episodic cluster headache. In only 10% of cases did the headache shift from one side to the other between bouts. Transitory partial Horner's syndrome occurred in two thirds of patients examined during cluster attacks. Toshniwal[84] described a patient with cluster headaches who developed an anterior ischemic optic neuropathy, and he suggested a possible mechanism. It is thought that during cluster attacks, increased intraocular pressure rises owing to intraocular vasodilation and increased blood flow, which could compromise optic disk circulation, causing blockade of axoplasmic flow and disk edema, setting the stage for anterior ischemic optic neuropathy. Hardebo[85] and Joseph and Rose[86] both described patients whose cluster headaches appeared to be associated with the occurrence of cold sores, one of whom ceased having any headaches after a course of acyclovir on two different occasions. All three authors felt that reactivation of the latent virus in the trigeminal system could trigger cluster headaches.

New information on possible mechanisms of cluster attacks has appeared. Boiardi et al.[87] studied visual evoked potentials in patients with cluster headache in pain-free periods and found that the P100 amplitudes were significantly lower and only on the side of the pain. Bussone et al.[88] demonstrated asymmetric conduction in the acoustic pathways of patients with cluster headache during and between clusters. Lithium abolished the asymmetry. These articles support central pathway alterations due to anatomic lesions or abnormalities in neurotransmitter functions. A review by Solomon[89] discusses the role of the central nervous system in the cyclical recurrences of cluster headache and the nervus intermedius as the pathway of the dysfunction in cluster headache. He theorizes that central autonomic dysregulation could cause vasodilation of the internal carotid artery, resulting in partial Horner's syndrome and possibly increasing permeability of the blood vessels with extravasation of inflammatory polypeptides and mediators causing the headache. Raskin[1] considers that the biologic clock is felt to be serotoninergically modulated and has been connected anatomically to the eye. Many of the drugs used for treating cluster headaches enhance serotoninergic neurotransmission, and this suggests that altered serotoninergic neurotransmission balance may be the etiology. He also reviews evidence that the alterations of cerebral blood flow seen in cluster headache may be due to neural mechanisms.

Trigeminal Neuralgia

Raskin[1] and Dubner et al.[90] have reviewed the possible mechanisms and pathophysiology of trigeminal neuralgia and believe that the majority of patients have a disinhibition of central pain gating mechanisms due to vascular compression of sensory roots of the trigeminal nerve as it enters the pons. Magnetic resonance imaging is necessary to rule out tumors of the cerebellopontine angle, which may be present in up to 5% of patients with this syndrome. Vessel impingement, arteriovenous malformations, and demyelinative lesions may also cause this pain syndrome. A central pathogenesis for the syndrome is suggested by the latency between stimulation of the trigger point and pain occurrence, by pain continuing after the trigger point is stimulated, by spontaneous remissions and refractory periods, and by the fact that it is rarely nocturnal.

Bullitt et al.,[91] in reviewing 2,000 patients with facial pain, found 16 with intracranial tumors, mostly posterior and middle fossa tumors. Several had been treated medically with pain relief before the tumors were found. Brisman[92] reviewed patients with trigeminal neuralgia treated with radiofrequency electrocoagulation of the gasserian ganglion and retrogasserian rootlets either alone or with glycerol. Results were divided by patients with multiple sclerosis and those without. Those patients with multiple sclerosis were more likely to be young and have bilateral facial pain. These patients responded well to radiofrequency electrocoagulation alone or with glycerol, though they tended to have a higher rate of reoperation.

Raskin[1] reviewed the several drugs that can be used in the treatment of trigeminal neuralgia, such as carbamazepine, phenytoin, baclofen, valproic acid, and clonazepam, as well as their side effects. These agents may be used alone or in combination, though some believe that carbamazepine in divided daily doses of 600 to 800 mg has been so consistently effective that, if it is not at least partially effective, doubt should be cast on the diagnosis of trigeminal neuralgia.[93] Recently, tocainide[94] was compared with carbamazepine in a double-blind crossover study and was felt to be equal in efficacy for the 2-week trial period. Sweet[93] noted a personal experience of problems with carbamazepine, especially in older patients, causing loss of energy and decreased mental performance, though it was effective in the pain syndrome. He also found only 2 reported deaths in 14,000 published cases of electrocoagulation, but reported personal communications of intracranial hemorrhage developing in 7 cases during operation, causing death in 6 and permanent hemiplegia in 1. Other complications included meningitis, aseptic meningeal reaction, temporal lobe abscess, oculomotor paresis (transient), and minor carotid cavernous fistulas. The procedure offered virtually complete relief, as only 7% needed another operation. Dysesthesias were felt to be the most serious complication. Glycerine instillation into the trigeminal rootlets has had encouraging results in five groups, but seven other groups have stopped using it because of too many initial failures, major sensory losses, or dysesthesias.[95, 96]

Microvascular decompression procedures are popular and reportedly have a 1% operative mortality, with recurrences ranging from 17% to 26%, but Sweet[93] noted that a private poll of major neurosurgical services performing the decompression techniques showed mortality and morbidity to be higher among less experienced surgeons. Burchiel et al.[97] showed major recurrence of pain after microvascular decompression at a rate of 3.5% annually. Those who had arterial compression of the nerve had longer pain relief. Zakrzewska and Nally[98] evaluated cryotherapy of branches of the trigeminal nerve using intraoral approaches and found 85% of patients gained immediate relief of their symptoms. Fifty-six percent had pain control for under 1 year and 25% had pain control for 1 to 2 years. After studying corneal reflexes, early and late blink reflexes, and masseter muscles with electromyograms, Cruccu et al.[99] felt that trigeminal function was less impaired by microcompression balloon techniques and recovered earlier than after thermocoagulation techniques.

Other Types of Facial Pain

A good review of different types of facial pain and their treatment was produced by Raskin.[1] Vascular compression of cranial nerves IX and X at the nerve root entry zone is probably the most common cause of glossopharyngeal neuralgia, but other causes such as nasopharyngeal carcinoma, peritonsillar abscesses, carotid aneurysm, cerebellopontine angle tumors, and ossified stylohyoid ligaments occur. Magnetic resonance imaging may supplement the thorough physical examination in identifying treatable causes. Barbash[100] reviewed a patient with glossopharyngeal neuralgia and repeated episodes of asystole lasting for 20 to 45 seconds associated with syncope, each event being preceded by the typical pain. It was felt that pain stimulation excited the vagus nerves, causing asystole and simultaneously abolishing sympathetic tone. For medical therapy, carbamazepine and other drugs usually used for trigeminal neuralgia are currently the most used. Good results using baclofen have been reported.[101] If medical treatment fails, glossopharyngeal nerve sectioning plus the sectioning of the upper three or four rootlets of the vagus nerve has been the standard surgical treatment.

Other cranial neuralgias such as sphenopalatine neuralgia (Sluder's neuralgia, pterygopalatine neuralgia, and greater superficial petrosal neuralgia), geniculate neuralgia, superior laryngeal neuralgia, and carotodynia have been reviewed by Raskin[1] and Bruyn.[102, 103] Cepero et al.[104] described 12 patients who underwent sphenopalatine ganglionectomy. All had complete and immediate resolution of neuralgia, but it was temporary in all but one patient. They felt that although there was a high recurrence of pain, it was less severe and was easily managed by medications. Jaeger et al.[105] reported two cases with reflex sympathetic dystrophy of the face who were helped by a stellate ganglion block with a local anesthetic. Hypothetical mechanisms of reflex sympathetic dystrophy are briefly reviewed, including formation of synapses between somatic afferent and sympathetic efferent fibers, self-exciting neuronal loops due to irritative foci in the periphery, dysfunction of central mechanisms, as well as abnormal membrane properties.

Raskin[1] and Cawson[106] discussed controversies between temporomandibular joint dysfunction and facial pain, noting that the four necessary signs and symptoms for diagnosis have been pain, tenderness, clicking, and limitation of jaw movement, though often there is no radiologic evidence for temporomandibular joint disease. Cawson does not believe that condylar displacement is the cause, and it may be that masseter muscle spasm and fatigue is the initiating event. A number of poorly defined treatments have been advocated, including relaxational techniques, soft diets, nonsteroidal anti-inflammatory drugs, and surgical procedures.

Kashihara et al.[107] described a patient with Raeder's syndrome who had an aneurysm of the intracranial carotid artery, thus indicating the need for thorough workup in this syndrome. Loeser[108] and Raskin[1] have produced excellent reviews of the pathophysiology and treatment of herpetic pain syndrome. For acute herpes zoster, Burrows' solution, as well as aspirin or narcotics if necessary, continue to be used for the pain. Acyclovir may help in reducing healing time and may help in decreasing postherpetic neuralgia, as may amantadine and steroids. Other treatments have included nerve blocks, tranquilizers, anticonvulsants, tricyclic antidepressants, analgesics, and ergot derivatives. Loeser[108] suggests that for herpes zoster, patients who are immunologically intact and under the age of 50 should have only symptomatic therapy, such as analgesics and topical treatments. Older patients or those who are immunologically compromised should have systemic steroids, topical idoxuridine, or systemic acyclovir. For treating postherpetic neuralgia, he feels it is best to begin with such therapy as transcutaneous electrical stimulation or tricyclic antidepressants, with or without a phenothiazine, and if these are unsuccessful, sympathetic or somatic nerve blocks may be of help. He feels that surgical therapy is of use only when the patient is disabled by the pain. Certain patients may also be candidates for thalamic stimulation therapy. Esmann et al.[109] showed that prednisolone treatment could reduce the period of acute pain if started within 4 days of ictus but had no effect on the development of postherpetic pain. Buck and Burks[110] have used capsaicin cream for the treatment of postherpetic neuralgia. The mainstay of treatment, however, appears to be amitriptyline with flunarizine or perphenazine added as second-line drugs. Addition of valproic acid combinations may also help.

Temporal Arteritis

Excellent reviews of temporal arteritis or giant cell arteritis are given by McDonnell et al.[111] and Raskin[1] McDonnell et al.[111] have noted the high frequency of false-negative biopsies in the literature, ranging from 9% to 61%, and that there were no clear pathologic criteria for diagnosis after temporal artery biopsy. They give their histopathologic criteria for active arteritis, healed arteritis, and atherosclerosis with representative slides from patients used in their article and give results of interobserver comparisons. Owing to the occurrence of false-negative biopsies and skip lesions, some patients will have to be diagnosed on clinical grounds.

In the study of Vilaseca et al.,[112] the simultaneous presence of recent-onset headache, jaw claudication, and abnormalities of the temporal arteries on physical examination had a specificity of 94.8% compared with the histologic diagnosis and 100% with respect to the final diagnosis. The diagnostic criteria included age greater than 55 years, a positive response to steroid therapy within 48 hours, history greater than 2 weeks in length, positive temporal artery biopsy, proximal symmetric muscle pain in the arms or stiffness or tenderness, jaw claudication, tenderness, thickening or redness of the temporal artery, constitutional symptoms such as malaise, anorexia, weight loss, or elevated temperature or anemia, recent onset of headache, and visual disturbances such as diplopia, blurring, or vision loss. Rosenfeld et al.[113] described an elderly woman with temporal arteritis who continued to experience progressive retinal ischemia with visual loss in the second eye after high-dose steroid treatment; however, the use of intravenous methylprednisolone reversed the progressive loss of vision of the second eye.

Solomon and Cappa[114] point out that the headache of temporal arteritis may not involve only the temporal area. In their study pain was often felt in the temporal, frontal, vertex, and occipital areas, and two patients had generalized headaches. The headache did not involve the temporal area in seven patients, and two patients, ultimately diagnosed with temporal arteritis, did not have headaches. They noted that blurring and nonspecific impairment of vision was frequently found as well as decreased visual acuity and diplopia and the symptoms of polymyalgia rheumatica with fever, myalgias, arthralgias, weight loss, fever, and anorexia. Allen and Studenski[115] also point out the occurrence of other signs and symptoms such as extremity claudication, jaw and tongue claudication, ear pain, stroke, and angina as well as systemic panarteritis involving the peripheral nervous system and abdominal or pelvic viscera. Patients under age 50 and with erythrocyte sedimentation rates less than 50 mm/hr have been reported to have this syndrome. A 3- to 5-cm arterial segment is optimal for a pathologic specimen because of skip lesions.

Lisak[116] discusses the possible pathogenetic mechanisms of temporal arteritis, such as immune complex deposition and cell-mediated immune reactions and antigenically modified vessel constituents. Raskin,[1] Allen and Studenski,[115] and others believe steroid therapy should start immediately, before confirmation by laboratory and pathologic determinations. They suggest that in very ill patients, intravenous methylprednisolone may be better. De Silva and Hazleman[117] reported a study of patients with giant cell arteritis or polymyalgia rheumatica showing that azathioprine could reduce the maintenance prednisolone requirement in these patients.

In an excellent review, Carlow[118] notes that the eye and periorbital regions are common points of headache but that the eye is rarely responsible if ophthalmic signs are not obvious. He also believes that refractive disorders and muscle imbalance are overemphasized as the cause of headache, and that correction of these problems seldom provides resolution, the exception being convergence insufficiency. Ocular neurosis is the usual cause of eye strain headache that begins abruptly with use of the eyes in which there is a normal ophthalmologic examination. There are several ocular lesions that are important and treatable as causes of headache, including conjunctivitis, corneal lesions, anterior uveitis, angle closure glaucoma, optic neuritis, metastatic orbital tumors, orbital pseudotumors, and the

Tolosa-Hunt syndrome. The symptoms of paratrigeminal syndrome, oculomotor nerve paralysis, small-vessel disease, carotid cavernous fistulas, and nasopharyngeal carcinomas may all have eye pain as a presenting symptom. Dissection of the internal carotid artery can also present with eye pain. Photophobia is often seen with subarachnoid hemorrhage, meningitis, retrobulbar neuritis, and migraine and probably has its basis in central cortical and brain-stem reflexes.[118]

THERAPY

A large number of articles relate to therapy for various types of vascular headaches, including a good "viewpoint" article about an overall approach to the treatment of vascular headaches by Daroff and Whitney.[119] The review provides a listing of drugs and dosages for treatments of various types of headaches, such as acute migraine and chronic cluster, assuming a correct diagnosis has been made.

Calcium Channel Blocking Drugs

Three calcium channel blocking drugs, nifedipine, verapamil, and nimodipine, are those most commonly used in the acute and chronic treatment of vascular headache. These three drugs were compared by Jonsdottir and colleagues[120] in separate prophylactic trials that they reviewed. These investigators reported that nifedipine provided symptomatic improvement in 65% of patients with common migraine and 77% of patients with classic migraine. Verapamil improved control of symptoms in 81% of patients with common migraine, 72% of those with classic, 67% of those with mixed, and 79% of those with cluster. Nimodipine was reported to be beneficial in 84% of patients with common migraine, 73% of those with classic, and 53% with chronic cluster but was much less effective for the treatment of mixed headache. The authors suggested that each one of the three calcium channel blockers showed different and specific therapeutic efficacies, which differed according to the clinical classification. The authors concluded that nifedipine appeared to be more effective than the other two drugs tested during treatment of classic migraine, whereas verapamil was most effective for controlling mixed headache and cluster headache.

Nimodipine was compared with flunarizine in an Italian study with 30 patients.[121] In this small group, the two drugs seemed to have similar efficacy, although nimodipine seemed to have a shorter latency, with onset of action within the first month. Nimodipine was compared with the serotonin antagonist pizotyline in a 4-week double-blind study, which suggested equal efficacy.[122] It was suggested that they were equally effective in both classic and common migraine and that they were both better than placebo. Once again, there were relatively few patients. The investigators did report that nimodipine had wider actions than were originally realized, influencing presynaptic transmitter release and reuptake, but also having an inhibitory effect on serotonin activity. Another prospective study[123] suggested clear benefit over placebo. Another calcium entry blocker, flunarizine, was the subject of three reports.[124–126] Again, this calcium channel blocking drug was equally effective when compared with pizotyline[124] and was effective when given sublingually,[125] being equal to ergotamine in this study from Italy. In the single case report, flunarizine, in addition to helping migraine, seemed to reduce seizures that were associated with complex visual hallucinations.[126]

Despite the flurry of reports that continue about calcium channel blocking drugs, beta-blocker therapy is still one of the mainstays of migraine prophylaxis. Propranolol was compared with amitriptyline by Ziegler et al.[127] and was found to be equally effective in a double-blind, placebo-controlled crossover design study of 30 patients. Many regard amitriptyline to be the drug of choice in mixed headache, particularly when there is a muscle contraction and depression factor. Time and experience will indicate whether tricyclic antidepressants are really as effective as the beta-blocking drugs in pure vascular headaches. "The ideal prophylactic agents for the therapy of migraines should be early active, possess long-term efficacy with few side effects and a convenient dosing schedule, and truly prevent attacks from occurring rather than merely decreasing their severity."[128] The fact is that no such ideal agent has been found, but long-acting propranolol (propranolol is still the drug of choice in migraine prophylaxis) may be a significant breakthrough. A retrospective chart review of 200 patients suggested that the long-acting form was as safe and efficacious as regular propranolol in the prophylaxis of migraine.[128] Other beta-blocking drugs that are reported to be better because of their more selective action were metoprolol[129] and atenolol.[130] Metoprolol (Lopressor) in a dose of 50 to 100 mg twice a day was better than the 40% response to placebo in one study.[129] Atenolol (Tenormin) in a dose of 100 mg daily appeared to be safe and effective in 70% of the 63 patients studied with classic and/or common migraine.[130] A combination drug with acetaminophen, the antihistamine buclizine, and codeine phosphate was slightly more effective than placebo in 30 subjects with vascular headaches.[131] A technique of vigorous bilateral compression and massage of the frontal branch of the superficial temporal artery started at the first sign of visual aura was successful in blocking 81% of attacks in 15 patients.[132] The authors speculated that the blood vessels of the extracranial circulation, as well as those of the circle of Willis, have perivascular nerve fibers of trigeminal origin, and it may well be that these nerve fibers, rather than the dilation of blood vessels with accumulation of vasoactive substances, mediate the pain of migraine. Digital massage might stimulate the nerve endings and for some reason stop the ensuing pain phase of the headache.

In an acute migraine or intractable migraine, parenteral dihydroergotamine (DHE) is reported to be effective. Callaham and Raskin[133] treated patients with 5 mg of prochlorperazine (Compazine) intravenously (to prevent the nausea often seen with 0.75 mg of intravenous DHE). Repetitive intravenous therapy for intractable migraine was reported by Raskin,[134] in which 49 of 55 treated patients became headache free within 48 hours, and 39 of them sustained benefits at a mean follow-up of 16 months. In this study, a test dose of 0.5 mg of DHE was given with 10 mg of metoclopramide (Reglan). If nausea was reported or if head pain ceased within 1 hour, no additional DHE was given for 8 hours. Then, another 0.5-mg dose was administered and repeated every 8 hours thereafter for 2 days. If there was nausea, the DHE dose was decreased to 0.3 mg, but if there was no nausea, the DHE dose could be increased to 1.0 mg with 10 mg of metoclopramide every 8 hours for 2 days. Gallagher[135] reported a study in which patients were treated with meperidine, promethazine, and dexamethasone in an emergency department of a large community hospital, suggesting that it was better than intravenous DHE.

Nonsteroidal anti-inflammatory drugs such fenoprofen (Nalfon) and naproxen sodium (Anaprox) have also been useful in the prophylaxis of migraine.[136–138] It appears in particular that naproxen sodium was as efficacious as ergotamine and associated with fewer side effects.[130, 138]

Other therapies for common and classic migraine include cyclandelate[139] and diet.[140] The diet was a carbohydrate-rich diet low in protein and tryptophan. Others believe that carbohydrate in the diet may be a cause of migraine.[141] Stellate ganglion blocks were reported useful in the treatment of unilateral migraine headache in a retrospective study of patients referred to an anesthesiology pain clinic.[142] Patients were said to have been treated with a variety of narcotics, sedatives, tranquilizers, and antidepressants before the stellate ganglion block, but there was no specific mention of antimigrainous therapy.

Chronic paroxysmal hemicrania, which usually responds to indomethacin, is also treated with steroids.[143] Steroids were also reported to help paroxysmal headache associated with a right-sided abducens palsy, a form of ophthalmoplegic migraine, in a 42-year-old man who had attacks from the age of 1½ years.[144] Initiation of prednisone within 4 hours of headache onset resulted in decreased severity and duration of headache and prevented or markedly ameliorated the ophthalmoparesis.

Cluster Headache

Cluster headache is usually treated medically, but when it is intractable, surgical therapies have been increasingly attempted. Diamond and colleagues[145] report a new study of histamine sensitization in a group of patients with intractable cluster headache. Of note is the fact that Horton first described this in 1939. It appears that there may be some patients who do respond. The authors only achieved 40% excellent response but point out that these were patients who had had prior treatment with corticosteroids, methysergide, ergotamine tartrate, lithium carbonate, and a variety of calcium channel blocking drugs.

Calcium channel blocking drugs such as nimodipine may be useful in episodic cluster headaches, as described in a new small open trial.[146] Butapine, a competitive reverse inhibitor of monoamine oxidase, has been reported in Europe to be useful in the management of Parkinson's disease. One report describes its use in cluster headache in an open study in Europe.[147] This should be regarded as a preliminary report, as the drug has not been tested in double-blind fashion nor is it available in the United States.

Onofrio and Campbell[148] reported surgical treatment of chronic cluster headache in 26 patients who were reportedly completely refractory to medical therapy. Fifty-four percent were said to have an excellent result and 31% had poor results. It should be noted that the group with poor results included some patients with persistent facial dysesthesia or numbness. Percutaneous radiofrequency trigeminal gangliorhizolysis was reported in treatment of disabling chronic cluster headache by Mathew and Hurt[149] in an open study. These authors concluded that the surgical procedures were reasonable in patients who had severe cluster headache and were totally resistant to medical therapy and had a strictly unilateral headache. An additional surgical treatment reported by Solomon and Apfelbaum[150] is surgical decompression of the facial nerve. These authors reasoned that the nervus intermedius appears to be a conduit for some of these symptoms of cluster headache, including tearing, injection of the conjunctiva, and nasal congestion. Similar to the concept that trigeminal neuralgia and hemifacial spasm are caused by microvascular decompression, these authors believe that a similar mechanism affecting the nervus intermedius could be part of the mechanism of cluster headache. Five patients with chronic cluster headache unresponsive to medication underwent surgical decompression of the root exit-entry zone of the facial nerve. In 2 patients the pain syndrome was markedly relieved for as long as 2 years, and in 1 patient initial improvement was obscured by narcotic condition. In 2 patients the operation was a failure. We would agree with the authors' conclusion that the association of cluster headache with cross compression of the nervus intermedius is an unproved theory or mechanism.

REFERENCES

1. Raskin NH: *Headache*. New York, Churchill Livingstone, Inc, 1988.

2. Olesen J: The pathophysiology of migraine, in Rose FC (ed): *Handbook of Clinical Neurology*, vol 48. New York, Elsevier North-Holland, Inc, 1986, pp 59–83.

3. Rose FC: *The Management of Headache*. New York, Raven Press, 1988.

4. Raskin NH: Migraine: Pathogenesis, in Raskin NH (ed): *Headache*. New York, Churchill Livingstone, Inc, 1988, pp 99–133.

5. Olesen J: The ischemic hypotheses of migraine. *Arch Neurol* 1987; 44:321–322.

6. Levin SR, Welch KMA, Ewing JR, et al: Asymmetric cerebral blood flow patterns in migraine. *Cephalalgia* 1987; 7:245–248.

7. Andersen AR, Friberg L, Olsen TS, et al: Delayed hyperemia following hypoperfusion in classic migraine. *Arch Neurol* 1988; 45:154–159.

8. Friberg L, Olsen TS, Lassen NA: Fast fluctuation of cerebrovascular tone causing focal ischemia in migraine patients. *Cephalalgia* 1987; 6(suppl):283–284.

9. Olsen TS, Friberg L, Lassen NA: Ischemia may be the primary cause of the neurologic deficits in classic migraine. *Arch Neurol* 1987; 44:156–161.

10. Olsen TS, Friberg L, Ronager J: Cerebrovascular reactivity is completely abolished during attacks of classic migraine. *Cephalalgia* 1987; 6(suppl):103–105.

11. Friberg L, Olsen TS, Roland PE, et al: Focal ischaemia caused by instability of cerebrovascular tone during attacks of hemiplegic migraine. *Brain* 1987; 110:917–934.

12. Solomon S, Harris PY, Lipton RB: Arterial stenosis in migraine: Spasm, edema, or inflammation? *Headache* 1988; 28:304–305.

13. Thie A, Spitzer K, Lachenmayer L, et al: Prolonged vasospasm in migraine detected by noninvasive transcranial Doppler ultrasound. *Headache* 1988; 28:183–186.

14. Meyer JS, Zetusky W, Jonsdottir M, et al: Cephalic hyperemia during migraine headaches. *Headache* 1986; 26:388–397.

15. Olesen J: Migraine and regional cerebral blood flow. *Trends Neurosci* 1985; 8:318–321.

16. Wahl M, Lauritzen M, Schilling L: Change of cerebrovascular reactivity after cortical spreading depression in cats and rats. *Brain Res* 1987; 411:72–80.

17. Sachs H, Wolf A, Russell JAG, et al: Effect of reserpine on regional cerebral glucose metabolism in control and migraine subjects. *Arch Neurol* 1986; 43:1117–1123.

18. Albe-Fessard D: Characteristics of spreading depression and of its progation: Their role in migraine. *Cephalalgia* 1987; 6(suppl):65–68.

19. Gloor P: Migraine and regional cerebral blood flow. *Trends Neurosci* 1986; 9:21.

20. De Noordhout AM, Timsit-Berthier M, Timsit M, et al: Contingent negative variation in headache. *Ann Neurol* 1986; 19:78–80.

21. Peroutka SJ: Antimigraine drug interactions with serotonin receptor subtypes in human brain. *Ann Neurol* 1988; 23:500–504.

22. Petraglia F, Martignoni E, Volpe A, et al: Involvement of serotonin in the central control of opoid secretion. *Cephalalgia* 1987; 6(suppl):506–513.

23. Muller-Schweinitzer E: Medication of migraine by pro-serotonergic drugs. *Cephalalgia* 1987; 6(suppl):138–140.

24. Hirsch AR: Neuroanatomic mechanisms: The limbic system and migraine. *Cephalalgia* 1987; 6(suppl):191–192.

25. Schoenen J: Central effects of beta-blocking drugs in migraineurs. *Cephalalgia* 1987; 6(suppl):536–538.

26. Raskin NH: On the origin of head pain. *Headache* 1988; 28:254–257.

27. Goadsby PJ, Piper RO, Lambert GA, et al: The effect of activation of the nucleus raphe dorsalis on carotid blood flow. *Am J Physiol* 1985; 248:257–262.

28. Edminson L, MacKenzie ET, Scatton B: Evidence for a central serotonergic projection to the cerebral resistance vessels: Possible functional implications. *Prog Appl Microcirc* 1985; 8:213–224.

29. Jacome DE: EEG features in basilar artery migraine. *Headache* 1987; 27:80–83.

30. Welch KMA: Migraine: A biobehavioral disorder. *Arch Neurol* 1987; 44:323–327.

31. Hanington E: Migraine is a platelet disorder. *Headache* 1987; 27:401–402.

32. Hanington E: The platelet and migraine. *Headache* 1986; 26:411–415.

33. D'Andrea G, Cananzi AR, Toldo M, et al: Platelet activation and migraine: A study with flunarizine. *Headache* 1986; 26:339–342.

34. Joseph R, Welch KMA: The platelet and migraine: A nonspecific association. *Headache* 1987; 27:375–380.

35. Steiner TJ, Rose FC: Migraine is not a platelet disorder. *Headache* 1987; 27:400.

36. D'Andrea G, Welch KMA, Grunfeld S, et al: Reduced platelet turnover of serotonin in diet restricted migraine patients. *Cephalalgia* 1987; 6(suppl):141–143.

37. Lanzi G, Grandi AM, Gamba G, et al: Migraine, mitral valve prolapse and platelet function in the pediatric age group. *Headache* 1986; 26:142–145.

38. Pfaffenrath V, Pollmann W, Autenriedth G, et al: Mitral valve prolapse and platelet aggregation in patients with hemiplegic and nonhemiplegic migraine. *Acta Neurol Scand* 1987; 75:253–257.

39. Rubin LS, Boyer J: A correlative study of immunoglobulin isotype expression in common migraine. *Headache* 1986; 26:137–141.

40. Levine SR, Welch KMA: The spectrum of neurologic disease associated with antiphospholipid antibodies: Lupus anticoagulants and anticardiolipin antibodies. *Arch Neurol* 1987; 44:876–883.

41. Colaco CB, Scadding GK, Lockhart S: Anti-cardiolipin antibodies in neurological disorders: Cross reaction with anti–single stranded activity. *Clin Exp Immunol* 1987; 68:313–319.

42. Ludwig CL, Stiller JW, Burns PJ, et al: Migraine headaches, migraine equivalents and anti–smooth muscle antibodies. *Headache* 1988; 28:332–336.

43. Visintini D, Trabattoni G, Manzoni GC, et al: Immunological studies in cluster headache and migraine. *Headache* 1986; 26:398–402.

44. Levine SR, Joseph R, D'Andrea G, et al: Migraine and the lupus anticoagulant: Case reports and review of the literature. *Cephalalgia* 1987; 7:93–99.

45. Gazzaniga PP, Ferroni P, Lenti L, et al: Identification of blood leukotrienes in classical migraine. *Headache* 1987; 27:211–215.

46. Selmaj K, de Belleroche J, Das I, et al: Leukotriene B4 generation by polymorphonuclear leukocytes: Possible involvement in the pathogenesis of headache. *Headache* 1986; 26:460–464.

47. Havanka-Kanniainen H, Tolenen U, Myllyla VV: Autonomic dysfunction in migraine. *Cephalalgia* 1987; 6:271–272.

48. Havanka-Kanniainen H, Juujarvi K, Tolenen U, et al: Cardiovascular reflexes and plasma noradrenaline levels in migraine patients before and during nimodipine medication. *Headache* 1987; 27:39–44.

49. Boiardi A, Munari L, Milanesi I, et al: Impaired cardiovascular reflexes in cluster headache and migraine patients: Evidence for an autonomic dysfunction. *Headache* 1988; 28:417–422.

50. Drummond PD: Pupil diameter in migraine and tension headache. *J Neurol Neurosurg Psychiatry* 1987; 50:228–230.

51. Takeshima T, Takao Y, Takahashi K: Pupillary sympathetic hypofunction and asymmetry in muscle contraction headache and migraine. *Cephalalgia* 1987; 7:257–262.

52. Herman P: Migraine, large pupils, mitral valve prolapse and emotional disturbances: An autonomic disorder. *Headache* 1987; 27:340–344.

53. Solomon S, Cappa KG, Smith CR: Common migraine: Criteria for diagnosis. *Headache* 1988; 28:124–129.

54. Peatfield RC: Can transient ischaemic attacks and classical migraine always be distinguished? *Headache* 1987; 27:240–243.

55. Kaplan RD, Solomon GD, Diamond S, et al: The role of MRI in the evaluation of a migraine population: Preliminary data. *Headache* 1987; 27:315–318.

56. Andersen AR, Andersson PG, Gilhus NE, et al: The symptomatology of classic migraine: A prospective study. *Cephalalgia* 1987; 6(suppl):163–164.

57. Coppeto JR, Greco P: Unilateral internuclear ophthalmoplegia, migraine, and supratentorial arteriovenous malformation. *Am J Ophthalmol* 1987; 104:191–192.

58. Amit R, Benezra D: Oculomotor ophthalmoplegic migraine in an infant. *Headache* 1987; 27:390–391.

59. Tomsak RL, Jergens PB: Benign recurrent transient monocular blindness: A possible variant of acephalgic migraine. *Headache* 1987; 27:66–69.

60. Edmeads J: Monocular migraine. *Headache* 1987; 27:115.

61. Goodwin JA, Gorelick PB, Helgason CM: Symptoms of amaurosis fugax in atherosclerotic carotid artery disease. *Neurology* 1987; 37:829–832.

62. Kunkel RS: Acephalgic migraine. *Headache* 1986; 26:198–201.

63. Pietrini V, Terzano MG, D'Andrea G, et al: Acute confusional migraine: Clinical and electroencephalographic aspects. *Cephalalgia* 1987; 7:29–37.

64. Broderick JP, Swanson JW: Migraine-related strokes: Clinical profile and prognosis in 20 patients. *Arch Neurol* 1987; 44:868–871.

65. Featherstone HJ: Clinical features of stroke in migraine: A review. *Headache* 1986; 26:128–133.

66. Bogousslavsky J, Regli F: Ischemic stroke in adults younger than 30 years of age: Cause and prognosis. *Arch Neurol* 1987; 44:479–482.

67. Rothrock JF, Walicke P, Swenson MR, et al: Migrainous stroke. *Arch Neurol* 1988; 45:63–67.

68. Bardwell A, Trott JA: Stroke in migraine as a consequence of propranolol. *Headache* 1987; 27:381–383.

69. Ardila A, Sanchez E, Rosselli D: Paroxysmal neuropsychological symptoms in migraine. *Cephalalgia* 1987; 6(suppl):200–201.

70. Hooker WD, Raskin NH: Neuropsychologic alterations in classic and common migraine. *Arch Neurol* 1986; 43:709–712.

71. Shuaib A, Hachinski VC: Migraine and the risks from angiography. *Arch Neurol* 1988; 45:911–912.

72. Dion JE, Gates PC, Fox AJ: Clinical events following neuroangiography: A prospective study. *Stroke* 1987; 18:997–1004.

73. Van den Bergh V, Amery WK, Waelkens J: Trigger factors in migraine: A study conducted by the Belgian Migraine Society. *Headache* 1987; 27:191–196.

74. Goldenberg E, Arlazoroff A, Tauber T, et al: Transient focal headaches with persistent ipsilateral EEG disturbances. *Headache* 1986; 26:30–32.

75. Drake ME, Du Bois C, Huber SJ, et al: EEG spectral analysis and time domain descriptors in headache. *Headache* 1988; 28:201–203.

76. Narbone MC, D'Amico D, Di Perri R: Classic migraine and intercalated seizures in a young woman: Efficacy of flunarizine. *Headache* 1988; 28:209–211.

77. Sacquegna T, Cortelli P, Baldrati A, et al: Impairment of consciousness and memory in migraine: A review. *Headache* 1987; 27:30–33.

78. Terzano MG, Pietrini V, Parrino L, et al: Migraine and intercalated seizures with occipital EEG paroxysms: Observations on a family. *Headache* 1986; 26:509–512.

79. Wauquier A: Is there a common pharmacological link between migraine and epilepsy? *Funct Neurol* 1986; 1:515–520.

80. Miller JW, Yanigihara T, Petersen RC, et al: Transient global amnesia and epilepsy. *Arch Neurol* 1987; 44:629–633.

81. Kudrow L: Cluster headache: Diagnosis, management, and treatment, in Dalessio DJ (ed): *Wolff's Headache and Other Head Pain*. New York, Oxford University Press, 1987, pp 112–130.

82. Watson CPN, Evans RJ: Chronic cluster headache: Review of 60 patients. *Headache* 1987; 27:158–165.

83. Sacquegna T, de Carolis P, de Capoa D, et al: The natural history of episodic cluster headache. *Headache* 1987; 27:370–371.

84. Toshniwal P: Anterior ischaemic optic neuropathy secondary to cluster headache. *Acta Neurol Scand* 1986; 73:213–218.

85. Hardebo JE: An association between cluster headache and herpes simplex. *N Engl J Med* 1986; 314:316.

86. Joseph R, Rose FC: Cluster headache and herpes complex: An association? *Br Med J* 1985; 290:1625–1626.

87. Boiardi A, Carenini L, Frediani F, et al: Visual evoked potentials in cluster headache: Central structures involvement. *Headache* 1986; 26:70–73.

88. Bussone G, Sinatra MG, Boiardi A, et al: Brainstem auditory evoked potential (BAEPs) in cluster headache (CH): New aspects for a central theory. *Headache* 1986; 26:67–69.

89. Solomon S: Cluster headache and the nervus intermedius. *Headache* 1986; 26:3–8.

90. Dubner R, Sharav Y, Gracely RH, et al: Idiopathic trigeminal neuralgia: Sensory features and pain mechanisms. *Pain* 1987; 31:23–33.

91. Bullitt E, Tew JM, Boyd J: Intracranial tumors in patients with facial pain. *J Neurosurg* 1986; 64:865–871.

92. Brisman R: Trigeminal neuralgia and multiple sclerosis. *Arch Neurol* 1987; 44:379–381.

93. Sweet WH: The treatment of trigeminal neuralgia (tic douloureux). *N Engl J Med* 1986; 315:174–177.

94. Lindstrom P, Lindblom U: The analgesic effect of tocainide in trigeminal neuralgia. *Pain* 1987; 28:45–50.

95. Saini SS: Retrogasserian anhydrous glycerol injection therapy in trigeminal neuralgia: Observations in 552 patients. *J Neurol Neurosurg Psychiatry* 1987; 50:1536–1538.

96. Young RF: Glycerol rhizolysis for treatment of trigeminal neuralgia. *J Neurosurg* 1988; 69:39–45.

97. Burchiel KM, Clarke H, Haglund M, et al: Long-term efficacy of microvascular decompression in trigeminal neuralgia. *J Neurosurg* 1988; 69:35–38.

98. Zakrzewska JM, Nally FF: The role of cryotherapy (cryoanalgesia) in the management of paroxysmal trigeminal neuralgia: A six-year experience. *Br J Oral Maxillofac Surg* 1988; 26:18–25.

99. Cruccu G, Inghilleri M, Fraioli B, et al: Neurophysiologic assessment of trigeminal function after surgery for trigeminal neuralgia. *Neurology* 1987; 37:631–638.

100. Barbash GI, Keren G, Korczyn AD, et al: Mechanisms of syncope in glossopharyngeal neuralgia. *Electroencephalogr Clin Neurophysiol* 1986; 63:231–235.

101. Ringel RA, Roy EP: Glossopharyngeal neuralgia: Successful treatment with baclofen. *Ann Neurol* 1987; 21:514–515.

102. Bruyn GW: Glossopharyngeal neuralgia, in Rose FC, Vinkin PJ, Bruyn HL, et al (eds): *Handbook of Clinical Neurology*. New York, Elsevier North-Holland, Inc, 1986, vol 48, pp 459–473.

103. Bruyn G: Shenopalatine neuralgia (Sluder), in Vinkin PJ, Bruyn HL, Klawans GW, et al (eds): *Handbook of Clinical Neurology*. New York, Elsevier North-Holland, Inc, 1986, vol 48, pp 475–482.

104. Cepero R, Miller RH, Bressler KL: Long-term results of sphenopalatine ganglioneurectomy for facial pain. *Am J Otolaryngol* 1987; 8:171–174.

105. Jaeger B, Singer E, Kroening R: Reflex sympathetic dystrophy of the face. *Arch Neurol* 1986; 43:693–695.

106. Cawson RA: Temporomandibular cephalalgia, in Rose FC (ed): *Handbook of Clinical Neurology*. New York, Elsevier North-Holland, Inc, 1986, vol 48, pp 413–416.

107. Kashihara K, Ito H, Yamamoto S, et al: Raeder's syndrome associated with intracranial internal carotid artery aneurysm. *Neurosurgery* 1987; 20:49–51.

108. Loeser JD: Herpes zoster and postherpetic neuralgia. *Pain* 1986; 25:149–164.

109. Esmann V, Kroon S, Peterslund NA, et al: Prednisolone does not prevent post-herpetic neuralgia. *Lancet* 1987; 2:126–129.

110. Buck S, Burks TF: The neuropharmacology of capsaicin. *Pharmacol Rev* 1986; 38:179–226.

111. McDonnell PJ, Moore GW, Miller NR, et al: Temporal arteritis. *Ophthalmology* 1986; 93:518–530.

112. Vilaseca J, Gonzalez A, Cid MC, et al: Clinical usefulness of temporal artery biopsy. *Ann Rheum Dis* 1987; 46:282–285.

113. Rosenfeld SI, Kosmorsky GS, Klingele TG, et al: Treatment of temporal arteritis with ocular involvement. *Am J Med* 1986; 80:143–145.

114. Solomon S, Cappa KG: The headache of temporal arteritis. *J Am Geriatr Soc* 1987; 35:163–165.

115. Allen NB, Studenski SA: Polymyalgia rheumatica and temporal arteritis. *Med Clin North Am* 1986; 70:369–384.

116. Lisak RP: Neurologic manifestations of collagen-vascular disease, in Asbury AK, McKhann GM, McDonald WI (eds): *Diseases of the Nervous System*. Philadelphia, WB Saunders Co, 1986, pp 1499–1509.

117. De Silva M, Hazleman BL: Azathioprine in giant cell arteritis/polymyalgia rheumatica: A double blind study. *Ann Rheum Dis* 1986; 45:136–138.

118. Carlow TJ: Headache and the eye, in Dalessio DJ (ed): *Wolff's Headache and Other Head Pain*. New York, Oxford University Press, 1987, pp 304–320.

119. Daroff RB, Whitney CM: Treatment of vascular headaches. *Headache* 1986; 26:470–472.

120. Jonsdottir M, Meyer JS, Rogers RL: Efficacy, side effects and tolerance compared during head-ache treatment with three different calcium blockers. *Headache* 1987; 27:364–369.

121. Bussone G, Baldini S, D'Andrea G, et al: Nimodipine versus flunarizine in common migraine: A controlled pilot trial. *Headache* 1987; 27:76–79.

122. Havanka-Kanniainen H, Hokkanen E, Myllyla VV: Efficacy of nimodipine in comparison with pizotifen in the prophylaxis of migraine. *Cephalalgia* 1987; 7:7–13.

123. Stewart DJ, Gelston A, Hakim A: Effect of prophylactic administration of nimodipine in patients with migraine. *Headache* 1988; 28:260–262.

124. Rascol A, Montastruc JL, Rascol O: Flunarizine versus pizotifen: A double-blind study in the prophylaxis of migraine. *Headache* 1986; 26:83–85.

125. Bunoso S, Di Stasio E, Marano E, et al: Sublingual flunarizine: A new effective management of the migraine attack: A comparison versus ergotamine. *Headache* 1986; 26:227–230.

126. Narbone MC, D'Amico D, Di Perri R: Classic migraine and intercalated seizures in a young woman: Efficacy of flunarizine. *Headache* 1988; 28:209–211.

127. Ziegler DK, Hurwitz A, Hassanein RS, et al: Migraine prophylaxis: A comparison of propranolol and amitriptyline. *Arch Neurol* 1987; 44:486–489.

128. Diamond S, Solomon GD, Freitag FG, et al: Long-acting propranolol in the prophylaxis of mi-graine. *Headache* 1987; 27:70–72.

129. Steiner TJ, Joseph R, Hedman C, et al: Metoprolol in the prophylaxis of migraine: Parallel-groups comparison with placebo and dose-ranging follow-up. *Headache* 1988; 28:15–23.

130. Johannsson V, Nilsson LR, Widelius T, et al: Atenolol in migraine prophylaxis: A double-blind cross-over multicentre study. *Headache* 1987; 27:372–374.

131. Uzogara E, Sheehan DV, Manschreck TC, et al: A combination drug treatment for acute com-mon migraine. *Headache* 1986; 26:231–236.

132. Lipton SA: Prevention of classic migraine headache by digital massage of the superficial tempo-ral arteries during visual aura. *Ann Neurol* 1986; 19:515–516.

133. Callaham M, Raskin N: A controlled study of dihydroergotamine in the treatment of acute mi-graine headache. *Headache* 1986; 26:168–171.

134. Raskin NH: Repetitive intravenous dihydroergotamine as therapy for intractable migraine. *Neu-rology* 1986; 36:995–997.

135. Gallagher RM: Emergency treatment of intractable migraine. *Headache* 1986; 26:74–75.

136. Diamond S, Solomon GD, Freitag FG, et al: Fenoprofen in the prophylaxis of migraine: A dou-ble-blind, placebo controlled study. *Headache* 1987; 27:246–249.

137. Behan PO, Connelly K: Prophylaxis of migraine: A comparison between naproxen sodium and pizotifen. *Headache* 1986; 26:237–239.

138. Miller DS, Talbot CA, Simpson W, et al: A comparison of naproxen sodium, acetaminophen and placebo in the treatment of muscle contraction headache. *Headache* 1987; 27:392–396.

139. Nappi G, Sandrini G, Savoini G, et al: Comparative efficacy of cyclandelate versus flunarizine in the prophylactic treatment of migraine. *Drugs* 1987; 33:103–109.

140. Hasselmark L, Malmgren R, Hannerz J: Effect of a carbohydrate-rich diet, low in protein-tryptophan, in classic and common migraine. *Cephalalgia* 1987; 7:87–92.

141. Low R: *Migraine: The Breakthrough Study That Explains What Causes It and How It Can Be Completely Prevented Through Diet.* New York, Henry Holt & Co, 1987.

142. Parris WCV, Jamison RN, Harris RS, et al: Use of stellate ganglion blocks in treating unilateral migraine headaches. *Cephalalgia* 1987; 6(suppl):475–476.

143. Hannerz J, Ericson K, Bergstrand G: Chronic paroxysmal hemicrania: Orbital phlebography and steroid treatment. *Cephalalgia* 1986; 7:189–192.

144. Smith CD, Reeves AG: Amelioration of ophthalmoplegic migraine by prednisone: A case report. *Headache* 1986; 26:93–94.

145. Diamond S, Freitag FG, Prager J, et al: Treatment of intractable cluster. *Headache* 1986; 26:42–46.

146. De Carolis P, Baldrati A, Agati R, et al: Nimodipine in episodic cluster headache: Results and methodological considerations. *Headache* 1987; 27:397–399.

147. Kruger H, Kohlhepp W, Reimann G, et al: Prophylactic treatment of cluster headache with budipine. *Headache* 1988; 28:344–346.

148. Onofrio B, Campbell K: Can the pain of chronic cluster be cut out? *Mayo Clin Proc* 1986; 61:537–544.

149. Mathew NT, Hurt W: Percutaneous radiofrequency trigeminal gangliorhizolysis in intractable cluster headache. *Headache* 1988; 28:328–331.

150. Solomon S, Apfelbaum RI: Surgical decompression of the facial nerve in the treatment of chronic cluster headache. *Arch Neurol* 1986; 43:479–482.

PART SEVEN

DIAGNOSTIC METHODS

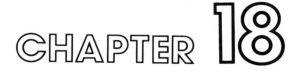

CHAPTER 18

The Visual Field

Hans Bynke, MD, PhD

Associate Professor, Neuro-Ophthalmology Unit; Department of Ophthalmology, University Hospital of Lund, Sweden

A great number of articles dealing with perimetry and other examination methods and with neurologic visual field defects and allied symptoms have been published in the past 2 years. As in the first volume of this series, I have restricted myself to reviewing and discussing publications of particular interest to the clinician.

METHODS OF EXAMINATION

Computerized Perimetry

Many automated perimeters are provided with advanced threshold programs, which is a prerequisite for an accurate examination of the visual field (VF). Such devices are the Octopus, Squid, and Humphrey perimeters, which use projected light spots as stimuli, and the Competer (Digilab) and Dicon perimeters, which use light-emitting diodes. An intelligible basic description of the Octopus perimeter was published in German.[1] Another group of automated perimeters, the suprathreshold screeners, conduct a more rapid but much less adequate test of the VF. Most ophthalmologists are probably aware of this fundamental difference between the instruments. Nevertheless, an interview of 137 practicing ophthalmologists showed that, in 1985, 41% of the automated perimeters used by this group

Curr Neuro Ophthalmol 2:333–350, 1989
© 1989, Year Book Medical Publishers, Inc.
0893–0147/89/02-333-350-$04.00

were suprathreshold screeners.[2] The situation can be expected to improve in the future, because industry has now moved from screening to threshold devices.

Computerized perimetry (CP) has at least three major advantages over manual perimetry (MP). First, because the operator's testing errors are eliminated, the examination can be delegated to technicians lacking all training in MP. Second, because the results may be obtained in numerical form, they can be subjected to exact calculations. Third, CP may be superior to *routine* MP for the detection and follow-up of small and shallow visual field defects (VFDs). This was recently confirmed in pseudotumor cerebri, Graves' disease, and alcohol amblyopia. Using MP, the incidence of VFDs in pseudotumor cerebri has not come up to 50%, excluding blind spot enlargement. Using CP in this disease, however, Smith and Baker[3] recorded VFDs in 68% of 44 eyes, and Wall and George[4] reported them in 77.5% of 40 eyes. In patients with Graves' disease and subnormal visual acuity, central scotomas and nerve fiber bundle defects may be recorded with MP, but Gasser and Flammer reported a patient with normal acuity in whom the Octopus revealed bilateral general constriction, which resolved after radiation therapy.[5] Using the Humphrey perimeter provided with a special grid, Brusini et al. found shallow centrocecal scotomas in no less than 13 of 33 chronic alcoholics with normal visual acuity and normal optic disks.[6]

Whereas threshold CP may be superior to *routine* MP, it is hardly more precise than a meticulous static MP performed by an experienced and highly motivated perimetrist,[7] and in pseudotumor cerebri, a modified Armaly-Drance strategy with Goldmann's perimeter is almost as efficient as CP.[4]

It is evident that CP misses scotomas located in areas between the given static test points.[8] When very small scotomas are suspected, I prefer the tangent screen. It should also be emphasized that CP is afflicted with disadvantages; these are important, particularly in neuro-ophthalmology. Many patients with cerebral disorders who can be tested with MP are unable to cooperate with automated machines. In addition, CP cannot differentiate functional from organic visual loss.[9] In such cases, MP may be the procedure of choice.

Although the automated technique eliminates the influence of the operator on the outcome of the examination, the subjective components remain. Both short-term and long-term fluctuations are inherent in the perimetric measurements of differential light sensitivity. The former represent the variations of the threshold values at any particular location during the examination. The latter represent the variations from one examination to another one. Both kinds of fluctuations are generally greater in pathological than in normal VFs.

Several investigations focused on the normal VF, which constitutes the basis for the analysis of pathologic changes. There is not only a gradual decline in differential light sensitivity from the fixation point toward the periphery, but also an increase of short-term fluctuations with eccentricity.[10-13] Various automated perimeters give similar but not identical results.[12, 14]

The VF is influenced by aging. Most investigators agree that differential light sensitivity decreases more at peripheral than central locations, i.e., that the hill of vision becomes not only depressed but also steeper with age.[10, 13, 15] Others state that the age-related depression is least in the pericentral area,[16] or that the slope does not change.[11] In addition, short-term fluctuations,[10, 11, 15-17] long-term fluctuations, and inter-individual variability[13] increase with aging and eccentricity. These phenomena, which start at the age of 20 or earlier and continue throughout life, may be caused by slowly progressive changes in the retina and in higher neurons.[15, 16] The periphery is suggested to be particularly vulnerable because of the lower density of neuronal elements.[15]

The age-related slope,[10, 13, 15, 16] short-term fluctuations,[10, 15] long-term fluctuations,[17] and differences between fellow eyes[11, 18] are more marked in superior than in inferior VF areas. This may be due to local alteration of the sensory system[16] and intermittent eyelid drooping.[10, 15, 18] The latter may be a problem in CP because of the randomized stimulus presentation.[18] In MP the patient usually anticipates when the superior VF is being tested and makes a conscious effort to elevate the lid.

As an effect of training, there is a tendency for the results to improve with serial examinations. This learning effect may be complete after the second session, develop over several sessions, or fail to appear. It is most pronounced in the peripheral and superior areas.[19]

The consequence of all these phenomena is that false-positive threshold values are common at peripheral and superior locations, particularly at the initial examination. Therefore, these areas may be hard to evaluate. However, the probability of pathology increases when low values appear close to the fixation point, involve two or more adjacent points, or can be reproduced.[12]

Using the Octopus, Neetens and Smets observed that VF defects produced by medullated retinal nerve fibers fluctuated during longitudinal follow-up.[20] It seems that these fluctuations represented nothing more than normal long-term fluctuations.

Surprisingly, alcohol at a blood concentration of about 0.08% has no substantial effect on the outcome of CP.[21] Similar results were previously demonstrated for diazepam.

The numerical data from CP and the opportunity for computer analysis have stimulated interest in the development of statistical methods to describe the probability that a given set of measurements represents normality or abnormality, or that sequentially obtained results represent stability or change. Such methods are the Delta program of the Octopus, linear regression analysis, and analysis of variance combined with trend analysis. In an excellent study of glaucoma VFs, Werner et al. demontrated that statistical models are superior to simple inspection of the automated VF charts.[22] The results would probably have been similar for neurologic VFDs.

Because threshold CP of the entire VF is a time-consuming and fatiguing procedure and the peripheral area may be hard to evaluate, the examination is usually confined to the area inside 20 to 30 degrees of eccentricity. Most hemianopic defects are detected by testing this area with MP. Accordingly, Wirtschafter stated that examination of the periphery is not required in most neuro-ophthalmologic cases.[23] Using the Competer, however, I found that in many cases the earliest hemianopic defects appear outside 20 degrees of eccentricity.[24] Using the Humphrey perimeter, Weber recently confirmed these findings.[25] The cause of this difference between MP and CP is obscure, but one possible explanation is that in these automated perimeters the sizes of the stimuli are too large for the most central area. Whatever the cause may be, the findings formed the basis for the design of a modified model, Competer 750, which can explore the VF out to 75 degrees on the temporal side and 45 degrees on the nasal side.[26] The duration of the test is not longer than with kinetic Goldmann perimetry. In my clinical work, Competer 750 has replaced Goldmann's instrument in about 60% of all neuro-ophthalmological perimetric examinations. MP is required in about 40%, usually because of inadequate patient cooperation (unpublished data).

It seems that the importance of the size of the stimuli is underestimated by designers of automated perimeters. As a rule, one and the same stimulus size is used for all eccentricities. I believe that adjustment of the size in relation to eccentricity would reduce many problems inherent in the automated technique. The linear cortical magnification factor (M) describes the extent of visual cortex, in millimeters, corresponding to 1 degree of arc in visual space. This factor, which is considered to be proportional to the square root of the retinal ganglion cell density in the receptive fields, is about 8 mm at the fixation point and decreases exponentially with eccentricity to less than 0.3 mm in the periphery. It has been proposed that if stimuli are sized in inverse proportion to M, sensitivity would become independent of eccentricity. The process, M-scaling, was tested on the Octopus[27] and Humphrey[28] perimeters. It was demonstrated that M-scaling alone does not result in the expected isosensitivity profile, indicating that additional factors are involved and that further research is required.

Ring Perimetry

On approaching an ordinary optotype from a long distance, this will first be detected. At closer distance it will also be identified and recognized. The closer distance is that used for testing visual acuity. If very low spatial frequencies, which do not contribute significantly to identification, are eliminated by means of a high-pass spatial frequency filter, detection and identification thresholds can be made almost identical. This was demonstrated in 1978 by Howland and co-workers,[29] who proposed the introduction of new optotypes to facilitate the conventional visual acuity test.

Frisén tested high-pass filtered optotypes[30] and concluded that specially designed rings of various sizes were best suited for perimetry.[31] Recently, he designed a VF screener in which the rings are generated by computer graphics and presented on a monitor.[32] The test is easily performed within 5 to 6 minutes and the results are supposed to express the number of functioning neuroretinal channels more directly than other kinds of perimetry. Preliminary results are promising.

Amsler Grid Tests

The Amsler grid is very quick and handy for exploration of the 10-degree area surrounding the fixation point, but because the standard grid is suprathreshold, relative scotomas may be missed. Wall and Sadun made the grid barely suprathreshold by using adjustable cross-polarizing filters in front of the eye tested.[33] In patients with optic neuropathies, they compared this method with standard Amsler, tangent screen, and Octopus examinations. A greater number of scotomas were detected with the modified Amsler test than with any of the other methods. A disadvantage not mentioned is that the results are more difficult to check than with the other methods.

Another modification was presented by Slavin.[34] A large and dense paracentral scotoma in the right eye was disclosed with Goldmann's perimeter in a man whose left VF was normal. Viewing a red Amsler grid on a black background with the right eye, the scotoma was found to be discrete. It disappeared at binocular testing with a red lens in front of the right eye and a green lens in front of the left eye. This demonstrated that the scotoma was spurious.

Oculokinetic Perimetry

Oculokinetic perimetry removes the need for the subject's eye to be kept immobile. Two methods will be considered.

Alvarez et al. use a white screen with a central black stimulus and 100 peripheral fixation points consisting of blue numbers.[35] The subject looks at each number in turn, and the numbers that are associated with disappearance of the test stimulus are crossed out. This method was compared with conventional MP and with CP in patients with neurologic VFDs. The results of the methods were identical or similar in all cases. The VFDs illustrated in the article are large and would probably have been disclosed with confrontation tests; but for recording, the method appears to be useful. According to the authors, it is more simple than conventional perimetry both for the patient and for the perimetrist.

A previously developed method for testing children aged 2 to 5 years was modified to be suited for infants.[36] The perimeter is hemispheric and provided with a central peephole. Central fixation is elicited by four red light-emitting diodes pulsing at a frequency of 1 Hz. The test stimuli consist of yellow light-emitting diodes pulsing at 10 Hz. When illuminated, the central diodes are extinguished and the infant looks at the peripheral stimulus. If the tested area is blind, the movement fails to appear. This technique was carefully evaluated in healthy infants aged 6 to 7 months and in healthy adults. The capacity was found to be high. The potential clinical utility was demonstrated in a child with severe hydrocephalus, in whom homonymous hemianopia was detected at the age of 14 months and subsequently confirmed.

Other Methods

A stimulus velocity of 5 degrees/sec has been recommended for kinetic examination of the peripheral VF, and 2 degrees/sec for the central 30-degree area. On the basis of a study performed with the Squid perimeter, which can also be used for kinetic testing, Johnson and Keltner concluded that a velocity of approximately 4 degrees/sec is optimal for all eccentricities.[37]

The conventional isometric projection of the VF gives a cramped representation of the informative central area. To bring about a relative magnification of this area various nonisometric scales have been designed. A Japanese group claimed that such a scale is advantageous for the evaluation of bitemporal defects caused by suprasellar tumors.[38] The results are partly convincing.

VISUAL FIELD DEFECTS IN INFRAGENICULATE LESIONS

Nonhemianopic Field Defects

The normal blind spot consists of an absolute scotoma and a surrounding narrow zone of relative sensitivity decrease. It is the latter which is enlarged in papilledema. This has been attributed to compression and displacement of the peripapillary photoreceptors and folding of the retina, resulting in a Stiles-Crawford effect. Corbett and co-workers found that the blind spot in papilledema can be reduced by adding suitable positive lenses to the refraction and concluded that elevation of the peripapillary sensory retina is an important cause of the enlargement.[39]

An idiopathic large blind spot syndrome was reported.[40] Seven patients aged 25 to 39 years experienced sudden impairment of monocular vision. Four of them also noticed photopsias. Visual acuity and color vision were normal. The scotomas were absolute, centered on the blind spots, and had steep geographic margins. The fundi were unremarkable, except in two patients who showed very mild peripapillary pigmentary abnormalities. All had clearing of the symptoms over 2 to 3 months. These features, prolonged photostress recovery tests, and positive multifocal electroretinography findings indicated a benign retinal dysfunction of unknown origin.

Physical exercise may result in transient worsening of the symptoms of multiple sclerosis (MS), including vision in acute optic neuritis (Uhthoff's phenomenon). This is due to slight hyperthermia, which inhibits conductivity in demyelinated nerve fibers. Conversely, slight hypothermia has been demonstrated to improve MS symptoms. The effect of a big icewater drink, which reduced body temperature by about 0.5°C, was studied using the Octopus perimeter in patients with optic nerve disease.[41] A significant improvement of the central VF was demonstrated in 14 of 18 eyes with acute optic neuritis and in 4 of 17 eyes with previous optic neuritis. No effect was found in 12 eyes with other kinds of optic neuropathy. The authors proposed this test for differential diagnosis. Optic neuritis can now be visualized on magnetic resonance imaging (MRI) with surface coils.[42] This more direct method can possibly be utilized for the same purpose.

Bilateral central scotomas developed in a case of Leber's optic neuropathy.[43] Remarkably, the patient presented with a large monocular subhyaloid hemorrhage presumed to originate from the initial peripapillary microangiopathy, which is typical for this disease.

Unilateral optic neuropathy with centrocecal scotoma occurred as the only clinical manifestation in a patient who was in remission from a non-Hodgkin's lymphoma.[44] Peripheral VF constriction and disk pallor developed over 2 months. Computed tomography (CT) scan showed diffuse enlargement of the intraorbital optic nerve. Following radiation therapy the peripheral VF improved but the scotoma remained. Confirmatory cerebrospinal fluid cytology did not occur until 6 months after the onset of eye symptoms.

Ocular and central nervous system complications are relatively frequent in acute leukemia but rare in chronic leukemia. In a comprehensive article, Currie and coworkers reported three patients in whom optic neuropathy was an early clinical manifestation of chronic lymphatic leukemia.[45] The first patient presented with monocular visual obscurations and enlargement of the blind spot from optic disk edema, thus simulating optic nerve sheath meningioma. The fellow eye was involved 10 months later. In the other two patients there were slowly progressive bilateral visual loss and central scotomas, but no optic disk edemas. In all three cases vision gradually decreased and optic atrophy with peripheral VF constriction developed. CT scans showed enlargement of the intraorbital optic nerves, and the VFs expanded after local radiation therapy. Surface marker studies of cerebrospinal fluid lymphocytes were useful for diagnosis. Leukemic infiltration of the optic nerves was confirmed at autopsy in the first case.

It is rare that occlusion of the internal carotid artery results in simultaneous ipsilateral anterior ischemic optic neuropathy (AION) and cerebral watershed infarction. This opticocerebral syndrome was reported in three patients with permanent monocular blindness or central scotoma.[46] I have seen this syndrome in one case.

Two women in whom cesarean section was performed under spinal anesthesia complained of black spots after surgery.[47] Both had a temporary drop of systemic blood pressure during the operation, which resulted in transient macular edema and permanent retinal pigmentary changes. Careful perimetry disclosed small bilateral ring scotomas, which did not resolve.

Ophthalmic migraine was reported in two women with previous attacks of classic migraine.[48] The symptoms, which included blindness preceded and followed by multiple scotomas, were ascribed to transient vascular optic neuropathy. One case also demonstrated optic disk edema. Vision normalized after 6 weeks and 10 days, respectively. I do not recognize this clinical picture.

The nitrosourea compound BCNU (carmustine) has a potential for causing acute and delayed side effects, particularly when infused into the carotid artery. Delayed toxicity usually takes the form of retinal vasculitis. However, Pickrell and Purvin reported a patient with a malignant glioma, who developed typical AION with pallid optic disk edema and inferior arcuate VF constriction in the ipsilateral eye 5 weeks after intracarotid infusion of BCNU.[49]

Because the arcuate optic nerve fiber bundles remain gathered all the way from the retina to the anterior optic chiasm, nerve fiber bundle VFDs are not pathognomonic for lesions of the retina and optic nerve head. A case report by Hupp and colleagues reminds us of this important fact.[50] Local constrictions and scotomas not respecting the vertical meridian were demonstrated in four patients with large intracranial tumors. An epidermoid cyst enveloping one optic nerve and the chiasm, and a chondroid chordoma involving one optic nerve, produced monocular defects. A meningioma extending into both posterior optic canals, and a pituitary adenoma, gave rise to binocular defects. Similar defects were recorded in a case of mediastinal and suprasellar sarcoidosis infiltrating the chiasm and adjacent structures.[51]

In cases of the kind just described, the history and follow-up are of great help, but diagnosis cannot be affirmed without CT scan and other methods. VFDs produced by tilted optic disks[52] and atypical retinitis pigmentosa[53] can mimic neurologic disorders, but are less problematic from a diagnostic point of view because a careful ophthalmologic examination is all that is required.

Various ophthalmic changes were found in 50 children shunted for congenital hydrocephalus.[54] Nonhemianopic defects were the most common VFDs. Homonymous hemianopias were recorded in two cases. The mechanisms were only partially discussed.

Complete excision of meningiomas involving the anterior visual pathway is not always possible without causing blindness and other neurologic deficits. The effect of radiation therapy was evaluated in 20 patients with progressive visual loss.[55] The VFs improved in 12 cases and stabilized in four. Repeat CT scans demonstrated reduced tumor size in only two cases. Another possible nonsurgical treatment is the antiestrogen tamoxifen citrate, which improved vision in a woman with meningioma.[50]

Gaze-evoked amaurosis is a transient monocular loss of vision occurring in a particular direction of eccentric gaze. This clinically useful symptom indicates the presence of an orbital tumor. It was recently described in three patients with optic nerve sheath meningiomas and in four patients with cavernous heman- giomas.[56, 57]

As a complication to internal carotid endarterectomy, a 73-year-old man devel- oped a carotid-cavernous fistula with ipsilateral acute glaucoma and blindness.[58] After balloon embolization of the fistula, the symptoms abated and vision was much improved. I have seen a younger man with a traumatic carotid-cavernous fistula and bilateral acute glaucoma who recovered after intracranial surgery of the fistula.

Other lesions of one or both optic nerves with blindness or various kinds of nonhemianopic VFDs were caused by giant cell arteritis,[59] sphenoethmoiditis,[60] syphilis in the acquired immune deficiency syndrome (AIDS),[61, 62] meningeal carcinomatosis,[63] postulated synergism between low-dose cranial irradiation and the nitrosourea compound CCNU (lomustine),[64] and self-inflicted gunshot wounds.[65]

Hemianopic Field Defects

Like gliomas originating within the anterior visual pathway, the less common hypothalamic gliomas are usually low-grade astrocytomas, and both may give rise to similar symptoms and signs. However, because hypothalamic gliomas merely distort the visual pathway, they can be subtotally removed without causing further visual damage. With very few exceptions, this is not possible with gliomas origi- nating within the visual pathway. Gillet and Symon[66] reported seven cases of ret- rochiasmatic hypothalamic glioma, and Coppeto et al.[67] one additional case. There were bitemporal hemianopias in three cases, homonymous hemianopias in three cases, and monocular temporal hemianopia in one case. In one patient, who presented with hemiparesis, the VFs were intact. Two patients exhibited endocrine symptoms. In most cases the radiologic diagnosis was craniopharyngioma. Vision normalized postoperatively in one case.[67]

Intrachiasmatic craniopharyngioma is a rare cause of chiasmal thickening, which can be separated from intrachiasmatic glioma using MRI.[68] In a young man with temporal hemianopia in one eye and central scotoma in the other eye, an in- traventricular craniopharyngioma with anterior extension into the chiasm and proximal optic nerves was found at craniotomy. Partial resection restored vision.

Thirteen cases of intrasellar arachnoid cysts were reported in an excellent pa- per.[69] In contrast to other arachnoid cysts, these appear to be acquired. Bitemporal hemianopia was recorded in six patients and junctional scotoma in one. The re- maining patients presented with endocrine symptoms and had normal VFs. All VFDs improved after transsphenoidal cyst excision. Recently, I saw a patient again who had presented with visual impairment in 1979. At the onset he had bi- lateral nonhemianopic arcuate scotomas. Four high-resolution CT scans taken be- tween 1980 and 1988 were interpreted as normal! Eventually, optic atrophy and bitemporal hemianopia developed, and a suprasellar arachnoid cyst was detected on MRI. The postoperative improvement was only moderate.

VFDs may occur in patients with the primary empty sella syndrome. The combination of empty sella and pseudotumor cerebri with papilledema and secondary VFDs is well known.[70] However, bitemporal superior hemianopia was recorded in a boy with normal optic disks in whom the chiasm was suggested to be dragged downward by an arachnoid diverticulum.[71]

In no fewer than 8 of 25 patients subjected to head trauma with indirect injury of the anterior visual pathway, the appearance of the VFDs indicated a lesion at or near the chiasm.[72] The paper should be read in original.

Rapidly occurring bitemporal hemianopia in two women was attributed to chiasmal neuritis.[73] There were no other symptoms consistent with MS, but examinations of the cerebrospinal fluid showed slight pleocytosis in both patients and increased protein content in one. CT scans were negative. MRI was not available. The VFs normalized over about 3 weeks and no new symptoms occurred during a follow-up period of 24 and 18 months, respectively.

Homonymous hemianopia is another less common manifestation of MS. In two cases of advanced MS and homonymous defects, optic tract involvement was documented on MRI, possibly for the first time.[74] One patient had right incongruous homonymous hemianopia, temporal hemianopic scotoma in the left VF, and slight pallor of the left optic disk. A demyelinated plaque was seen at the left optic tract-chiasm-nerve junction. In the other patient, who had remarkably congruous right homonymous scotomas and normal disks, the plaque was situated in the left optic tract and brain stem. Vision improved in the first case and normalized in the second.

VISUAL FIELD DEFECTS IN SUPRAGENICULATE LESIONS

Homonymous Hemianopic Defects

Homonymous horizontal sectoranopia may be produced both by geniculate and suprageniculate lesions. Four new patients with congruous sectoranopia and normal optic disks were reported.[75] Two had occipital infarctions and the other two arteriovenous malformations in the posterior temporal lobe.

Kölmel reported three cases of homonymous paracentral scotomas.[76] Severe photophobia was a prominent symptom. In two cases the probable mechanism was cerebral hypoxia induced by uterine hemorrhage and cardiac surgery, respectively, and in one case it could not be identified. The lesions could not be visualized on CT and MRI, but were suggested to be cortical. The scotomas resolved in two cases. I have seen transient homonymous paracentral scotomas associated with photopsia following cardiac surgery, and also agree with the author that nonsymptomatic VFDs of this kind may be found without a demonstrable cause.

In a patient with posttraumatic bilateral homonymous hemianopia with sparing of the central VF, spatial disorientation and memory deficits, CT showed bilateral occipital and mesial temporal infarctions with preservation of the occipital poles.[77] The mechanism was tentorial herniation with compression of both posterior cerebral arteries secondary to a frontal subdural hematoma.

According to previous authors, hemiparesis with aphasia, or hemiplegia, constituted delayed complications to indirect electrical contact. Four days after an electrical injury, which "burned" the hand and caused blurring of vision for several minutes, a 53-year-old hypertensive man sustained occipital infarction with homonymous hemianopia.[78]

Recent investigation indicates that in the future, positron emission tomography (PET) will give valuable information in cases of homonymous hemianopia. In one study, the baseline (nonstimulated) metabolic function of the denervated occipital cortex was assessed in 18 patients with extraoccipital neoplasms.[79] The metabolism was found to be decreased only in cases of homonymous defects, and mainly within the macular representation of the primary visual cortex. In another study, the metabolic function was assessed in five patients with dense homonymous defects due to ischemic lesions involving the suprageniculate visual pathway.[80] An initial PET was made shortly after the ictus, and a final PET between 1 and 10 months later. In two cases without primary involvement of the occipital lobe according to CT, the hemianopia abated and the striate metabolism improved. On the contrary, in three cases with primary damage of the occipital lobe, neither VF nor striate metabolism improved. Consequently, sparing of the striate cortex seemed to be a prerequisite for recovery. Although the number of cases was small and the follow-up period short in two patients without any improvement, these results are very interesting.

Homonymous defects caused by vascular lesions involving the suprageniculate pathway were followed up over 3 years.[81] Spontaneous regression was largely completed after 6 months, and more extensive VFDs were subjected to higher restoration ratios than less extensive VFDs. It is not entirely clear to me how the latter results were obtained.

Superficial temporal artery–middle cerebral artery (STA-MCA) microvascular bypass surgery may be beneficial not only in hemiparesis, but also in hemianopia. Earlier authors reported complete reversal of a 7-year-old hemianopia after this procedure. Recently, a man with complete homonymous hemianopia caused by middle cerebral artery stenosis was treated with STA-MCA only 3 weeks after the stroke.[82] The hemianopia improved immediately and resolved over the following month. Arteriography demonstrated parallel improvement of the vascular supply.

Another chapter of this volume is devoted to psychovisual disturbances. One of these, visual hemineglect, increases the disability of patients with homonymous hemianopia and will therefore be mentioned also in this context. Visual hemineglect is usually caused by a lesion in the parietal lobe or the posterior thalamus of the nondominant hemisphere and may occur in combination with left homonymous hemianopia. Patients with isolated dense homonymous defects notice their field defect and feel handicapped—but they soon learn to compensate by developing searching eye movements toward the blind side. On the contrary, patients with additional severe hemineglect are unaware of the hemianopia and often bump into objects on the blind side. In most cases, hemineglect recovers spontaneously within months. It is conventionally diagnosed with the line bisection test or by copying a complex figure. In an excellent paper, which should be read by all ophthalmologists, Meienberg et al. discussed these matters and demonstrated the superiority of infrared reflection oculography in two cases of homonymous hemianopia for an objective and quantitative diagnosis of additional visual hemineglect.[83]

The anterior choroidal artery syndrome combines the triad of hemiplegia, hemianesthesia, and homonymous hemianopia, but incomplete forms are more frequent than complete forms. This rare syndrome is caused by infarctions situated in the posterior limb of the internal capsule, sparing the thalamus medially and encroaching upon the tip of the globus pallidus laterally. The hemianopia is usually due to damage of the optic radiation, but can sometimes be caused by damage to the optic tract or lateral geniculate body, which are also supplied by this artery. In a report of 16 cases, Decroix and coworkers found hemiplegia or hemiparesis in 14 patients and hemianesthesia in 13, but hemianopia in only 3.[84] In two of them, the hemianopia was left-sided and associated with severe visual hemineglect. This symptom also occurred in a patient with right-sided infarction and normal VF.

In a preliminary study, automobile drivers with VFDs were tested in a driving simulator with respect to possible compensatory mechanisms.[85] The duration of the VFDs was at least 1 year. Only three of 22 drivers with homonymous hemianopia or quadrantanopia were able to compensate for their VFDs. Interestingly, the authors stated that the possibility of compensation could not be predicted from the results of perimetry. Therefore, I suggest that other disturbances were present and influenced driving performance. In another study, a battery of psychometric tests disclosed concealed psychovisual and mental deficits in patients subjected to closed head injury less than 2 years earlier. The deficits were most pronounced in cases of binocular VFDs.[86]

Cortical Blindness

In a comprehensive report of 25 adults with cortical blindness, Aldrich et al. found the most common causes to be ischemic stroke, cardiac surgery, and cerebral angiography.[87] Remarkably, only 7 patients denied their blindness or were unaware of it. Electroencephalography was superior to visually evoked potentials as a diagnostic adjuvant. No patient with bioccipital CT changes from any cause had good recovery of vision. The outcome was poor in all 8 patients with stroke, but fair or good in 11 of the other 17 cases. Three patients regained full vision. In 1 of these the blindness was secondary to head trauma, which is a more frequent cause in children. Sacher and Klöti reported spontaneous recovery of vision within 3 hours in 7 children subjected to closed head injury.[88]

Another cause of transient cortical blindness is the toxemia of pregnancy, which was reported in two women in whom vision recovered completely a few weeks after cesarean section.[89] CT scans showed transient occipital hypodensities, indicating altered vascular permeability with resulting plasma effusion.

Permanent cortical blindness was described after posterior fossa surgery, which produced spasm of cerebral arteries,[90] in acute demyelination consistent with Schilder's disease,[91] and in nonspecific dementia due to cortical amyloid angiopathy.[92]

SUMMARY

The advantages and disadvantages of CP in neuro-ophthalmology have become better defined in the past 2 years. Recent investigations confirm that for detecting and following up small and shallow VFDs CP may be superior to routine manual perimetry. CP can replace manual methods in the majority of neuro-ophthalmological examinations, but in cases of inadequate cooperation and functional visual loss, manual perimetry is still the procedure of choice. Many of the particular problems inherent in the automated technique will probably be solved in the future.

In neuro-ophthalmology, there is also a need for other examination methods, for example in patients with malfixation and in young children. New or modified methods were designed and evaluated.

A surprisingly large number of recent case reports deal with rare or less common causes of VFD . Many of these reports contain much interesting information, valuable also for experienced clinicians.

REFERENCES

1. Herbolzheimer WG: Die programmgesteuerte Perimetrie, ihre Vorzüge und ihre Nachteile. *Klin Mbl Augenheilk* 1986; 189:270–277.

2. Smith TJ, Goins KM: Standards of perimetry, in Greve EL, Heijl A (eds): *Seventh International Visual Field Symposium*. Dordrecht, Kluwer Academic Publishers, 1987, pp 551–555.

3. Smith TJ, Baker RS: Perimetric findings in pseudotumor cerebri using automated techniques. *Ophthalmology* 1986; 93:887–894.

4. Wall M, George D: Visual loss in pseudotumor cerebri. *Arch Neurol* 1987; 44:170–175.

5. Gasser P, Flammer J: Optic neuropathy in Graves' disease. *Ophthalmologica* 1986; 192:22–27.

6. Brusini P, Dal Mas P, Della Mea G, et al: Centro-coecal field examination in chronic alcoholism, in Greve EL, Heijl A (eds): *Seventh International Visual Field Symposium*. Dordrecht, Kluwer Academic Publishers, 1987, pp 639–644.

7. Sucs FE, Verriest G: Inter- and intraindividual sensitivity variations with manual and automated static perimeters. *Ophthalmologica* 1987; 195:209–214.

8. Stepanik J: Der blinde Fleck: Kritische Betrachtung rasterperimetrischer Aussage über ein Skotom bekannter Grösse. *Klin Mbl Augenheilk* 1986; 189:409–412.

9. Smith TJ, Baker RS: Perimetric findings in functional disorders using automated techniques. *Ophthalmology* 1987; 94:1562–1566.

10. Katz J, Sommer A: Asymmetry and variation in the normal hill of vision. *Arch Ophthalmol* 1986; 104:65–68.

11. Brenton RS, Phelps CD: The normal visual field on the Humphrey Field Analyzer. *Ophthalmologica* 1986; 193:56–74.

12. Lewis RA, Johnson CA, Keltner JL, et al: Variability of quantitative automated perimetry in normal observers. *Ophthalmology* 1986; 93:878–881.

13. Heijl A, Lindgren G, Olsson J: Normal variability of static perimetric threshold values across the central visual field. *Arch Ophthalmol* 1987; 105:1544–1549.

14. Brenton RS, Argus WA: Fluctuations on the Humphrey and Octopus perimeters. *Invest Ophthalmol Vis Sci* 1987; 28:767–771.

15. Jaffe GJ, Alvarado JA, Juster RP: Age-related changes of the normal visual field. *Arch Ophthalmol* 1986; 104:1021–1025.

16. Haas A, Flammer J, Schneider U: Influence of age on the visual fields of normal subjects. *Am J Ophthalmol* 1986; 101:199–203.

17. Katz J, Sommer A: A longitudinal study of the age-adjusted variability of automated visual fields. *Arch Ophthalmol* 1987; 105:1083–1086.

18. Brenton RS, Phelps CD, Rojas P, et al: Interocular differences of the visual field in normal subjects. *Invest Ophthalmol Vis Sci* 1986; 27:799–805.

19. Wood JM, Wild JM, Hussey MK, et al: Serial examination of the normal visual field using Octopus automated projection perimetry. Evidence for a learning effect. *Acta Ophthalmol* 1987; 65:326–333.

20. Neetens A, Smets RM: Medullated retinal nerve fibers. *Neuro-Ophthalmol* 1987; 7:329–334.

21. Zulauf M, Flammer J, Signer C: The influence of alcohol on the outcome of automated static perimetry. *Graefe's Arch Clin Exp Ophthalmol* 1986; 224:525–528.

22. Werner EB, Bishop KI, Koelle J, et al: A comparison of experienced clinical observers and statistical tests in detection of progressive visual field loss in glaucoma using automated perimetry. *Arch Ophthalmol* 1988; 106:619–623.

23. Wirtschafter JD: Examination of the peripheral visual field. *Arch Ophthalmol* 1987; 105:761–762.

24. Bynke H: A study of the depth of hemianopic field defects for optimizing computerized perimetry. *Neuro-Ophthalmol* 1984; 4:237–247.

25. Weber J: Computerized perimetry in neuro-ophthalmology: Comparison of different test patterns by an 'information index,' in Greve EL, Heijl A (eds): *Seventh International Visual Field Symposium*. Dordrecht, Kluwer Academic Publishers, 1987, pp 621–628.

26. Bynke H, Krakau CET, Öhman R, et al: A new computerized perimeter ('Competer 750') for examination of neuro-ophthalmic patients, in Greve EL, Heijl A (eds): *Seventh International Visual Field Symposium*. Dordrecht, Kluwer Academic Publishers, 1987, pp 249–256.

27. Wood JM, Wild JM, Drasdo N, et al: Perimetric profiles and cortical representation. *Ophthalmic Res* 1986; 18:301–308.

28. Wild JM, Wood JM, Flanagan JG: Spatial summation and the cortical magnification of perimetric profiles. *Ophthalmologica* 1987; 195:88–96.

29. Howland B, Ginsburg A, Campbell F: High-pass spatial frequency letters as clinical optotypes. *Vision Res* 1978; 18:1063–1066.

30. Frisén L: Vanishing optotypes. New type of acuity test letters. *Arch Ophthalmol* 1986; 104:1194–1198.

31. Frisén L: High-pass resolution targets in peripheral vision. *Ophthalmology* 1987; 94:1104–1108.

32. Frisén L: A computer-graphics visual field screener using high-pass spatial frequency resolution targets and multiple feedback devices, in Greve EL, Heijl A (eds): *Seventh International Visual Field Symposium.* Dordrecht, Kluwer Academic Publishers, 1987, pp 441–446.

33. Wall M, Sadun AA: Threshold Amsler grid testing. *Arch Ophthalmol* 1986; 104:520–523.

34. Slavin ML: The use of the red Amsler grid and red-green lenses in detecting spurious paracentral visual field defects. *Am J Ophthalmol* 1987; 103:338–339.

35. Alvarez E, Damato B, Wakakura M, et al: Oculo-kinetic perimetry. A visual field test for neuro-ophthalmic patients. *Neuro-Ophthalmol* 1988; 8:23–30.

36. Mayer DL, Fulton AB, Cummings MF: Visual fields of infants assessed with a new perimetric technique. *Invest Ophthalmol Vis Sci* 1988; 29:452–459.

37. Johnson CA, Keltner JL: Optimal rates of movement for kinetic perimetry. *Arch Ophthalmol* 1987; 105:73–75.

38. Haruta R, Kani K, Mimura O, et al: A new numerical representation of the visual field in cases of chiasmal tumor, in Greve EL, Heijl A (eds): *Seventh International Visual Field Symposium.* Dordrecht, Kluwer Academic Publishers, 1987, pp 613–617.

39. Corbett JJ, Jacobson DM, Mauer RC, et al: Enlargement of the blind spot caused by papilledema. *Am J Ophthalmol* 1988; 105:261–265.

40. Fletcher WA, Imes RK, Goodman D, et al: Acute idiopathic blind spot enlargement. *Arch Ophthalmol* 1988; 106:44–49.

41. Heider W, Gottlob I: Ein differentialdiagnostischer Test bei Neuritis nervi optici. *Klin Mbl Augenheilk* 1987; 190:420–423.

42. Miller DH, Johnson G, McDonald WI, et al: Detection of optic nerve lesions in optic neuritis with magnetic resonance imaging. *Lancet* 1986; 1:1490–1491.

43. Kerty E, Eide N, Hapnes R: A subhyaloid haemorrhage as the presenting symptom of bilateral optic neuropathy. *Acta Ophthalmol* 1987; 65(suppl 182):172–175.

44. Lanska DJ, Lanska MJ, Tomsak RL: Unilateral optic neuropathy in non-Hodgkin's lymphoma. *Neurology* 1987; 37:1563–1564.

45. Currie JN, Lessell S, Lessell IM, et al: Optic neuropathy in chronic lymphocytic leukemia. *Arch Ophthalmol* 1988; 106:654–660.

46. Bogousslavsky J, Regli F, Zografos L, et al: Optico-cerebral syndrome: Simultaneous hemodynamic infarction of optic nerve and brain. *Neurology* 1987; 37:263–268.

47. Stilma JS, De Lange JJ, Crezee FC: Bilateral central scotoma with preservation of central vision in 2 patients following caesarian section under spinal anesthesia. *Doc Ophthalmol* 1987; 67:59–68.

48. Pittke EC: Sehstörungen als Leitsymptome der okulären Migräne. *Klin Mbl Augenheilk* 1986; 189:317–322.

49. Pickrell L, Purvin V: Ischemic optic neuropathy secondary to intracarotid infusion of BCNU. *J Clin Neuro-Ophthalmol* 1987; 7:87–91.

50. Hupp SL, Savino PJ, Schatz NJ, et al: Nerve fibre bundle visual field defects and intracranial mass lesions. *Can J Ophthalmol* 1986; 6:231–235.

51. Ludmerer KM, Kissane JM: Visual impairment, pituitary dysfunction, and hilar adenopathy in a young man. *Am J Med* 1986; 80:259–268.

52. Giuffrè G: The spectrum of the visual field defects in the tilted disc syndrome. *Neuro-Ophthalmol* 1986; 6:239–246.

53. Heidemann DG, Beck RW: Retinitis pigmentosa: A mimic of neurologic disease. *Surv Ophthalmol* 1987; 32:45–51.

54. Mankinen-Heikkinen A, Mustonen E: Ophthalmic changes in hydrocephalus: A follow-up examination of 50 patients treated with shunts. *Acta Ophthalmol* 1987; 65:81–86.

55. Kupfersmith MJ, Warren FA, Newall J, et al: Irradiation of meningiomas of the intracranial anterior visual pathway. *Ann Neurol* 1987; 21:131–137.

56. Orcutt JC, Tucker WM, Mills RP, et al: Gaze-evoked amaurosis. *Ophthalmology* 1987; 94:213–218.

57. Manor RS, Ben Sira I: Amaurosis fugax at downward gaze. *Surv Ophthalmol* 1987; 31:411–416.

58. Brodsky MC, Hoyt WF, Halbach VV, et al: Recovery from total monocular blindness after balloon embolization of carotid-cavernous fistula. *Am J Ophthalmol* 1987; 104:86–87.

59. Kelly SP, Robertson DA, Rostron CK: Preventable blindness in giant cell arteritis. *Br Med J* 1987; 294:431–432.

60. Slavin ML, Glaser JS: Acute severe irreversible visual loss with sphenoethmoiditis—'posterior' orbital cellulitis. *Arch Ophthalmol* 1987; 105:345–348.

61. Zaidman GW: Neurosyphilis and retrobulbar neuritis in a patient with AIDS. *Ann Ophthalmol* 1986; 18:260–261.

62. Zambrano W, Perez GM, Smith JL: Acute syphilitic blindness in AIDS. *J Clin Neuro Ophthalmol* 1987; 7:1–5.

63. McCrary III JA, Patrinely JR, Font RL: Progressive blindness caused by metastatic occult signet-ring cell gastric carcinoma. *Arch Ophthalmol* 1986; 104:410–413.

64. Wilson WB, Perez GM, Kleinschmidt-Demasters BK: Sudden onset of blindness in patients treated with oral CCNU and low-dose cranial irradiation. *Cancer* 1987; 59:901–907.

65. Keane JR: Blindness from self-inflicted gunshot wounds. *J Clin Neuro-Ophthalmol* 1986; 6:247–249.

66. Gillett GR, Symon L: Hypothalamic glioma. *Surg Neurol* 1987; 28:291–300.

67. Coppeto JR, Monteiro MLR, Uphoff DF: Exophytic suprasellar glioma: A rare cause of chiasmatic compression. *Arch Ophthalmol* 1987; 105:28.

68. Brodsky MC, Hoyt WF, Barnwell SL, et al: Intrachiasmatic craniopharyngioma: A rare cause of chiasmal thickening. *J Neurosurg* 1988; 68:300–302.

69. Meyer FB, Carpenter SM, Laws ER Jr: Intrasellar arachnoid cysts. *Surg Neurol* 1987; 28:105–110.

70. De Vries-Knoppert WAEJ: Primary empty sella syndrome and benign intracranial hypertension. *Doc Ophthalmol* 1986; 61:319–325.

71. Fusco R, Magli A, Guacci P, et al: Empty sella syndrome. *Ophthalmologica* 1988; 196:92–97.

72. Noble MJ, McFadzean R: Indirect injury to the optic nerves and optic chiasm. *Neuro-Ophthalmol* 1987; 7:341–348.

73. Waespe W, Haenny P: Bitemporal hemianopia due to chiasmal optic neuritis. *Neuro-Ophthalmol* 1987; 7:69–74.

74. Rosenblatt MA, Behrens MM, Zweifach PH, et al: Magnetic resonance imaging of optic tract involvement in multiple sclerosis. *Am J Ophthalmol* 1987; 104:74–79.

75. Sato Y, Matusda S, Igarashi Y, et al: Horizontal homonymous sectoranopia due to a more proximal lesion than the lateral geniculate body. *Neuro-Ophthalmol* 1986; 6:407–416.

76. Kölmel HW: Homonymous paracentral scotomas. *J Neurol* 1987; 235:22–25.

77. Soza M, Tagle P, Kirkham T, et al: Bilateral homonymous hemianopia with sparing of central vision after subdural hematoma. *Can J Neurol Sci* 1987; 14:153–155.

78. Gans M, Glaser JS: Homonymous hemianopia following electrical injury. *J Clin Neuro-Ophthalmol* 1986; 6:218–221.

79. Fishbein DS, Chrousos GA, Di Chiro G, et al: Glucose utilization of visual cortex following extra-occipital interruptions of the visual pathways by tumor. *J Clin Neuro-Ophthalmol* 1987; 7:63–68.

80. Bosley TM, Dann R, Silver FL, et al: Recovery of vision after ischemic lesions: Positron emission tomography. *Ann Neurol* 1987; 21:444–450.

81. Messing B, Ganshirt H: Follow-up of visual field defects with vascular damage of the geniculo-striate visual pathway. *Neuro-Ophthalmol* 1987; 7:231–242.

82. Benzel EC, Mirfarkhraee M: Complete homonymous hemianopsia: Reversal with arterial bypass. *South Med J* 1987; 80:249–251.

83. Meienberg O, Harrer M, Wehren C: Oculographic diagnosis of hemineglect in patients with homonymous hemianopia. *J Neurol* 1986; 233:97–101.

84. Decroix JP, Graveleau P, Masson M, et al: Infarction in the territory of the anterior choroidal artery. *Brain* 1986; 109:1071–1085.

85. Hedin A, Lövsund P: Effects of visual field defects on driving performance, in Greve EL, Heijl A (eds): *Seventh International Visual Field Symposium.* Dordrecht, Kluwer Academic Publishers, 1987, pp 541–547.

86. Uzzell BP, Obrist WD, Dolinskas CA, et al: Relation of visual field defects to neuropsychological outcome after closed head injury. *Acta Neurochir (Wien)* 1987; 86:18–24.

87. Aldrich MS, Alessi AG, Beck RW, et al: Cortical blindness: Etiology, diagnosis, and prognosis. *Ann Neurol* 1987; 21:149–158.

88. Sacher P, Klöti J: Die transitorische posttraumatische zerebrale Blindheit. *Schweiz Med Wochenschr* 1987; 117:656–659.

89. Lau SPC, Chan FL, Yu YL, et al: Cortical blindness in toxaemia of pregnancy: Findings on computed tomography. *Bri J Radiol* 1987; 60:347–349.

90. Brau RH, Lameiro J, Llaguno AV, et al: Metamorphopsia and permanent cortical blindness after a posterior fossa tumor. *Neurosurgery* 1986; 19:263–266.

91. Sedwick LA, Klingele TG, Burde RM, et al: Schilder's (1912) disease: Total cerebral blindness due to acute demyelination. *Arch Neurol* 1986; 43:85–87.

92. Nadeau SE, Bebin J, Smith E: Nonspecific dementia, cortical blindness, and Congophilic angiopathy: A clinicopathological report. *J Neurol* 1987; 234:14–18.

CHAPTER 19

The Visual Evoked Potential in Clinical Neuro-Ophthalmology

W. I. M. Verhagen, M.D., Ph.D.

Department of Neurology and Clinical Neurophysiology, Canisius Wilhelmina Hospital, Nijmegen, The Netherlands

G. P. M. Horsten, M.D., Ph.D.

Eye Clinic, Academic Medical Center, Amsterdam, The Netherlands

Measurement of the visual evoked potential (VEP) is now one of the most frequently used diagnostic investigations in neuro-ophthalmology. Of the many reports that have appeared on this subject, we review here those that are of clinical importance and a few others that mention interesting results.

In the early 1960s, only flash stimuli were used, but Hubel and Wiesel[1] had found that brain cortex neurons also respond to more complex visual patterns. Pattern stimuli became especially popular after a study by Halliday et al.[2] in 1972.

The pattern VEP (PVEP) is dependent on many parameters, such as contrast level, type and orientation of the pattern, field size, method, and rate of presentation.[3] Small patterns (gratings and checks) will predominantly stimulate the contrast and spatial-frequency detectors in the fovea and visual cortex.[4]

The VEP is a response of the visual system from the retina to the cerebral cortex, but factors influencing retinal luminance such as ptosis, miosis, lens and media opacities, and refractive errors are important too. Retinal disorders may affect both the latency and the amplitude—for example, maculopathies,[5-8] central serous choroidopathy,[9, 10] macular holes,[11, 12] tilted disks and oblique entrance of the optic nerve,[13, 14] and optic nerve drusen.[15, 16]

The PVEP is not particularly useful in the diagnosis of glaucoma; only a few patients are reported to have shown greatly increased latencies.[17-20] Good et al.[21] suggested that a reduction of the P1 amplitude of the flash VEP might be useful in early diagnosis and assessment of chronic glaucoma. Additional information on macular function can be obtained by measuring the PVEP after the macular photo stress test; delayed recovery may occur in retinal vascular disease and intoxication[22] with antimalarial drugs. In interpreting VEPs, the patient's age must be taken into account.[23, 24] Maturational changes in children[25-28] can be documented with the aid of the VEP. The development of the VEP has been shown to be altered in infants with prenatal disorders.[29] Neonates of 22 to 23 weeks gestational age had no identifiable waves, but in all infants a large negative wave was seen after about 300 msec at 24 weeks.[28] Between 30 and 35 weeks of gestational age, a small positive wave (P200) was seen in over one third, and after 36 weeks it was seen in all infants.[28, 30]

Taylor et al.[28] suggest from their longitudinal studies that rapid changes of the VEP, such as that waveforms emerge earlier than they do in cross-sectional data, occur because development of the visual cortex may be accelerated postnatally. Norcia et al.[31] suggest the same for the development of visual acuity as indicated by the VEP.

MULTIPLE SCLEROSIS

The diagnosis of multiple sclerosis (MS) depends primarily on clinical criteria, but evoked potentials (EP), especially the VEP, are very important for detecting clinically silent lesions. Many articles have confirmed the results of Halliday et al.[2, 32] on the delayed PVEP in optic neuritis and MS. Lowitzsch[33] reviewed the literature on MS. In the definite group, the prevalence of disturbed PVEP was 90% to 100%, in the probable group 60%, and in the possible group 30%, amounting to PVEP change in about 40% of all patients with MS. The use of stimuli of high and low spatial frequencies is of great importance because different subsystems may be affected.[34-36] Pattern orientation is also important.[37, 38]

Sanders et al.[39] studied the disparity between visual function (visual acuity, color vision, visual field, contrast sensitivity) and PVEP in optic neuritis; several stimulus configurations were used. The VEP amplitudes were associated with the outcome of all clinical tests independently of check size, luminance, or the presentation method used. The VEP latencies showed poor correlation with the clinical tests. Neima and Regan,[36] however, reported that reduced contrast sensitivity at high spatial frequencies was associated with reduced visual acuity and amplitude reduction in small check tests. Harrison et al.[40] also found a significant correlation between an abnormal PVEP latency and a color vision deficit.

During serial recordings, a very poor correspondence is reported between the changes in EP and the variation in overall clinical disability, as well as among EP modalities.[41, 42]

Several studies compared the sensitivity of multimodal EP with magnetic resonance imaging (MRI) and cerebrospinal fluid (CSF) analysis in MS. Giesser et al.[43] state that combined EP testing had a higher sensitivity than MRI in confirming the diagnosis of ME, but five other studies found MRI to be more sensitive than EP or CSF analysis.[44-48] The inclusion criteria for the study as well as the methods and criteria for the investigations may have influenced these results. It is clear, however, that using high and low spatial frequencies in PVEP testing results in a higher detection rate.[46]

A rise of temperature is known to lead to increase of symptoms in MS, but the hot bath test does not give additional information in PVEP testing.[49, 50]

Abnormal VEP have predictive value for the diagnosis of definite MS, when clinical doubt exists.[51, 52] Bøttcher and Trojaborg[53] noted a shift in clinical diagnosis to the definite group in patients who had initially shown abnormal EP.[53]

ANTERIOR VISUAL PATHWAY LESIONS

The PVEP is useful in detecting anterior visual pathway compression by pituitary tumors.[54, 55] The most important disturbance is a reduced response over the hemisphere ipsilateral to the visual field defect. Because amplitude asymmetry to full-field stimulation is often found in normal humans, inclusion of half-field stimulation is important.[54, 55-58] However, amplitude differences are also present after left- and right-hemifield stimulation, with greater responses over the ipsilateral hemisphere after right-hemifield stimulation, and with marked differences between transient and steady-state VEPs. This probably reflects activities of different populations of cortical neurons.[59, 60] This is compatible with neuroanatomic asymmetries of the striate cortex.

In temporal arteritis, PVEP amplitude and latency abnormalities that returned to normal after treatment have been reported.[61] Hannerz et al.[62] recorded PVEP in patients with orbital phlebopathy; among 12 patients with visual dysfunction, only two showed markedly prolonged latencies and four reduced amplitudes, suggesting a predominantly axonal degeneration. A number of abnormal VEP patterns may be found in anterior ischemic optic neuropathy, correlating with the type of visual field defect. It is therefore only possible to detect these with multichannel recordings and different types of visual field stimulation. No significant changes were observed in time, indicating no significant recovery.[63]

In amblyopia, abnormal PVEP amplitudes and increased latencies are well known.[64-66] Teping et al.[66] observed that amblyopic eyes lack pattern selectivity;

peak latency delay and amplitude reductions were only prominent when checks smaller than 40 min. of arc were used, and not with large checks. Srebro[67] noted that PVEP were nearly five times as large in eccentrically fixating amblyopic eyes as in centrally fixating eyes, in comparison with the fellow, nonamblyopic eye. The two groups of amblyopes had comparably poor visual acuity. Moschos et al. [68] noted more delayed PVEP in amblyopic eyes with eccentric fixation as compared with central fixation, but they did not report the amplitudes, and moreover there were remarkable differences in visual acuity between the two groups tested.

RETROCHIASMAL LESIONS

Only when there is a marked visual field defect does the PVEP seem useful in the diagnosis of retrochiasmal visual pathway lesions. Blumhardt et al.[69, 70] in particular found an amplitude asymmetry more pronounced after hemifield stimulation, even in patients without a visual field defect. Holder[71] noted definitely abnormal VEP in only 55% of his patients.

In patients suffering from transient ischemic attacks, Thorwirth et al.[72] found only amplitude differences between the two hemispheres. Verma et al.[73] investigated PVEP in a group of patients with stroke, comparing them with age-matched controls. The mean interocular P100 latency difference was greater in the stroke group. The same was true of the left-right amplitude ratio difference.

EXTRAPYRAMIDAL DISORDERS

Parkinson's Disease

Bodis-Wollner and Yahr[74] found a delay of the PVEP P100 in Parkinson's disease (PD). This was confirmed by others, using sine-wave gratings[75] or checkerboard stimuli.[75, 76] The PVEP latencies have been reported to become normal after levodopa treatment and to correlate with the severity of the disease.[77] Some others observed normal PVEP[78, 79]; this was presumably due to the low spatial frequency that they used, as Tartaglione et al.[80] have demonstrated that the delay of the transient VEP depends on the spatial frequency used. The VEP abnormalities became most evident with spatial frequencies greater than 2 cycles per degree. Using spatial frequencies of 2 to 3 cycles per degree, Marx et al.[81] tested several input modulation frequencies. They found that more abnormalities became evident with a frequency of 4.19 Hz rather than with 8.41 or 1 Hz. Transient VEP latency alterations showed no correlation with age or PD duration.

Skrandies and Gottlob[82] noted a general reduction in contrast sensitivity in patients with PD. Herishanu et al.[83] stated that significantly higher contrast thresholds for patients with PD are more important than the spatial frequency for the differences in VEP latency in comparison with controls. Review of their data showed that when spatial frequencies of 4.6 and 16 cycles per degree were used, the P100 latencies were most pronounced (but not statistically significant) at 6 cycles per degree, whatever contrast level was used. It is also clear that their spatial frequencies were all higher than the lower limit described by Tartaglione et al.[80] Gottlob et al.[84] confirmed the PVEP latency increase in PD for patterns of high contrast only, but they used a reversal frequency of 2 Hz and a larger checkerboard size than Tartaglione et al.[80]

Huntington's Disease

Significant reduction of the amplitude of PVEP is mentioned in several studies of patients with Huntington's disease.[85, 86] Peak latencies were normal except in the study of Ehle et al.[87] Hennerici et al.[88] noted an absence of asymmetric hemisphere lateralization to half-field pattern stimulation and large amplitude distortion of the VEP complex in patients and their offspring.

MISCELLANEOUS DISORDERS

Ataxia

In most patients with Friedreich's ataxia (FA), PVEP amplitudes are normal or mildly decreased, whereas 65% to 75% have increased latencies.[89–94] By measuring the N75-P100 interval, an increase of temporal dispersion was seen.[90, 94] There is a good correlation between VEP anomalies and clinical visual disturbances, especially visual acuity.[95] In the visual system of patients with FA, nerve fiber depletion, cell loss, and paranodal degeneration have been reported.

Increased latencies are uncommon, but low-amplitude or absent VEP have been reported in ataxia telangiectasia,[93–96] which is probably caused by axonal loss. In late-onset ataxia, Nousiainen et al.[97] reported a 40% rate of PVEP disturbances, especially increased latency. The patients with the most delayed responses had markedly reduced amplitudes. Abnormal PVEP were also observed in patients with spastic ataxia; some had increased latencies,[92] others had reduced amplitudes with normal latencies.[95–98] Patients with vitamin E deficiency due to cystic fibrosis may develop spinocerebellar degeneration. Ten patients were examined by Kaplan et al.[99]; three had altered vision whereas only two of them had increased

P100 latencies. Messenheimer et al.[100] found similar results. The abnormalities decreased during vitamin E supplementation.

Dementia

In senile dementia of the Alzheimer type, an increase in latency of the late PVEP components has been observed. The P100 latencies, however, did not distinguish these patients from other groups of patients studied by Visser et al.[101] Several studies reported significant differences between normal subjects and patients with dementia in the major positive peak latency of the Flash-Vep (FVEP).[102-104]

Kidney Failure

The PVEP were studied in patients following kidney transplantation; 10 weeks after the transplantation, P100 latencies were significantly shortened. The P100 latency increased significantly with increasing spatial frequency before and after transplantation.[105]

Phenylketonuria

In phenylketonuric children, PVEP correlated well with metabolic control; 5 of 8 children that started after 2 months of age with a low phenylalanine diet, as well as only 1 of the 6 with an early dietary regimen and 6 of 9 with high mean phenylalanine plasma levels (during 1 year), showed abnormal responses, whereas all children with good metabolic control had normal responses.[106] In phenylketonuria, anomalous metabolism of neurotransmitters, as well as incomplete myelination, is described[107, 108]; both can be responsible for the presented PVEP abnormalities.

Macroglobulinemia

Barbieri et al.[109] studied PVEP in patients with neuropathy and macroglobulinemia. The P100 was increased bilaterally in 5 of the 6 patients whose IgM M-proteins reacted with myelin-associated glycoprotein; intraneural injection of serum containing anti–myelin-associated glycoprotein M-protein induced focal demyelination.[110] It is also interesting that only 1 of the 5 patients with IgM that did not bind to myelin-associated glycoprotein had an abnormal PVEP.

REFERENCES

1. Hubel DM, Wiesel TN: Receptive fields of single neurons in the cat's striate cortex. *J Physiol* 1959; 148:574–591.

2. Halliday AM, McDonald WI, Mushin J: Delayed visual evoked responses in optic neuritis. *Lancet* 1972; 1:982–985.

3. Arden GB, Bodis-Wollner I, Halliday AM, et al: Methodology of patterned visual stimulation, in Desmedt JE (ed): *Visual Evoked Potentials in Man: New Developments.* Oxford, England, Clarendon Press, 1977, pp 3–15.

4. Maffei L: Electroretinographic and visual cortical potentials in response to alternating gratings. *Ann NY Acad Sci* 1982; 388:1–10.

5. Lennerstrand G: Delayed visual evoked cortical potentials in retinal disease. *Acta Ophthalmol* 1982; 60:497–504.

6. Bodis-Wollner I, Feldman R: Old perimacular pathology causes VEP delays in man. *Electroencephalogr Clin Neurophysiol* 1982; 53:38–39P.

7. Bodis-Wollner I, Feldman RG, Guillory SL, et al: Delayed visual evoked potentials are independent of pattern orientation in macular disease. *Electroencephalogr Clin Neurophysiol* 1987; 68:172–179.

8. Celesia GG, Kaufman D: Pattern ERGs and visual evoked potentials in maculopathies and optic nerve diseases. *Invest Ophthalmol Vis Sci* 1985; 26:726–735.

9. Papakostopoulos D, Hart CD, Cooper R, et al: Combined electrophysiological assessment of the visual system in central serous retinopathy. *Electroencephalogr Clin Neurophysiol* 1984; 59:77–80.

10. Folk JC, Thompson HS, Han DP, et al: Visual function abnormalities in central serous retinopathy. *Arch Ophthalmol* 1984; 102:1299–1302.

11. Bass SJ, Sherman J, Bodis-Wollner I, et al: Visual evoked potentials in macular disease. *Invest Ophthalmol Vis Sci* 1985; 26:1071–1074.

12. Johnson LN, Yee RD, Hepler RS, et al: Alteration of the visual evoked potential by macular holes: Comparison with optic neuritis. *Graefes Arch Clin Exp Ophthalmol* 1987; 225:123–128.

13. Wijngaarde R, van Lith GHM: Electrodiagnostics of the tilted disc syndrome. *Doc Ophthalmol* 1981; 50:697–706.

14. Bass SJ, Sherman J: Visual evoked potential (VEP) delays in tilted and/or oblique entrance of the optic nerve head. *Neuro Ophthalmology* 1988; 8:109–122.

15. Brudet-Wickel CLM, van Lith GHM, Graniewski-Wijnands HS: Drusen of the optic disc and occipital transient pattern reversal responses. *Doc Ophthalmol* 1981; 50:243–248.

16. Mustonen E, Sulg I, Kallanranta T: Electroretinogram (ERG) and visual evoked response (VEP) studies in patients with optic disc drusen. *Acta Ophthalmol* 1980; 58:539–549.

17. Huber C, Wagner T: Electrophysiological evidence for glaucomatous lesions in the optic nerve. *Ophthalmol Res* 1978; 10:22–29.

18. Towle VL, Moskowitz A, Sokol S, et al: The visual evoked potential in glaucoma and ocular hypertension: Effects of check size, field size, and stimulation rate. *Invest Ophthalmol Vis Sci* 1983; 24:175–183.

19. Papst N, Bopp M, Schnaudigel OE: Pattern electroretinogram and visual evoked cortical potentials in glaucoma. *Graefes Arch Clin Exp Ophthalmol* 1984; 222:29–33.

20. Rouland JF, Hache JC: Les potentiels évoqués visuels dans le glaucome et l'hypertension oculaire. *J Fr Ophtalmol* 1987; 10:225–232.

21. Good PA, Marsters JB, Mortimer MJ: Flash stimulation evoked potentials in diagnosis of chronic glaucoma. *Lancet* 1987; 1:1259–1260.

22. Franchi A, Magni R, Lodigiani L, et al: VEP pattern after photostress: An index of macular function. *Graefes Arch Clin Exp Ophthalmol* 1987; 225:291–294.

23. Barnet AB, Friedman SL, Weiss IP, et al: VEP development in infancy and early childhood: A longitudinal study. *Electroencephalogr Clin Neurophysiol* 1980; 49:476–489.

24. Celesia GC, Daly RF: Effects of aging on visual evoked responses. *Arch Neurol* 1979; 34:403–407.

25. Ellingson RJ: Variability of visual evoked responses in the human newborn. *Electroencephalogr Clin Neurophysiol* 1970; 29:10–19.

26. Watanabe K, Iwase K, Hara K: Maturation of visual evoked responses in low-birthweight infants. *Dev Med Child Neurol* 1972; 14:425–435.

27. Hrbek A, Mareš P: Cortical evoked responses to visual stimulation in full-term and premature newborns. *Electroencephalogr Clin Neurophysiol* 1964; 16:575–581.

28. Taylor MJ, Menzies R, MacMillan LJ, et al: VEPs in normal full-term and premature neonates: Longitudinal versus cross-sectional data. *Electroencephalogr Clin Neurophysiol* 1987; 68:20–27.

29. Hakamada S, Watanabe K, Hara K, et al: The evolution of visual and auditory evoked potentials in infants with perinatal disorders. *Brain Dev* 1981; 3:339–344.

30. Placzek M, Mushin J, Dubowitz LMS: Maturation of the visual evoked response and its correlation with visual acuity in preterm infants. *J Dev Med Child Neurol* 1985; 27:448–454.

31. Norcia AM, Tyler CW, Piecuch R, et al: Visual acuity development in normal and abnormal preterm human infants. *J Pediatr Ophthalmol Strabismus* 1987; 24:70–74.

32. Halliday AM, McDonald WI, Mushin J: Visual evoked response in diagnosis of multiple sclerosis. *Br Med J* 1973; 4:661–664.

33. Lowitzsch K: Visuell evozierte Potentiale (VEP) bei der Multiplen Sklerose. *Aktuele Neurol* 1982; 9:170–174.

34. Regan D, Silver R, Murray TJ: Visual acuity and contrast sensitivity in multiple sclerosis: Hidden visual loss. *Brain* 1977; 100:563–579.

35. Bodis-Wollner I, Hendly CD, Mylin LH, et al: Visual evoked potentials and the visuogram in multiple sclerosis. *Ann Neurol* 1979; 5:40–47.

36. Neima D, Regan D: Pattern visual evoked potentials and spatial vision in retrobulbar neuritis and multiple sclerosis. *Arch Neurol* 1984; 41:198–201.

37. Camissa J, Mylin LH, Bodis-Wollner I: The effect of stimulus orientation on the visual evoked potential in multiple sclerosis. *Ann Neurol* 1981; 10:532–539.

38. Coupland SG, Kirkham TH: Orientation-specific visual evoked potential deficits in multiple sclerosis. *Can J Neurol Sci* 1982; 9:331–337.

39. Sanders EACM, Volkers ACW, van der Poel JC, et al: Visual function and pattern visual evoked response in optic neuritis. *Br J Ophthalmol* 1987; 71:602–608.

40. Harrison AC, Becker WJ, Stell WK: Colour vision abnormalities in multiple sclerosis. *Can J Neurol Sci* 1987; 14:279–285.

41. De Weerd AW: Variability of central conduction in the course of multiple sclerosis: Serial recordings of evoked potentials in the evaluation of therapy. *Clin Neurol Neurosurg* 1987; 89:9–15.

42. Anderson DC, Slater GE, Sherman R, et al: Evoked potentials to test a treatment of chronic multiple sclerosis. *Arch Neurol* 1987; 44:1232–1236.

43. Giesser BS, Kurtzberg D, Vaughan HG, et al: Trimodal evoked potentials compared with magnetic resonance imaging in the diagnosis of multiple sclerosis. *Arch Neurol* 1987; 44:281–284.

44. Farlow MR, Markand ON, Edwards MK, et al: Multiple sclerosis: Magnetic resonance imaging, evoked responses, and spinal fluid electrophoresis. *Neurology* 1986; 36:828–831.

45. Kirschner HS, Tsai SI, Runge VM, et al: Magnetic resonance imaging and other techniques in the diagnosis of multiple sclerosis. *Arch Neurol* 1985; 42:859–863.

46. Guérit JM, Monje Argiles A: The sensitivity of multimodal evoked potentials in multiple sclerosis: A comparison with magnetic resonance imaging and cerebrospinal fluid analysis. *Electroencephalogr Clin Neurophysiol* 1988; 70:230–238.

47. Cutler JR, Aminoff MJ, Brant-Zawadzki M: Evaluation of patients with multiple sclerosis by evoked potentials and magnetic resonance imaging: A comparative study. *Ann Neurol* 1986; 20:645–648.

48. Gebarski SS, Gabrielsen TO, Gilman S, et al: The initial diagnosis of multiple sclerosis: Clinical impact of magnetic resonance imaging. *Ann Neurol* 1985; 17:469–474.

49. Matthews WB, Read DJ, Pountney E: Effect of raising body temperature on visual and somatosensory evoked potentials in patients with multiple sclerosis. *J Neurol Neurosurg Psychiatry* 1979; 42:250–255.

50. Rolak LA, Ashizawa T: The hot bath test in multiple sclerosis: Comparison with visual evoked responses and oligoclonal bands. *Acta Neurol Scand* 1985; 72:65–67.

51. Matthews WB, Wattam-Bell JRB, Pountney E: Evoked potentials in the diagnosis of multiple sclerosis: A follow up study. *J Neurol Neurosurg Psychiatry* 1982; 45:303–307.

52. Hamburger HA, Leutcher WM, Thompson R: Visual evoked potentials in the diagnosis of multiple sclerosis. *Ann Ophthalmol* 1984; 16:752–755.

53. Bøttcher J, Trojaborg W: Follow-up of patients with suspected multiple sclerosis: A clinical and electrophysiological study. *J Neurol Neurosurg Psychiatry* 1982; 45:809–814.

54. Halliday AM, Halliday F, Kriss A, et al: The pattern-evoked potential in compression of the anterior visual pathways. *Brain* 1976; 99:357–374.

55. Camacho LM, Wenzel W, Aschoff J: Klinische Anwendung der visuell evozierten Potentialen zur Untersuchung von chiasmatischen und post-chiasmatischen Läsionen. *Arch Psychiatr Nervenkr* 1981; 230:243–256.

56. Rowe MJ: The clinical utility of half-field pattern-reversal visual evoked potential testing. *Electroencephalogr Clin Neurophysiol* 1982; 53:73–77.

57. Holder GE: The effects of chiasmal compression of the pattern visual evoked potential. *Electroencephalogr Clin Neurophysiol* 1978; 45:278–280.

58. Staudacher T, Reuther R, Rittmann M, et al: Die Wertigkeit der visuell evozierten Potentiale (VEP) bei Kompression der vorderen Sehbahn, speziell in der Chiasmaregion. *Nervenarzt* 1985; 56:560–561.

59. Kuroiwa Y, Celesia GG, Toghi H: Amplitude difference between pattern-evoked potentials after left and right hemifield stimulation in normal subjects. *Neurology* 1987; 37:795–799.

60. Milner BA, Regan D, Heron JR: Theoretical models of the generation of steady-state evoked potentials, their relation to neuroanatomy and their relevance to certain clinical problems, in Arden GB (ed): *The Visual System: Neurophysiology, Biophysics and Their Clinical Application.* New York, Plenum Publishing Corp, 1971, pp 157–169.

61. Hamburger HA, Beckman H, Thompson R: Visual evoked potentials as an aid in the diagnosis and treatment of temporal arteritis. *Ann Ophthalmol* 1984; 16:330–332.

62. Hannerz J, Persson HE, Wanger P: Optic nerve involvement in patients with orbital phlebopathy: Pattern-reversal electroretinograms and visual evoked cortical potentials. *Neuro Ophthalmology* 1988; 8:151–159.

63. Thompson PD, Mastaglia FL, Carroll WM: Anterior ischaemic optic neuropathy: A correlative clinical and visual evoked potential study of 18 patients. *J Neurol Neurosurg Psychiatry* 1986; 49:128–135.

64. Arden GB, Barnard WM, Mushin J: Visual evoked responses in amblyopia. *Br J Ophthalmol* 1974; 58:183–192.

65. Wanger P, Persson HE: Visual evoked responses to pattern-reversal stimulation in childhood amblyopia. *Acta Ophthalmol* 1980; 58:697–706.

66. Teping C, Kau T, Vomberg E, et al: VECP-Befunde bei amblyopen Kindern. *Fortschr Ophthalmol* 1987; 84:283–286.

67. Srebro R: Visually evoked potentials in eccentrically and centrally fixing amblyopes. *Br J Ophthalmol* 1984; 68:468–471.

68. Moschos M, Iliakis E, Theodosiadis G: VER changes in amblyopia. *Fortschr Ophthalmol* 1987; 84:280–282.

69. Blumhardt LD, Halliday AM: Cortical abnormalities and the visual evoked response. *Doc Ophthalmol Proc Ser* 1981; 27:347–365.

70. Blumhardt LD, Barrett G, Kriss A, et al: The pattern-evoked potential in lesions of the posterior visual pathways. *Ann NY Acad Sci* 1982; 388:264–289.

71. Holder GE: Pattern visual evoked potential in patients with posteriorly situated space-occupying lesions. *Doc Ophthalmol* 1985; 59:121–128.

72. Thorwirth VV, Volles E, Lossi C, et al: Auditorisch evozierte Hirnstammpotentiale, visuell musterevozierte und somatosensibel evozierte Potentiale bei transitorisch ischämischen Attacken (TIA). *Schweiz Arch Neurol Neurochir Psychiatr* 1983; 132:41–54.

73. Verma NP, Kooi KA, Gilroy J: Monocular pattern-shift visual evoked potentials in hemispheric strokes. *Electroencephalogr Clin Neurophysiol* 1984; 58:205–210.

74. Bodis-Wollner I, Yahr MD: Measurements of visual evoked potentials in Parkinson's disease. *Brain* 1978; 101:661–671.

75. Bodis-Wollner I, Yahr MD, Thorton J: Visual evoked responses and the severity of Parkinson's disease, in Clifford RF, Calpideo R (eds): *Progress in Parkinson's Disease*. New York, Pitman Medical, 1981, pp 126–137.

76. Gawel MJ, Das P, Vincent S, et al: Visual and auditory evoked responses in patients with Parkinson's disease. *J Neurol Neurosurg Psychiatry* 1981; 44:227–232.

77. Bodis-Wollner I, Yahr MD, Mylin L, et al: Dopaminergic deficiency and delayed visual evoked potentials in humans. *Ann Neurol* 1982; 11:478–483.

78. Ehle AL, Stewart RM, Lellelid NE, et al: Normal checkerboard pattern reversal evoked potentials in parkinsonism. *Electroencephalogr Clin Neurophysiol* 1982; 54:336–338.

79. Hansch EC, Syndulko K, Cohen SN, et al: Cognition in Parkinson's disease: An event-related potential perspective. *Ann Neurol* 1982; 11:599–607.

80. Tartaglione A, Pizio N, Bino G, et al: VEP changes in Parkinson's disease are stimulus dependent. *J Neurol Neurosurg Psychiatry* 1984; 47:305–307.

81. Marx M, Bodis-Wollner I, Bobak P, et al: Temporal frequency-dependent VEP changes in Parkinson's disease. *Vision Res* 1986; 26:185–193.

82. Skrandies W, Gottlob I: Alterations of visual contrast sensitivity in Parkinson's disease. *Hum Neurobiol* 1986; 5:255–259.

83. Herishanu YO, Louzoun Z, Garlik T: Contrast grating sensitivity and visual evoked potentials in parkinsonian patients. *Neuro Ophthalmology* 1986; 6:43–48.

84. Gottlob I, Schneider E, Heider W, et al: Alteration of visual evoked potentials and electroretinograms in Parkinson's disease. *Electroencephalogr Clin Neurophysiol* 1987; 66:349–357.

85. Oepen G, Doerr M, Thoden U: Visual (VEP) and somatosensory (SSEP) evoked potentials in Huntington's chorea. *Electroencephalogr Clin Neurophysiol* 1981; 51:666–670.

86. Josiassen RC, Shagass C, Mancall EL, et al: Auditory and visual evoked potentials in Huntington's disease. *Electroencephalogr Clin Neurophysiol* 1984; 57:113–118.

87. Ehle AL, Stewart RM, Lellelid NA, et al: Evoked potentials in Huntington's disease. *Arch Neurol* 1984; 41:379–382.

88. Hennerici M, Hömberg V, Lange HW: Evoked potentials in patients with Huntington's disease

and their offspring: II. Visual evoked potentials. *Electroencephalogr Clin Neurophysiol* 1985; 62:167–176.

89. Carroll WM, Kriss A, Baraitser M, et al: The incidence and nature of visual pathway involvement in Friedreich's ataxia: A clinical and visual evoked potential study of 22 patients. *Brain* 1980; 103:411–434.

90. Livingstone IR, Mastaglia FL, Edis R, et al: Visual involvement in Friedreich's ataxia and hereditary spastic ataxia. *Arch Neurol* 1981; 38:75–79.

91. Nuwer MR, Perlman SL, Packwood JW, et al: Evoked potential abnormalities in the various inherited ataxias. *Ann Neurol* 1983; 13:20–27.

92. Ghezzi A, Montanini R: Comparative study of visual evoked potentials in spinocerebellar ataxias and multiple sclerosis. *Acta Neurol Scand* 1985; 71:252–256.

93. Taylor MJ, Chan-Lui WY, Logan WJ: Longitudinal evoked potential studies in hereditary ataxias. *Can J Neurol Sci* 1985; 12:100–105.

94. Pinto F, Amantini A, Scisciolo G, et al: Visual involvement in Friedreich's ataxia: PERG and VEP study. *Eur Neurol* 1988; 28:246–251.

95. Sridharan R: Visual evoked potentials in spinocerebellar degenerations. *Clin Neurol Neurosurg* 1983; 85:235–243.

96. Taylor MJ, Logan WJ: Multimodal electrophysiological assessment of ataxia telangiectasia. *Can J Neurol Sci* 1983; 10:261–265.

97. Nousiainen U, Partanen J, Laulumaa V, et al: Involvement of somatosensory and visual pathways in late onset ataxia. *Electroencephalogr Clin Neurophysiol* 1987; 67:514–520.

98. Livingstone IR, Mastaglia FL, Edis R, et al: Pattern visual evoked responses in hereditary spastic paraplegia. *J Neurol Neurosurg Psychiatry* 1981; 44:176–178.

99. Kaplan PW, Rawal K, Erwin CW, et al: Visual and somatosensory evoked potentials in vitamin E deficiency with cystic fibrosis. *Electroencephalogr Clin Neurophysiol* 1988; 71:266–272.

100. Messenheimer JA, Greenwood RS, Tennison MB, et al: Reversible visual evoked potential abnormalities in vitamin E deficiency. *Ann Neurol* 1984; 15:499–506.

101. Visser SL, van Tilburg W, Hooijer C, et al: Visual evoked potentials (VEPs) in senile dementia (Alzheimer type) and in non-organic behavioural disorders in the elderly: Comparison with EEG parameters. *Electroencephalogr Clin Neurophysiol* 1985; 60:115–121.

102. Visser SL, Stam FC, van Tilburg W, et al: Visual evoked response in senile and presenile dementia. *Electroencephalogr Clin Neurophysiol* 1976; 40:385–392.

103. Harding GFA, Doggett CE, Orwin A, et al: Visual evoked potentials in presenile dementia. *Doc Ophthalmol Proc Ser* 1981; 27:193–202.

104. Wright CE, Harding GFA, Orwin A: Presenile dementia: The use of the flash and pattern VEP in diagnosis. *Electroencephalogr Clin Neurophysiol* 1984; 57:405–415.

105. Brown JJ, Sufit RL, Sollinger HW: Visual evoked potential changes following renal transplantation. *Electroencephalogr Clin Neurophysiol* 1987; 66:101–107.

106. Landi A, Ducati A, Villani R, et al: Pattern-reversal visual evoked potentials in phenylketonuric children. *Child Nerv Syst* 1987; 3:278–281.

107. McKean CM: The effects of high phenylalanine concentrations on serotonin and catecholamine metabolism in the human brain. *Brain Res* 1972; 4:469–476.

108. Shah SN, Peterson A, McKean CM: Lipid composition of human cerebral white matter and myelin in PKU. *J Neurochem* 1972; 19:2369–2376.

109. Barbieri S, Nobile-Orazio E, Baldini L, et al: Visual evoked potentials in patients with neuropathy and macroglobulinemia. *Ann Neurol* 1987; 22:663–666.

110. Hays AP, Latov N, Takatsu M, et al: Experimental demyelination of nerve induced by serum of patients with neuropathy and an anti-MAG IgM M-protein. *Neurology* 1987; 37:242–256.

CHAPTER 20

Orbital Computed Tomography

Martin L. Leib, M.D.

Director, Orbit and Ophthalmic Plastic Surgery Service, The Edward S. Harkness Eye Institute, Columbia-Presbyterian Medical Center; Assistant Professor of Clinical Ophthalmology, Columbia University College of Physicians and Surgeons, New York, New York

Mandes R. Kates, Ph.D., M.D.

Clinical Assistant, Manhattan Eye, Ear, and Throat Hospital, New York, New York

Computed tomography (CT) is a mainstay of diagnostic imaging of the orbit and is indispensible to the orbital specialist. It is clearly the most cost-effective method for investigating orbital disease, even in comparison with magnetic resonance imaging (MRI). The quantity of information and the variety of clinical applications of CT are enormous, especially when viewed in relation to the relatively low cost, the ready availability, and the relatively short time required for most studies. Only with increased sensitivity of surface receiver coils and reduced scanning time can MRI approach CT in clinical efficacy.

The technology of CT scanning has not changed significantly over the past 2 years. Rather, advances have been made in the utilization of third- and fourth-generation scanners to maximize the information obtained. In addition, our growing experience with pathologic correlation of CT findings is permitting even more precise diagnosis.

The most dramatic advances have come in our understanding of orbital trauma.

Curr Neuro Ophthalmol 2:363–372, 1989
© 1989, Year Book Medical Publishers, Inc.
0893–0147/89/02-363-372-$04.00

Computed tomography has not only allowed more accurate diagnosis of orbital injuries; it has played a vital role in our understanding of the pathophysiologic mechanisms involved by enhancing our appreciation of the local anatomy. Significant strides have also been made in the diagnosis of a variety of ocular motility disorders, including, of course, Graves' disease but also a number of inflammatory conditions affecting the extraocular muscles.

To exploit the power of CT fully requires, at a minimum, precise positioning of the patient with the head oriented appropriately for the condition at hand. Also, more than ever before, the results depend on the skill and knowledge of the radiologist.

TECHNIQUE

For a number of years, efforts have been under way to accurately measure the volumes of the orbit itself and its various tissues.[1, 2] The most recent of these efforts is that of Manson and co-workers.[3] Theirs might be called the "region of interests" method. The investigator outlines a region of interest in the CT image with an electronic stylus; a computer then computes the area of this region and determines the volume by multiplying by the slice thickness. In this manner the authors determined the soft-tissue orbital volume, the bony orbital volume, the retrobulbar volume, the fat volume, and the globe volume. The accuracy of volume measurements reported for phantoms of known volumes approached 98%. Orbital volumes were also determined by alternative methods, and in relation to these measurements the region of interest method also is reportedly 98% accurate. Diametric measurements were used to analyze a series of trauma cases.

Considerable attention has been paid to the importance of proper patient positioning for orbital CT. The coronal scan is frequently the most important position, especially in trauma cases. However, the parasagittal plane, which is not new to orbital imaging,[1] is becoming more popular.[4–6] Koornneff and Zonneveld[4, 6] routinely use the sagittal scan plane for injuries involving the orbital floor and orbital roof. This plane is most valuable in assessing pathology of the inferior rectus, superior rectus, and levator palpebrae muscles. A variation of this technique, the direct oblique sagittal scan, has been introduced by Ball.[5] This plane is approximately perpendicular to the orbital floor, which normally slopes inferiorly going from medial to lateral. Both of these groups emphasize that the sagittal plane complements, but does not replace, the direct coronal image. Furthermore, there is a growing preference expressed by both of these groups for use of the direct coronal imaging technique, rather than reformatting. Reformatting should probably be limited to situations where patient positioning is a problem, for the best reformation images are inferior to those obtained by the direct techniques.[7]

Mafee and co-workers[8] have continued to advocate dynamic CT as applied to the orbital region. This is a technique that is analogous to angiography and is used to determine the vascularity of a lesion. In brief, a rapid sequence of scans of a previously identified lesion are obtained immediately following the intravenous injection of contrast material. The radiodensity of the lesion in Hounsfield units is then measured as a function of time over the 30 to 40 seconds following the injection. The rate of increase, the maximum, and the rate of decrease in this radiodensity are characteristic for different types of lesions. The great advantage of this method is that it is much safer than angiography. The classic use of dynamic CT in the orbit is to distinguish between the highly vascular capillary hemangioma and the poorly vascular cavernous hemangioma.

ANATOMIC STUDIES

The most important anatomic development in the orbit has been the investigations, led by Koornneff and Zonneveld, into the structure and function of the connective tissue system of the orbit. The findings of these investigations, which have been ongoing throughout the 1980s, have been reviewed.[4] More recently, with "state-of-the art" CT, it has been possible to generate images of this connective tissue system in normal and pathologic situations,[4, 9] particularly in the coronal plane. With extremely high-quality imaging technique it is possible to visualize the connective tissue septa that interconnect the extraocular muscles with each other, with the globe, and with the periorbita.

Considerable attention has also been given to the normal anatomy of the extraocular muscles as revealed by CT scanning. Miller and Mafee[10] and Haik et al.[11] have reviewed the techniques and findings of CT scanning of the extraocular muscles. Both groups have reviewed the optimal scanning technique and patient positioning for viewing the extraocular muscles. They recommend taking 1.5-mm sections at 2- to 4-mm intervals. Direct coronal imaging is preferred in virtually all cases, supplemented by axial or sagittal views, depending on which muscle or muscles are being investigated. The normal anatomy of all of the extraocular muscles was reviewed.

NON-NEOPLASTIC PROCESSES

Idiopathic Inflammations

Our understanding of idiopathic orbital inflammatory disease, formerly referred to as pseudotumor, is the result of CT. Specifically, it is now well known that most orbital inflammations are not generalized but are limited to one or more specific orbital tissues as noted in our previous review.[1] Computed tomography has revealed no fewer than six variations of orbital inflammation: myositis, perineuritis, dacryoadenitis, scleritis, lymphoid hyperplasia, and trochleitis. Though no new subsets of orbital inflammation have come to light in the past 2 years, variations on the previously mentioned conditions have been discovered. For example, Lahoud and co-workers[12] have reported a case of orbital myositis confined to the inferior oblique muscle with pathologic correlation.

Frohman et al.[13] have reported three cases of biopsy-proved idiopathic orbital inflammation in which there was bone destruction. This finding, which was evident on CT scan in all three cases, is usually thought to be indicative of malignant neoplasia but apparently can also occur in severe inflammatory disease as well. Several other idiopathic, but not necessarily inflammatory, orbital conditions have been discussed in the recent literature as well. The CT findings in the extremely rare primary amyloidosis of the lacrimal gland have been reported by Levine and Buckman.[14] This lesion, for the most part, follows the contour of the surrounding normal structures, but there was some evidence of compressive changes in the orbital bone. Calcifications were also noted. These findings are suggestive but not specific for this rare condition, and CT does not distinguish it from benign mixed tumor, retinoblastoma, or meningioma.[14] A second case of biopsy-proved primary orbital amyloidosis has also been reported.[15] This was the first reported case of primary orbital amyloidosis confined to an extraocular muscle. Computed tomography showed a fusiform thickening of the left medial rectus muscle, not easily distinguishable from the muscle enlargement seen in Graves' orbitopathy. An idiopathic inflammation impinging on the orbit from without has been reported by Chen and co-workers.[16] In this one patient with an orbital apex syndrome, the cause was shown by CT to be a sphenoid sinus mucocele. Typical of mucoceles, there was bone erosion but no postcontrast enhancement.

Computed tomographic scanning has been used to give the first inkling of an understanding of a very rare benign condition called acquired hyperopia with choroidal folds. Using technically superior CT technique, Stimac et al.[17] have identified the following characteristics of this condition on CT:

1. Flattening of the posterior part of the globe.
2. Enlargement of the optic nerve and optic nerve head.
3. In some cases, a visible space between the nerve sheath and optic nerve.

These findings suggest that an accumulation of cerebrospinal fluid in the subarachnoid space of the optic nerve may play a role in the pathogenesis of this condition. Before these CT findings, we had essentially no clue as to the cause of this condition.[17-19]

Graves' Orbitopathy

The most important contribution in the area of CT scanning in Graves' disease has been that of Glatt and co-workers.[20] This group investigated the CT findings in cases of optic neuropathy in Graves' disease. They devised a simply measured numerical index based on the relative diameters of the extraocular muscles and the orbit that indicates whether a patient is at risk for optic nerve compression. The beauty of the method is that it does not require any sophisticated computer interface. The measurement can be made from either a direct or reformatted coronal image, and the measurements are done manually. The authors also discuss the value of coronal imaging in these patients and discuss situations in which the diagnosis of optic neuropathy can be made on clinical grounds and in which situations CT scanning is necessary.

Rootman and co-workers[21] performed CT scans on a series of patients who were to have excisions of Müller's muscle for lid retraction. Pathologic studies were performed on the specimens that revealed minimal morphologic involvement of Müller's muscle in these patients. However, they also noted that the presence of lid retraction was qualitatively, if not quantitatively, correlated with enlargement of the superior rectus and levator muscles demonstrated on CT scan. On the basis of these findings, they suggest that striated, not smooth muscle is implicated in the lid retraction seen in Graves' orbitopathy.

Computed tomography of the orbit has been used to follow the response to intravenous methylprednisolone therapy in patients with Graves' orbitopathy.[22] However, repeated CT scanning of patients receiving steroid therapy to follow their response is not appropriate in the routine clinical setting.

Trauma

Manson and co-workers[3] have used CT scanning to enhance our understanding of the pathogenesis of traumatic enophthalmos. As noted above, they have devised the region of interest method for measuring the volumes of the various tissue compartments in the orbit. They showed consistently that in patients with traumatic enophthalmos there was an increase in the volume of the bony orbit. In contrast, there was no consistent decrease in the volume of orbital fat. This demonstrates, at least in their series, that fat atrophy is not a cause of enophthalmos. In fact, they showed that, if anything, the soft-tissue volumes in the orbit were increased, not decreased. Furthermore, they performed the study after repair of the bony orbital defect and found that successful correction of enophthalmos was correlated with restoration of the normal bony orbital volume.

Koornneff and Zonneveld[4] have used high-resolution multiplanar CT, as noted above, to acquire a detailed understanding of the mechanisms of posttraumatic ocular motility disturbances. They have identified four possible causes of motility problems after orbital injuries:

1. Posttraumatic edema.
2. Ocular motor nerve injury.
3. Severe enophthalmos.
4. Scar tissue formation affecting the orbital connective tissue septa.

The use of CT thus has enabled them to decide intelligently whether surgical repair of an orbital injury is necessary. Thus, if enophthalmos or scar tissue is the cause of the motility problem, surgical repair may be beneficial. Furthermore, in cases with scar formation, an accurately performed CT scan can show the precise location of the pathology and thereby guide the surgical repair. They emphasize that they rarely, if ever, see actual entrapment of an extraocular muscle in a blowout fracture. Though true incarceration of a muscle may be rare, others have reported what they believe is a CT finding diagnostic of this situation. Anda et al.[23] believe that the disappearance of the inferior rectus muscle at the level of an orbital floor fracture in a coronal image is diagnostic of entrapment.

Koornneff and Zonneveld[4] also report a number of cases in which ocular motility was abnormal because of a retained intraorbital foreign body. Computed tomographic scanning was essential in diagnosing these situations and in guiding the surgical correction. Several unusual diagnoses by CT have been reported recently. Conrad and Freedman[24] report a CT scan showing complete transection of the inferior rectus muscle caused by an assailant. Mono et al.[25] report two cases of intracranial penetration via an orbital route. The clinical findings in both these cases were confusing, but CT scanning clearly showed injuries to the brain in both instances.

Vascular Disease

Johnson and co-workers[26] report a clinicopathologic study of an individual who suffered bilateral blindness after a severe hemorrhage and hypotension. Although this syndrome is well known, it is poorly understood, and this report includes the first orbital CT abnormality in this condition. The axial scan showed bilateral enlargement of the optic nerves. The pathologic correlate of this CT finding is hemorrhagic infarction of both optic nerves. The probable pathogenesis of this optic nerve infarction is discussed.

NEOPLASTIC PROCESSES

It has been long established that CT revolutionized orbital tumor diagnosis. This follows from the great variety of information that CT provides: location, size, shape, boundary characteristics, radiodensity, contrast enhancement, dynamic contrast enhancement, attachments to other intraorbital structures, the presence or absence of calcification and cystic spaces, the effect on adjacent bone (none, expansion, erosion), and the involvement of adjacent structures (such as the globe, sinuses, and cranium).[1] When this information is combined with clinical data, such as age, visual function, the degree of exophthalmos, and the natural history, it is often possible to make a diagnosis without obtaining a tissue specimen, though biopsy is often imperative.

Clearly this is not always the case, however. The most critical situation may be in the diagnosis of lacrimal gland lesions. Approximately half of all cases of lacrimal gland enlargement are epithelial tumors, and the majority of these are benign to mixed tumors. The very act of performing a biopsy on a benign mixed tumor has an adverse effect on the prognosis, since the likelihood of recurrence, even after an apparently complete excision, is increased when an incisional biopsy has been done previously. Thus, the ability to diagnose these lesions preoperatively is of the utmost importance. Mafee and Haik[27] have reviewed CT scanning of lacrimal gland lesions. They describe in great detail the characteristics of inflammatory lesions of the lacrimal gland, benign and malignant lymphoid tumors of the lacrimal gland, and benign and malignant epithelial tumors of the lacrimal gland. Epithelial tumors are less likely to be compressed by the surrounding normal tissues; rather, they displace or compress the globe, for example. In addition, enlargement of the lacrimal fossa is more common than an epithelial tumor. The benign mixed tumor is usually well encapsulated, with a smooth contour, whereas malignant tumors have irregular borders and satellite lesions. There are other benign and malignant lesions that need to be considered in the differential diagnosis of lacrimal gland enlargement. They include lacrimal gland cyst, dermoid cyst, hematic cyst, sarcoidosis, idiopathic inflammation, reactive lymphoid hyperplasia, Wegener's granulomatosis, lymphoma, and adenoid cystic carcinoma.

Benign and malignant lymphoid tumors can occur primarily in the extraocular muscles, as recently reported by Hornblass et al.[28] The clinical and CT findings in seven patients were described. In six of seven, the predominant finding was enlargement of the superior rectus and levator muscles. In some cases the two muscles were distinguishable anteriorly. In the one remaining case, the rectus muscle was predominantly involved. Tumors in five of the seven cases were shown to be benign pathologically, and in the remaining two they were malignant.

It is important to emphasize the limitations of CT in the diagnosis of orbital tumors. For the most part, these limitations are related to the resolution of CT scanning. For example, in cases of retinoblastoma, CT can delineate many features of the tumor but it does not reveal whether the tumor has spread from the eye into the optic nerve.[29] Similarly, there is a case report of a large orbital melanoma easily identified by CT; however, CT did not show the small primary choroidal melanoma.[30] The choroidal melanoma was, however, detected by ultrasonography. Finally, when the clinical findings are misleading, the interpretation of the CT scan is more difficult. For example, Harnett and co-workers[31] reported a case of an orbital mass that occurred following enucleation for a choroidal melanoma. Because of the history, this mass was thought to be a recurring melanoma. However, pathologic examination revealed that it was a cavernous hemangioma.

SUMMARY

Computed tomography remains a highly sophisticated diagnostic instrument of great speed, resolution, flexibility, availability, and cost-effectiveness; only with increased sensitivity of surface receiver coils and reduced scanning time can MRI approach CT in clinical efficacy. Nonetheless, there are several areas of orbital disease where MRI surpasses CT. Further enhancement of the resolution element and the mathematical dissection of the orbit and adenexa are still the awaited frontiers in diagnostic imaging.

REFERENCES

1. Leib M, Kates MR: Orbital computer-assisted tomography, in Lessell S, van Dalen JTW (eds): *Neuro-ophthalmology*. Chicago, Year Book Medical Publishers, 1988, vol 1, pp 323–335.
2. Leib ML, Cooper WC, Wai PM, et al: Volume determination of the orbit with high resolution CT scans and quantitative digital image analysis. *Orbit* 1982; 1:150.
3. Manson PN, Grivas A, Rosenbaum A, et al: Studies on enophthalmos: II. The measurement of orbital injuries and their treatment by quantitative computed tomography. *Plast Reconstr Surg* 1986; 77:203–214.
4. Koornneff L, Zonneveld FW: The role of direct multiplanar high resolution CT in the assessment and management of orbital trauma. *Radiol Clin North Am* 1986; 25:753–766.
5. Ball JB Jr: Direct oblique sagittal CT of orbital wall fractures. *AJR* 1987; 148:601–608.
6. Zonneveld FW, Koornneff L: Patient positioning for direct sagittal CT of the orbit parallel to the optic nerve. *Radiology* 1986; 158:547–549.
7. Leib ML: Computerized tomography of the orbits, in Halk B: Advanced Imaging Techniques in Ophthalmology. *Int Ophthalmol Clin* 1986; 26:103–121.
8. Mafee MF, Miller MT, Tan W, et al: Dynamic computed tomography and its application to ophthalmology. *Radiol Clin North Am* 1987; 25:715–731.
9. Koornneff L, Zonneveld FW: Orbital anatomy: The direct scanning of the orbit in three planes and their bearings on the treatment of motility disturbances of the eye after orbital "blow-out" fractures. *Acta Morphol Neerl Scand* 1985; 23:229–246.
10. Miller MT, Mafee MF: Computed tomography scanning in the evaluation of ocular motility disorders. *Radiol Clin North Am* 1987; 25:733–752.
11. Haik BG, Saint-Louis LA, Smith ME: Computed tomography of extraocular muscle abnormalities. *Int Ophthalmol Clin* 1986; 26:123–150.
12. Lahoud S, Brownstein S, Barsoun-Homsy M: Inferior oblique myositis presenting as superior oblique muscle palsy. *Can J Ophthalmol* 1988; 23:124–127.
13. Frohman LP, Kupersmith MJ, Lang J, et al: Intracranial extension and bone destruction in orbital pseudotumor. *Arch Ophthalmol* 1986; 104:380–384.
14. Levine MR, Buckman G: Primary localized orbital amyloidosis. *Ann Ophthalmol* 1986; 18:165–167.
15. Holmstrom GE, Nyman KG: Primary orbital amyloidosis localized to an extraocular muscle. *Br J Ophthalmol* 1987; 71:32–33.
16. Chen HJ, Kao LY, Lui CC: Mucocele of the sphenoid with the apex orbitae syndrome. *Surg Neurol* 1986; 25:101–104.
17. Stimac GK, Mills RP, Dailey RA, et al: CT of acquired hyperopia with choroidal folds. *Am J Neuroradiol* 1987; 8:1107–1111.
18. Kalina RE, Mills RP: Acquired hyperopia with choroidal folds. *Ophthalmology* 1980; 87:44–50.

19. Dailey RA, Mills RP, Stimac GKL, et al: The natural history and CT appearance of acquired hyperopia with choroidal folds. *Ophthalmology* 1986; 93:1336–1342.

20. Glatt HJ, Burde RM, Gado MH: Optic nerve dysfunction in thyroid eye disease: CT. *Radiology* 1988; 167:503–507.

21. Rootman J, Patel S, Berry K, et al: Pathological and clinical study of Müller's muscle in Graves' ophthalmopathy. *Can J Ophthalmol* 1987; 22:32–36.

22. Nagaya Y, Isumi M, Kiriyama T, et al: Treatment of Graves' ophthalmopathy with high-dose intravenous methylprednisolone pulse therapy. *Acta Endocrinol* 1987; 116:513–518.

23. Anda S, Elsas T, Harstad HK: The missing rectus: A CT observation from blow-out fracture of the orbital floor. *J Comput Assist Tomogr* 1987; 11:895–897.

24. Conrad MR, Freedman HL: Transection of orbital rectus muscle demonstrated by computed tomography. *J Comput Assist Tomogr* 1987; 11:359–360.

25. Mono J, Hollenberg RD, Harvey JT: Occult transorbital intracranial penetrating injuries. *Ann Emerg Med* 1986; 15:589–591.

26. Johnson MW, Kincaid MC, Trobe JD: Bilateral retrobulbar optic nerve infarctions after blood loss and hypotension: A clinicopathologic case study. *Ophthalmology* 1987; 94:1577–1584.

27. Mafee MF, Haik BG: Lacrimal gland and fossa lesions: Role of computed tomography. *Radiol Clin North Am* 1987; 25:767–779.

28. Hornblass A, Jakobiec FA, Reifler DM, et al: Orbital lymphoid tumors located predominately within extraocular muscles. *Ophthalmology* 1987; 94:688–697.

29. John-Mikolajewski V, Messmer E, Sauerwein W, et al: Orbital computed tomography: Does it help in diagnosing the infiltration of choroid, sclera, and/or optic nerve in retinoblastoma? *Ophthalmic Paediatr Genet* 1987; 8:101–104.

30. Rochels R, Nover A: Small choroidal melanoma with diffuse orbital involvement detected and differentiated with standardized echography: With special reference to the reliability of sonography in predicting scleral tumoral infiltration. *Ophthalmologica* 1986; 192:39–45.

31. Harnett AN, Thorpe P, Hungerford J: Cavernous haemangioma presenting as an orbital mass after enucleation for a choroidal melanoma: Case report. *Br J Ophthalmol* 1988; 72:618–620.

CHAPTER 21

Neuroradiology

Jin S. Leo, M.D.

Professor of Radiology, Texas Tech University Health Sciences Center, Lubbock, Texas

J. T. W. Van Dalen, M.D., Ph.D.

Associate Professor of Ophthalmology, The University of Arizona Health Sciences Center, Tucson, Arizona

Joel S. Dunnington, M.D.

Assistant Professor of Radiology, Department of Radiology, Texas Tech University Health Sciences Center, Lubbock, Texas

The clinical application of magnetic resonance imaging (MRI) in neurologic disorders has almost reached maturity. The recent development and guidelines for MRI in clinical practice will be discussed. We will also review some important issues in this chapter, including the current role of computed tomography (CT) in neuroophthalmology, low osmolality contrast for CT, and duplex sonography—a highly accurate, noninvasive method for evaluating patients with vascular occlusive disease.

OPTIC NERVE

CT has been the primary imaging test in orbital disorders. MRI is now being applied to diseases of the orbit. The advantages of CT are more rapid scan times, thinner sections, and higher spatial resolution. CT, at the present time, is superior to MRI in the evaluation of small optic meningiomas. Relative insensitivity to calcifications, as well as motion and chemical shift artifacts, may limit the ability of MRI to delineate these lesions. Orbital MRI may be most useful, providing information not available on CT, in (1) identifying lesions in the orbital apex and optic canal, (2) defining the posterior extents of optic pathway gliomas, and (3) characterizing lesions containing hemorrhage or other paramagnetic material.[1] The ability to obtain images easily in three orthogonal planes is a distinct advantage of MRI. The relationship between CT and MRI is still evolving.

MRI is highly sensitive in detecting lesions in the brain in patients with multiple sclerosis (MS). Brain lesions on MRI similar to those of MS are found in 50% to 70% of adult patients with idiopathic isolated optic neuritis.[2, 3] A majority of this group of patients will eventually progress to MS.[4] Initial efforts to detect optic neuritis with MRI were unsuccessful. The major problem with the commonly used T_1- and T_2-weighted spin-echo sequences is chemical shift artifacts between optic nerve and orbital fat, preventing a clear image of the optic nerve. This problem is largely overcome by using a short time inversion recovery (STIR) sequence; which suppresses the orbital fat signal and reduces chemical shift artifacts. Miller et al. performed MRI of the optic nerve using STIR in 37 adult patients with recent or past attacks of optic neuritis.[5] MRI revealed high-signal lesions in 84% of symptomatic and 20% of asymptomatic nerves. Slow or poor visual recovery was associated with more extensive lesions, or lesions within the optic canal. They recorded no false positive results in 15 normal subjects whose MRI images with STIR sequence were reviewed blindly in conjunction with those of 18 optic neuritis patients.

High-resolution CT scanners enable the visualization in vivo of structures in the orbits that were previously unobservable. Regardless of the cause of increased intracranial pressure, three features were noted repeatedly by Jinkins in the study group of patients with papilledema, as compared with normal subjects.[6] These features included (1) a dilated optic nerve sheath that was seen in all 20 patients, (2) a "bulging" of the terminal optic nerve sheath subarachnoid space into the posterior aspect of the globe at the optic nerve head in 18 of 20 patients, and (3) depressed perfusion of the optic disk/nerve junction as measured by dynamic CT with intravenous contrast injection in all 6 patients with chronic symptomatic papilledema.

OPTIC CHIASM AND JUXTASELLAR REGION

The investigation of suprasellar masses can be difficult, as a great variety of lesions with similar clinical manifestations are found in this region. CT scanning has been well established as the primary imaging tool for the region. But CT is usually unsatisfactory in determining the relationship between tumors and surrounding structures, and in evaluating possible vascular anomalies. MRI enabled characterization of lesions containing hemorrhage, fat, flowing blood, mucus, and cyst and allowed more specific diagnosis than CT in 6% of cases.[7] MRI was equivalent to CT in allowing lesions to be detected.[7-9] In many cases the posterior extension of the tumor and its relationship to adjacent structures were shown better by MRI.[7, 8] Absent signals on T_1 and T_2-weighted images caused by rapidly flowing blood, or absent signals on T_1-weighted images with increased signals on T_2-weighted images from slow or turbulent flow, are findings that allow confident diagnosis of aneurysms and arteriovenous malformations. Vascular abnormalities can be better evaluated with MRI, and angiography can be avoided in some cases.[7]

High-resolution CT has clearly become the mainstay in the diagnosis of space-occupying lesions of the juxtasellar region, but is not without deficiencies. The most important deficiencies are the difficulty of obtaining direct scans in more than one plane, bone artifacts, the difficulty of separating tumor from vascular anomalies, and the frequent need for administration of intravenous contrast media.

MRI has been used and compared with CT for this region by many authors.[10-13] While MRI and CT were found to be equally sensitive, MRI was superior in further delineating and characterizing lesions.[10, 11] MRI was superior to CT and angiography in depicting the relationship of tumors to adjacent blood vessels, and equally effective as angiography in showing vascular encasement by tumors with narrowing of vessel's lumina.[12] Provided there are no contraindications, MRI should be the primary radiologic screening test in suspected lesions of the juxtasellar region.[10]

Imaging of pituitary microadenomas is still evolving. Microadenomas may reveal few or no abnormalities on high-resolution CT. In an earlier comparative study CT was found to be superior to MRI in detecting microadenomas.[14] Medium magnetic field strength (0.5 T) and 5.0-mm slice thicknesses were used for that study. In a recent comparative prospective study, however, MRI was better than CT in detecting pituitary microadenomas.[15] MRI detected a microadenoma at its correct location in all eight proven cases, while CT showed a focal abnormality in the correct location in only four of the eight patients. In this study MRI detected a focal pituitary signal abnormality in 83% and CT demonstrated a focal density abnormality in 42% of patients who were clinically and endocrinologically considered to harbor microadenomas. The improved MRI results are probably due to better resolution with high-strength magnetic fields (1.5 T), thinner slices (3 mm), and cardiac gating. Cardiac-gated spin-echo images reduced the phase-encoding artifacts generated by intracavernous carotid and cerebrospinal fluid (CSF) pulsation. Gadolinium–diethylenetriamine pentaacetic acid (Gd-DTPA), a newly available MRI contrast agent, was found to improve the contrast between the lesion and the pituitary, and hence increase detectability of pituitary microadenomas.[16, 17] Thus, MRI will probably replace CT as a screening method for suspected pituitary microadenomas.[15]

With the advent of high-resolution CT, the pathologic processes responsible for the Tolosa-Hunt syndrome (THS) can be imaged directly by CT.[18, 19] High-resolution CT in patients with THS usually demonstrates soft tissue infiltration in either the orbital apex or the cavernous sinus, with no associated bone destruction or hyperostosis.[18, 19] Symptomatic improvement following steroids in a patient with painful ophthalmoplegia is an essential feature of THS, but is not proof of the diagnosis. Painful ophthalmoplegia caused by cavernous sinus lesions, including lymphoma, metastasis, and meningioma, has also been reported to respond symptomatically to steroids initially.[20] Kwan et al. proposed that resolution of soft tissue inflammation in the orbital apex and cavernous sinus on CT while a patient is asymptomatic and not taking steroids (Fig 1) should be an additional clinical criterion for THS.[18]

Distinguishing patients with third cranial nerve palsy secondary to ischemia from those with structural lesions is a common clinical problem.[22] Sixty-three patients with third cranial nerve palsies, either isolated or in association with other neurologic deficits, were reviewed by Kwan et al.[21] They found that microvascular infarction secondary to diabetes mellitus and/or hypertension was the most common cause in patients with isolated third cranial nerve palsy, and extensive neuroradiologic evaluation is not indicated in this subgroup. The overall diagnostic yield of high-resolution CT for isolated third nerve palsy was low (30%), but improved (to 60%) if diabetes and hypertension were excluded. However, the yield of CT was very high (90%) in patients with third nerve palsies associated with additional neurologic deficits. The status of the pupil in and of itself cannot be the sole determinant as to whether angiography is indicated to exclude an aneurysm. Careful ophthalmologic observation is mandatory to determine the logical

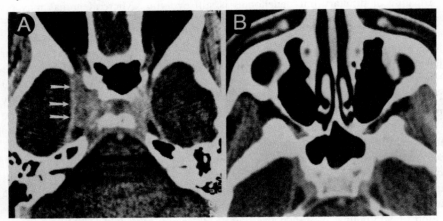

FIG 1.
Tolosa-Hunt syndrome. **A,** axial CT scan shows enlargement of right cavernous sinus with enhancement *(arrows)* before steroid therapy. **B,** follow-up CT scan 7 months later shows normal symmetric cavernous sinus. (From Kwan ES, Wolpert SM, Hedges TR III, et al: Tolosa-Hunt syndrome revisited: Not necessarily a diagnosis of exclusion. *AJNR* 1987; 8:1067–1072. Used by permission.)

sequence of radiologic evaluation. Angiography is indicated in patients with pupil-sparing third nerve palsy who are young and have no clinical history of diabetes and/or hypertension, and in patients in whom the ophthalmoplegia is accompanied by pupillomotor dysfunction.[21]

Clinical experience with MRI has demonstrated its superiority over CT in the evaluation of brain tumors, including suprasellar lesions, due to its superior contrast resolution and multiplanar capabilities. However, craniopharyngiomas are different from most tumors in that their diagnosis depends heavily on detection of calcification and cysts. The variable histologic appearances of craniopharyngiomas and the difficulty in identifying calcifications with MRI have cast doubt on its efficacy in suspected craniopharyngiomas.

Comparison between CT and MRI for craniopharyngiomas has been made recently.[23, 24] MRI was found to be superior or equal to CT in demonstrating the tumor (sensitivity).[23, 24] CT was superior to MRI in detecting the presence of calcification, which, with the clinical history, correctly suggested the diagnosis of craniopharyngioma (specificity).[23, 24] The extent of the lesion was more clearly seen with MRI using sagittal and coronal views than with high-resolution CT. The relationship of these lesions to the optic chiasm, hypothalamus, and midbrain was clearly seen on sagittal MRI. Coronal MRI provided the best view of the relationship of craniopharyngioma to the cavernous sinus and third ventricle. MRI was the preferred method for detecting the presence of recurrent tumor because of its superior contrast resolution; since the tissue diagnosis has been made, detection of tumor calcification is not essential. The appearance of craniopharyngioma on T_1-weighted images ranged from hypointense (fluid or ossification) to hyperintense (cholesterol crystal or methemoglobin) in comparison to surrounding brain parenchyma. It is uniformly bright on T_2-weighted images, except for rare lesions with ossification or heavy calcification.[23, 24] Giant cystic craniopharyngiomas can extend into the lateral ventricle and posterior cranial fossa. They are more common in children, and calcification usually occurs.[25]

An intrasellar and suprasellar cystic mass without calcification may be difficult to diagnose. The differential diagnosis should include cystic pituitary adenoma, craniopharyngioma, Rathke's cleft cyst, and arachnoid cyst. Rathke's cleft cysts are usually small and rarely cause symptoms. These cysts can enlarge and cause symptoms secondary to compression of the pituitary gland, optic chiasm, and hypothalamus. The most common clinical manifestions of an enlarged Rathke's cleft cyst include pituitary dysfunction, visual disturbance, and headache. There was considerable variation in the CT density and MRI intensity patterns.[26] A typical Rathke's cleft cyst would be a simple cyst with CT density and MRI intensity similar to that of CSF with no contrast enhancement. The cysts were located in the anterior sella turcica and/or the anterior suprasellar cistern, in the midline.[26] Intrasellar arachnoid cysts are rare lesions that can cause headache, vision loss, and pituitary dysfunction. The visual field loss was most frequently a bitemporal hemianopia indicative of suprasellar extension and chiasmal compression.[27] CT and

MRI typically showed a cystic lesion within the sella, often with suprasellar extension, and with density and intensity identical to CSF.[27]

The advent of CT scanners during the past decade has provided progressively more reliable and informative images of chiasmal gliomas. A survey of 22 cases was reported by Fletcher et al.[28] CT documents the broad spectrum of these tumors. Three CT patterns of chiasmal gliomas are diagnostic: tubular thicking of the optic nerve and chiasm, a suprasellar tumor with contiguous optic nerve expansion, and a suprasellar tumor with optic tract involvement. Tubular optic nerve and chiasmal thickening was observed only in patients with neurofibromatosis. Chiasmal gliomas with contiguous intraorbital optic nerve expansion were found predominantly in patients with neurofibromatosis. The diagnosis of chiasmal glioma cannot be made on the basis of CT criteria alone if a suprasellar mass without optic nerve or tract involvement is found. The diagnosis may require a biopsy to obtain histologic confirmation. This type of tumor was observed primarily in patients who did not have neurofibromatosis. Tumor growth was documented by CT in only a few globular-type chiasmal gliomas, with most chiasmal gliomas remaining the same size for many years.[28]

Early diagnosis and steroid treatment are important because of the high mortality in untreated cases of pituitary apoplexy. The diagnosis is often delayed or unrecognized because the majority of hemorrhages occur in unsuspected pituitary adenomas. CT scanning has been shown to be effective in the detection of pituitary adenomas with acute hemorrhage. Lacomis et al. reported three cases of pituitary apoplexy, with CT and MRI.[29] The MRI scans obtained at least 5 days after the onset of symptoms suggested pituitary hemorrhage in all three cases, whereas CT indicated pituitary hemorrhage in only one case. Increased intensity on the T_1-weighted images was the hallmark on MRI in all three cases. Initially a blood clot is hyperdense on a CT scan, but over time its attenuation diminishes and the blood clot appears isodense. Eventually the clot may appear hypodense. Hemorrhage is difficult to identify during the isodense stage on a CT scan. MRI may be superior to CT in identifying pituitary apoplexy, at least in the subacute phase.

POSTERIOR VISUAL PATHWAYS

Despite the excellent display of anatomy and pathology on MRI, it was apparent early on that MRI could benefit from a contrast agent to help assess the vascularity of lesions and the compromised blood-brain barrier. The first available contrast agent for MRI is Gd-DTPA. Gadolinium-DTPA is a poor activator of the complement system and is not expected to produce anaphylactoid reactions.[30] Clinical trials have proven that Gd-DTPA has extremely low toxicity.[31-34] At the clinical dosage of 0.1 mmol/kg, no renal or hepatic toxic effects have been noted. A transient rise in serum iron level has been reported quite commonly,[31-33] but the effect is not considered to be significant. Following intravenous injection, Gd-

DTPA is distributed throughout the intravascular and extracellular spaces of the body, except in the brain, and is rapidly excreted by the kidneys. When the blood-brain barrier is disrupted, the contrast molecules diffuse into the interstitial compartment and produce high signals on T_1-weighted images.

In general, the enhancement patterns of Gd-DTPA on MRI are similar to those observed on CT with contrast, except that rapidly flowing blood does not enhance on MRI. The T_2-weighted MRI images without contrast are still more sensitive than T_1-weighted images with contrast in detecting intra-axial lesions, including tumors, multiple sclerosis, occult arteriovenous malformations, and infectious processes.[33] Gadolinium-DTPA may not improve sensitivity of MRI in the detection of intra-axial lesions; however, useful information, such as the presence of perfusion of a lesion and active breach of the blood-brain barrier, are well depicted with Gd-DTPA. The benefit of Gd-DTPA is even more apparent in extra-axial lesions such as meningiomas.[34, 35] These lesions may be isointense to the adjacent brain on both T_1- and T_2-weighted nonenhanced images. The majority of meningiomas demonstrate bright, homogenous enhancement with Gd-DTPA. Contrast-enhanced MRI is more sensitive than T_2-weighted nonenhanced images for detecting metastatic foci, especially meningeal carcinomatoses.[36, 37]

Identifying clinical symptoms and signs remains the standard method of diagnosing MS, since no laboratory tests are yet specific and sensitive for the disease. It was found that MRI is the most sensitive technique for diagnosing MS, in comparison with the findings of CSF and visually evoked potential.[38, 39] MRI, using balanced images and T_2-weighted images, has dramatically increased the detection of MS, but fails to enable separation of active from quiescent lesions. Gadolinium-enhanced MRI appears to be more sensitive than high-dose-contrast CT in the detection of the transient abnormalities of the blood-brain barrier that occur in patients with active MS, and to be capable of distinguishing active lesions that may be responsible for abnormal clinical findings.[40] At the clinical dosage of 0.1 mmol/kg, Gd-DTPA is much safer than high-dose iodinated contrast, which may cause fluid overload, kidney damage, and other adverse reactions. Cerebral atrophy is known to be present in some patients with MS, and it may be related to the dementia of MS. It was found that neither the number of lesions nor the extent of generalized cerebral atrophy was significantly greater in demented compared with nondemented patients; however, atrophy of the corpus callosum was significantly more extensive on MRI in demented patients.[41] Diffuse moderate to severe atrophy of the corpus collosum was noted in 40% of patients with a confirmed diagnosis of MS.[42]

As more radiotherapeutic regimens have been implemented, long-term effects of neurotoxicity in the surviving patients have been recognized. The majority of patients without evidence of tumor recurrence showed demyelination with variable clinical expression, including confusion, ataxia, and psychomotor retardation.[43] In addition to supratentorial white matter demyelination, radiotherapy may cause focal damage to critical structures. Beyer et al. reported three cases of occlusion of major arteries with a moyamoya pattern after irradiation for glioma of the optic chiasm.[44] The effectiveness of radiotherapy for optic chiasm glioma remains unproven. This treatment should be used sparingly, at best, in view of the potentially severe side effects, especially in the pediatric population. The authors recommended irradiating only when rapid tumor growth[51] occurs or when the patient is clinically deteriorating.

The advent of CT afforded a marked improvement in demonstrating the abnormalities of tuberous sclerosis. MRI has also recently been reported to be very useful in evaluation of this disease.[45–48] Based on the findings on CT and/or MRI, often the radiologist can establish or confirm the clinical diagnosis of tuberous sclerosis. The MRI findings consist of subependymal nodules projecting into the lateral ventricle on T_1-weighted images, distortion of the normal cortical architecture on T_1-weighted images, and increased signal on T_2-weighted images for parenchymal hamartomas. The more severely affected patients appear to have more cerebral parenchymal hamartomas. MRI is better than CT for the detection of parenchymal hamartomas.[45–48] Calcifications must be present in subependymal nodules or parenchymal hamartomas in order to diagnose tuberous sclerosis. CT is extremely sensitive for detecting small calcifications, and it is easy to demonstrate these lesions using CT. MRI, on the other hand, has been shown to be extremely poor at demonstrating calcifications. Once the MRI and CT findings are understood, the choice of modality is clear. In the initial examination of a child with seizures, CT and MRI are probably equal in effectiveness. MRI should be used for follow-up because of the lack of ionizing radiation.[45]

Malignant melanoma to the brain is the third most common metastasis in humans; its incidence is surpassed only by lung and breast carcinoma. MRI is a sensitive diagnostic modality for intracranial neoplasms, but signal intensity characteristics of these lesions are often nonspecific. Intracranial melanoma metastases lend themselves to study by MRI, since these lesions are often paramagnetic with melanin and hemorrhage. Most malignant melanomas are hyperintense to normal white matter on T_1-weighted images and hypointense to normal white matter on T_2-weighted images due to decreased T_1 and T_2 relaxation times (Fig 2).[49, 50] Hemorrhage in the lesion may have a greater influence on this unique appearance than does melanin.[49] These MRI findings are opposite to those of most brain lesions. The diagnosis of metastatic malignant melanoma should be considered for lesions that contain regions of increased signal intensity on T_1-weighted images and decreased signal intensity on T_2-weighted images.

In the presence of an intracranial hematoma, CT is of limited use in delineating hemorrhagic brain tumors, because the hematoma often obliterates any evidence of the underlying neoplasm. It is often impossible on CT to distinguish hemorrhagic neoplasm from non-neoplastic hematoma. Twelve patients with 15 separate spontaneously hemorrhagic intracranial malignant lesions (7 primary gliomas, 8 metastatic lesions) were reported by Atlas et al.[51] Compared with non-neoplastic hematomas, the MR images of hemorrhagic intracranial malignancies showed (1) notable nonhemorrhagic tissue corresponding to tumor; (2) diminished, or (3) absent, irregular hemosiderin deposition; and pronounced or persistent edema. Al-

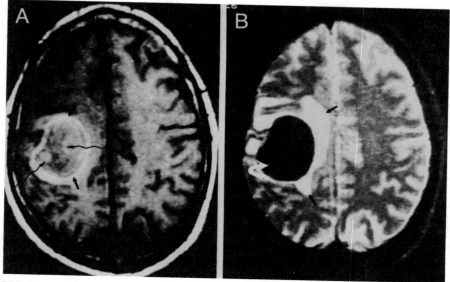

FIG 2.
Metastatic melanoma. **A,** T_1-weighted MRI image demonstrates increased signal intensity along the periphery *(short arrows)* and in the center *(long arrows)* of a right parietal lesion. **B,** T_2-weighted image demonstrates decreased signal intensity within the lesion *(white arrow)*. Increased signal intensity at the periphery of the lesion *(black arrows)* represents edema. (From Woodruff WW, Djang WT, McLendon RE, et al: Intracerebral malignant melanoma: High-field-strength MR imaging. *Radiology* 1987; 165:209–213. Used by permission.)

though not all of these MR findings were uniformly present in all cases, and it is likely that none of these features are diagnostic of malignancy, the demonstration of these characteristics in the appropriate clinical setting may suggest malignancy as the cause of an intracranial hematoma.[51]

The results from neuroimaging for migraine have been variable. MRI has been found to be very useful in detecting parenchymal changes of migraine. Soges et al. reported 11 (46%) of the patients (7 with classic or common and 4 with complicated migraine) showed well-defined high-signal lesions on T_2-weighted images.[52] The lesions associated with classic migraine were focal and predominantly distributed in the periventricular white matter. In the group with complicated migraine, larger cortical abnormalities similar to infarcts were seen in 3 patients. The focal periventricular white matter lesions were not necessarily associated with neurologic deficits, but the cortical lesions were. The white matter lesions encountered in patients with migraine resemble those of MS, and leukoencephalopathies of other etiologies. They are occasionally referred to as "unidentified bright objects" (UBOs) because of their nonspecificity. UBOs are fairly common in the normal elderly; however, they are rarely found in normal individuals under 45 years of age.

Blindness is an uncommon premonitory symptom of eclampsia. It is mainly attributed to retinal abnormalities, especially retinal vascular thrombosis, retinal edema, and detachment. Visual loss can sometimes be cortical in origin. Two cases of cortical blindness in toxemia of pregnancy have been reported.[53] CT scans showed edema with bilateral hypodense areas in the occipital lobes. There was gradual and complete recovery of vision, together with CT documentation of resolution of the cerebral changes on both cases, after termination of pregnancy. In the evaluation of sudden visual loss in toxemia of pregnancy, CT is helpful in showing the characteristic features of cortical blindness, as well as excluding other intracranial lesions such as pituitary adenoma with hemorrhage or cerebral hematoma.

BRAIN STEM AND CEREBELLUM

MRI is known to be a highly sensitive imaging technique for detecting MS plaques, and is the technique of choice for evaluating brain stem disorders. MRI is

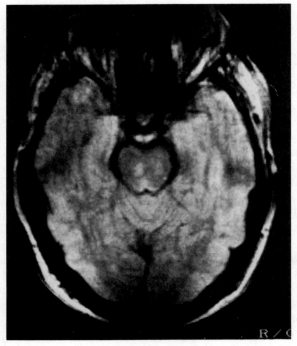

FIG 3.
A 61-year-old patient with internuclear ophthalmoplegia from a recent stroke. A CT scan was normal. The T$_2$-weighted MRI image shows an increased signal intensity in the central portion of the mesencephalon, just to the right of the midline. (Courtesy of J Seeger.)

thus ideally suited to evaluate gaze disorders attributable to brain stem dysfunction, such as internuclear ophthalmoplegia (INO). Atlas et al.[54] studied 11 patients with INO (9 with clinical multiple sclerosis, 2 with clinical infarction), using MRI and CT. MRI showed focal or nodular areas of high signal intensity on T_2-weighted images in the region of medial longitudinal fasciculus in 10 of 11 patients. CT failed to show the lesions in all 9 patients examined (Fig 3). In 1 patient with a clinical diagnosis of infarction, no lesion was detected on MRI. In 1 of 4 patients who had MRI after intravenous Gd-DTPA, an enhancing ring lesion was seen in the region of the medial longitudinal fasciculus on T_1-weighted images, indicating active blood-brain barrier disruption. This correlated with the patient's recent-onset INO.

Subcortical arteriosclerotic encephalopathy (SAE) is characterized pathologically by a spectrum of lesions that includes loss of myelin, loss of axon, gliosis, and infarction within deep portions of the white matter resulting from arteriosclerosis of the penetrating arteries. MRI is well known to be very sensitive in detecting UBOs of cerebral white matter diseases, including SAE. Brain stem abnormalities frequently accompanied supratentorial SAE and were seen as multiple, fairly symmetric areas of poorly defined increased signal intensities on T_2-weighted MR images (Fig 4).[55] Abnormal signals were not seen within the superficial pons, medulla, or cerebellar white matter, including the cerebellar peduncles.[55] Since the pons is the widest part of the brain stem, it derives its central blood supply from the longest of the basilar penetrating arteries. The central pons may therefore be at particular risk for ischemic damage, just as deep portions of the cerebral white matter are the most common sites of supratentorial SAE.

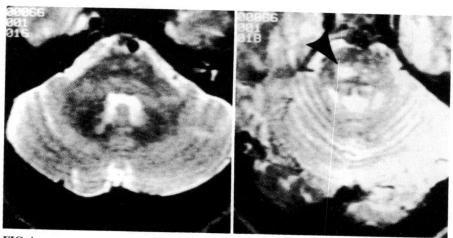

FIG 4.
Brain stem subcortical arteriosclerotic encephalopathy. T_2-weighted MRI images through the middle and upper pons show multiple areas of poorly defined increased signal (*arrowhead*) in the central portion of the pons. (From Salomon A, Yeates AE, Burger PC, et al: Subcortical arteriosclerotic encephalopathy: Brain stem findings with MR imaging. *Radiology* 1987; 165:625–629. Used by permission.)

Because of the small size and relatively long course of the aqueduct, it represents a vulnerable site at which blockage of CSF flow can produce obstructive hydrocephalus. Because MRI can delineate the fine structure of the brain stem, it is a desirable technique for examination of the cerebral aqueduct. The cerebral aqueducts of 70 patients and 20 normal controls was evaluated with MRI by Kemp et al.[56] In these normal subjects the aqueduct was always well visualized on a sagittal T_1-weighted image with a signal void within the aqueduct. Hydrocephalus caused by obstruction at the aqueduct level is frequently, but not always, associated with loss of the flow-related signal void. Sixty percent of patients with distortion or compression of the aqueduct and hydrocephalus had a signal flow void within the aqueduct.

MISCELLANEOUS

Duplex sonography is a highly accurate noninvasive method for evaluating patients with occlusive vascular disease.[57-60] This technique consists of B-mode ultrasound imaging and Doppler spectrum analysis. High-resolution real-time ultrasound imaging allows the demonstration of vascular anatomy and assessment of the risk of embolism through plaque characterization, and Doppler spectrum analysis provides quantification of flow characteristics to determine the degree of stenosis. Studies using duplex sonography followed by angiography demonstrate a 95% agreement between duplex sonography and angiography in identifying carotid stenosis of greater than 50%.[59] It is important to emphasize that the accuracy of duplex sonography will depend on the expertise of the operator. When the test is carefully performed by qualified personnel, duplex sonography is the best available noninvasive technique. Its accuracy is close to that of invasive studies, including intra-arterial angiography for carotid occlusive disease. MRI angiography with various techniques is being developed, and preliminary results have been reported (Fig 5).[61-63] This procedure is a noninvasive test with great potential. One is encouraged to think that this modality may replace arteriography for the investigation of vascular diseases.

Calcification can occur in a wide range of conditions. The presence, distribution, and morphologic features of this finding are of major importance in radiologic diagnosis. CT is highly sensitive in detecting calcifications. The highly utilized spin-echo T_1- and T_2-weighted MR imaging is the most sensitive imaging technique for detection of most intracranial diseases, but its inability to detect calcification consistently is well recognized.[64, 65] The most common finding of calcification on MRI is a focus of diminished signal, which is better demonstrated on a T_2-weighted image. This negative contrast is less conspicuous than the positive contrast of calcification on CT. Atlas et al. reported that a new MR technique, using reduced flip-angle gradient-echo acquisition can improve the sensitivity of detecting calcification on MRI.[66] They studied 17 patients with partially calcified

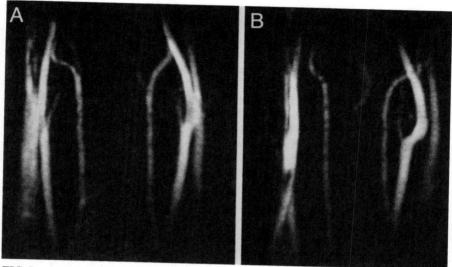

FIG 5.
MRI angiograph. **A,** anteroposterior and **B,** oblique projections of the vascular structure in the neck of a young, healthy volunteer. (From Dumoulin CL, Hart HR: Magnetic resonance angiography. *Radiology* 1986; 161:717–720. Used by permission.)

intracranial lesions, as documented by CT with MRI at 1.5 tesla field strength. In all 17 patients MR images with this technique showed marked hypointensity throughout the entire area of calcification, matching the calcified region as seen on CT. The hypointensity due to calcification on MR images is very nonspecific; non-contrast CT is required to confirm its presence.[66]

How safe is MRI? The safety of MRI is excellent as expected, according to the report by Gangarosa et al.[67] These researchers obtained information from Food and Drug Administration (FDA) summaries of medical devices, accounts published in the medical literature, and discussions with the FDA. Significant incidents in their report included one death, two cardiac arrests, and one unilateral visual loss due to a previously unrecognized intraocular iron foreign body. Two incidents (one death, one cardiac arrest) were probably not caused by MRI, because both patients were critically ill. One cardiac arrest was due to pacemaker malfunction during MRI scanning. The FDA has specifically alerted the MRI community to the dangers of implanted cardiac pacemakers and neurostimulators; patients with such prostheses should be excluded from the vicinity of the magnet. Patients placed in high-strength magnetic fields with undetected intraocular ferromagnetic foreign bodies are at risk for severe eye injury. No satisfactory screening method currently exists to identify such patients. History, plain radiography, and CT of the orbit would be helpful, but they are not sufficiently sensitive and specific for detection of undiscovered small ferromagnetic objects.

Iodinated contrast is used almost routinely for all CT scans, including brain and orbit. The search for the ideal radiopaque contrast material for intravascular use has continued since the discovery of the x-ray. Currently used water-soluble iodinated contrast media are hyperosmolar compounds, relatively safe, low in cost, and in use for over 30 years. They are called high-osmolality contrast media (HOCM). Recently, a new generation, low-osmolality contrast media (LOCM), has been introduced into the marketplace. Approximately 5% to 8% of all intravascular injections with HOCM are complicated by adverse reactions, most of which are mild or moderate in degree and not life-threatening.[68-70] Older patients tend to have more severe, occasionally fatal, reactions to HOCM. Deaths from HOCM administration are variably reported to occur in 1 of 12,500 to 1 of 66,502.[69, 70] Considerable improvement in patient tolerance and in safety of LOCM has been proven by scientific study and clinical use.[71] The new contrast agents cost at least 10 times more than the old ones. Under the current atmosphere of cost controls and consumerism in medicine, the higher cost prohibits LOCM from routine universal usage. LOCM are recommended for high-risk patients (old age, cardiovascular disease, allergy/asthma, dehydration, diabetes mellitus, anxiety), and for patients who previously would have been considered to have a contraindication (previous mild to moderate reaction to contrast media, renal failure, sickle cell disease, multiple myeloma, kidney transplantation).[71]

CONCLUSION

At present, MRI is recommended as the first diagnostic study in evaluating diseases of the optic chiasm, juxtasellar region, optic radiation, brain stem, and posterior cranial fossa, as well as suspected demyelinating diseases and metastatic brain tumors. MRI and CT are complementary in investigating diseases of the orbit. The use of Gd-DTPA contrast will increase the sensitivity of MRI for detecting extra-axial lesions and metastatic foci, and may provide useful information leading to diagnosis for intra-axial lesions. MRI is contraindicated when there is any possibility of a metallic foreign body in the orbit and when there are intracranial metallic clips for aneurysm, implanted cardiac pacemakers, and neurostimulators.

REFERENCES

1. Atlas SW, Bilaniuk LT, Zimmerman RA, et al: Orbit: Initial experience with surface coil spin-echo MR imaging at 1.5 T. *Radiology* 1987; 164:501–509.

2. Ormerod IEC, McDonald WI, du Boulay EPGH, et al: Disseminated lesions at presentation in patients with optic neuritis. *J Neurol Neurosurg Psychiatry* 1986; 49:124–127.

3. Jacobs L, Kinkel PR, Kinkel WR: Silent brain lesions in patients with isolated idiopathic optic neuritis. *Arch Neurol* 1986; 43:452–455.

4. Francis DA, Compston DAS, Batchelor JR, et al: A reassessment of the risk of multiple sclerosis developing in patients with optic neuritis after extended follow-up. *J Neurol Neurosurg Psychiatry* 1987; 50:758–765.

5. Miller DH, Newton MR, van der Poel JC, et al: Magnetic resonance imaging of the optic nerve in optic neuritis. *Neurology* 1988; 38:175–179.

6. Jinkins JR: "Papilledema": Neuroradiologic evaluation of optic disk protrusion with dynamic orbital CT. *AJNR* 1987; 8:681–690.

7. Karnaze MG, Sartor K, Winthrop JD, et al: Suprasellar lesions: Evaluation with MR imaging. *Radiology* 1986; 161:77–82.

8. Patronas NJ, Dwyer AJ, Papathanasiou M, et al: Contributions of magnetic resonance imaging in the evaluation of optic gliomas. *Surg Neurol* 1987; 28:367–371.

9. Hahn FJ, Leibrock LG, Huseman CA, et al: The MR appearance of hypothalamic hamartoma. *Neuroradiology* 1988; 30:65–68.

10. Sartor K, Karnaze MG, Winthrop JD, et al: MR imaging in infra-, para- and retrosellar mass lesions. *Neuroradiology* 1987; 29:19–29.

11. Sze G, Uichanco III LS, Brant-Zawadzki MN, et al: Chordomas: MR imaging. *Radiology* 1988; 166:187–191.

12. Young SC, Grossman RI, Goldberg HI, et al: MR of vascular encasement in parasellar masses: Comparison with angiography and CT. *AJNR* 1988; 9:35–38.

13. Yeakley JW, Kulkarni MV, McArdle CB, et al: High-resolution MR imaging of juxtasellar meningiomas with CT and angiographic correlation. *AJNR* 1988; 9:279–285.

14. Davis PC, Hoffman JC, Spencer T, et al: MR imaging of pituitary adenoma: CT, clinical, and surgical correlation. *AJNR* 1987; 8:107–112.

15. Kulkarni MV, Lee KF, McArdle CB, et al: 1.5-T MR imaging of pituitary microadenomas: Technical considerations and CT correlation. *AJNR* 1988; 9:5–11.

16. Davis PC, Hoffman JC Jr, Malko JA, et al: Gadolinium-DTPA and MR imaging of pituitary adenoma: A preliminary report. *AJNR* 1987; 8:817–823.

17. Dwyer AJ, Frank JA, Doppman JL, et al: Pituitary adenomas in patients with Cushing disease: Initial experience with Gd-DTPA-enhanced MR imaging. *Radiology* 1987; 163:421–426.

18. Kwan ES, Wolpert SM, Hedges III TR, et al: Tolosa-Hunt syndrome revisited: Not necessarily a diagnosis of exclusion. *AJNR* 1987; 8:1067–1072.

19. Thomas DJB, Charlesworth MC, Afshar F, et al: Computerized axial tomography and magnetic resonance scanning in the Tolosa-Hunt syndrome. *Br J Ophthalmol* 1988; 72:299–302.

20. Spector RH, Fiandaca MS: The "sinister" Tolosa-Hunt syndrome. *Neurology* 1986; 36:198–203.

21. Kwan ES, Laucella M, Hedges III TR, et al: A cliniconeuroradiologic approach to third cranial nerve palsies. *AJNR* 1987; 8:459–468.

22. Wykes WN: Prolactinoma presenting with intermittent third nerve palsy. *Br J Ophthalmol* 1986; 70:706–707.

23. Pusey E, Kortman KE, Flannigan BD, et al: MR of craniopharyngiomas: Tumor delineation and characterization. *AJNR* 1987; 8:439–444.

24. Freeman MP, Kessler RM, Allen JH, et al: Craniopharyngioma: CT and MR imaging in nine cases. *J Comput Assist Tomogr* 1987; 11:810–814.

25. Young SC, Zimmerman RA, Nowell MA, et al: Giant cystic craniopharyngiomas. *Neuroradiology* 1987; 29:468–473.

26. Kucharczyk W, Peck WW, Kelly WM, et al: Rathke cleft cysts: CT, MR imaging, and pathologic features. *Radiology* 1987; 165:491–495.

27. Meyer FB, Carpenter SM, Laws Jr. ER: Intrasellar arachnoid cysts. *Surg Neurol* 1987; 28:105–110.

28. Fletcher WA, Imes RK, Hoyt WF: Chiasmal gliomas: Appearance and long-term changes demonstrated by computerized tomography. *J Neurosurg* 1986; 65:154–159.

29. Lacomis D, Johnson LN, Mamourian AC: Magnetic resonance imaging in pituitary apoplexy. *Arch Ophthalmol* 1988; 106:207–209.

30. Weinmann HJ, Brasch RC, Press WR, et al: Characteristics of gadolinium-DTPA complex: A potential NMR contrast agent. *AJR* 1984; 142:619–624.

31. Graif M, Steiner RE: Contrast-enhanced magnetic resonance imaging of tumours of the central nervous system: A clinical review. *Br J Radiol* 1986; 59:865–873.

32. Niendorf HP, Laniado M, Semmler W, et al: Dose administration of gadolinium-DTPA in MR imaging of intracranial tumors. *AJNR* 1987; 8:803–815.

33. Brant-Zawadzki M, Berry I, Osaki L, et al: Gd-DTPA in clinical MR of the brain: 1. Intraaxial lesions. *AJNR* 1986; 7:781–788.

34. Haughton VM, Rimm AA, Czervionke LF, et al: Sensitivity of Gd-DTPA-enhanced MR imaging of benign extraaxial tumors. *Radiology* 1988; 166:829–833.

35. Berry I, Brant-Zawadzki M, Osaki L, et al: Gd-DTPA in clinical MR of the brain: 2. Extraaxial lesions and normal structures. *AJNR* 1986; 7:789–793.

36. Russell EJ, Geremia GK, Johnson CE, et al: Multiple cerebral metastases: Detectability with Gd-DTPA-enhanced MR imaging. *Radiology* 1987; 165:609–617.

37. Healy ME, Hesselink JR, Press GA, et al: Increased detection of intracranial metastases with intravenous Gd-DTPA. *Radiology* 1987; 165:619–624.

38. Paty DW, Oger JJF, Kastrukoff LF, et al: MRI in the diagnosis of MS: A prospective study with comparison of clinical evaluation, evoked potentials, oligoclonal banding, and CT. *Neurology* 1988; 38:180–185.

39. Uhlenbrock D, Seidel D, Gehlen W, et al: MR imaging in multiple sclerosis: Comparison with clinical, CSF, and visual evoked potential findings. *AJNR* 1988; 9:59–67.

40. Grossman RI, Gonzalez-Scarano F, Atlas SW, et al: Multiple sclerosis: Gadolinium enhancement in MR imaging. *Radiology* 1986; 161:721–725.

41. Huber SJ, Paulson GW, Shuttleworth EC, et al: Magnetic resonance imaging correlates of dementia in multiple sclerosis. *Arch Neurol* 1987; 44:732–736.

42. Simon JH, Holtas SL, Schiffer RB, et al: Corpus callosum and subcallosal-periventricular lesions in multiple sclerosis: Detection with MR. *Radiology* 1986; 160:363–367.

43. Curnes JT, Laster DW, Ball MR, et al: Magnetic resonance imaging of radiation injury to the brain. *AJNR* 1986; 7:389–394.

44. Beyer RA, Paden, Sobel DF, et al: Moyamoya pattern of vascular occlusion after radiotherapy for glioma of the optic chiasm. *Neurology* 1986; 36:1173–1177.

45. Altman NR, Purser RK, Donovan Post MJ: Tuberous sclerosis: Characteristics at CT and MR imaging. *Radiology* 1988; 167:527–532.

46. McMurdo SK Jr, Moore SG, Brant-Zawadzki M, et al: MR imaging of intracranial tuberous sclerosis. *AJNR* 1987; 8:77–82.

47. Roach ES, Williams DP, Laster DW: Magnetic resonance imaging in tuberous sclerosis. *Arch Neurol* 1987; 44:301–303.

48. Martin N, de Broucker T, Cambier J, et al: MRI evaluation of tuberous sclerosis. *Neuroradiology* 1987; 29:437–443.

49. Woodruff WW, Djang WT, McLendon RE, et al: Intracerebral malignant melanoma: High-field-strength MR imaging. *Radiology* 1987; 165:209–213.

50. Atlas SW, Grossman RI, Gomori JM, et al: MR imaging of intracranial metastatic melanoma. *J Comput Assist Tomogr* 1987; 11:577–582.

51. Atlas SW, Grossman RI, Gomori JM, et al: Hemorrhagic intracranial malignant neoplasms: Spin-echo MR imaging. *Radiology* 1987; 164:71–77.

52. Soges LJ, Cacayorin ED, Petro GR, et al: Migraine: Evaluation by MR. *AJNR* 1988; 9:425–429.

53. Lau SPC, Chan FL, Yu YL, et al: Cortical blindness in toxaemia of pregnancy: Findings on computed tomography. *Br J Radiol* 1987; 60:347–349.

54. Atlas SW, Grossman RI, Savino PJ, et al: Internuclear ophthalmoplegia: MR-anatomic correlation. *AJNR* 1987; 8:243–247.

55. Salomon A, Yeates AE, Burger PC, et al: Subcortical arteriosclerotic encephalopathy: Brain stem findings with MR imaging. *Radiology* 1987; 165:625–629.

56. Kemp SS, Zimmerman RA, Bilaniuk LT, et al: Magnetic resonance imaging of the cerebral aqueduct. *Neuroradiology* 1987; 29:430–436.

57. Acker JD, Cole CA, Mauney KA, et al: Duplex carotid ultrasound. *Neuroradiology* 1986; 28:608–617.

58. Walsh J, Markowitz I, Kerstein MD: Carotid endarterectomy for amaurosis fugax without angiography. *Am J Surg* 1986; 152:172–174.

59. Lo LY, Ford CS, McKinney WM, et al: Asymptomatic bruit, carotid and vertebrobasilar transient ischemic attacks: A clinical and ultrasound correlation. *Stroke* 1986; 17:65–68.

60. Langlois YE, Roederer GO, Strandness DE: Ultrasonic evaluation of the carotid bifurcation. *Echocardiography* 1987; 4:141–159.

61. Dumoulin CL, Hart HR: Magnetic resonance angiography. *Radiology* 1986; 161:717–720.

62. Gullberg GT, Wehrli FW, Shimakawa A, et al: MR vascular imaging with a fast gradient refocusing pulse sequence and reformatted images from transaxial sections. *Radiology* 1987; 165:241–246.

63. Laub GA, Kaiser WA: MR angiography with gradient motion refocusing. *J Comput Assist Tomogr* 1988; 12:377–382.

64. Oot RF, New PFJ, Pile-Spellman J, et al: The detection of intracranial calcifications by MR. *AJNR* 1986; 7:801–809.

65. Tsuruda JS, Bradley WG: MR detection of intracranial calcification: A phantom study. *AJNR* 1987; 8:1049–1055.

66. Atlas SW, Grossman RI, Hackney DB, et al: Calcified intracranial lesions: Detection with gradient-echo-acquisition rapid MR imaging. *AJNR* 1988; 9:253–259.

67. Gangarosa RE, Minnis JE, Nobbe J, et al: Operational safety issues in MRI. *Magn Reson Imaging* 1987; 5:287–292.

68. Shehadi WH: Contrast media adverse reactions: Occurrence, recurrence, and distribution patterns. *Radiology* 1982; 143:11–17.

69. Ansell G, Tweedie MCK, West CR, et al: The current status of reactions to intravenous contrast media. *Invest Radiol* 1980; 15:532–539.

70. Hartman GW, Hattery RR, Witten DM, et al: Mortality during excretory urography: Mayo Clinic experience. *AJR* 1982; 139:914–922.

71. McClennan BL: Low-osmolality contrast media: Premises and promises. *Radiology* 1987; 162:1–8.

Index